Surviving In the Kitchen

Recipes for life, love, and a full stomach.

Amanda Blackwood

MANDOLIN PUBLISHING

Published by the Mandolin Publishing Group
Amanda Blackwood, LLC
For more information, write to:
Amanda Blackwood
AuthorAmandaBlackwood@gmail.com
Or find us on Facebook
https://www.facebook.com/Mandolinpublishing

Chat with the Chef!

facebook.com/AmandaBlackwoodSurvivor

instagram.com/detailedpieces

linkedin.com/in/authoramandablackwood

Learn more:

detailedpieces.com

growthfromdarkness.com

To my husband Kyle,

The most devoted guinea pig I could've ever asked for.

Thank you for always being so willing to try my newest creations, and for being honest, even when the things I make are honestly terrible!

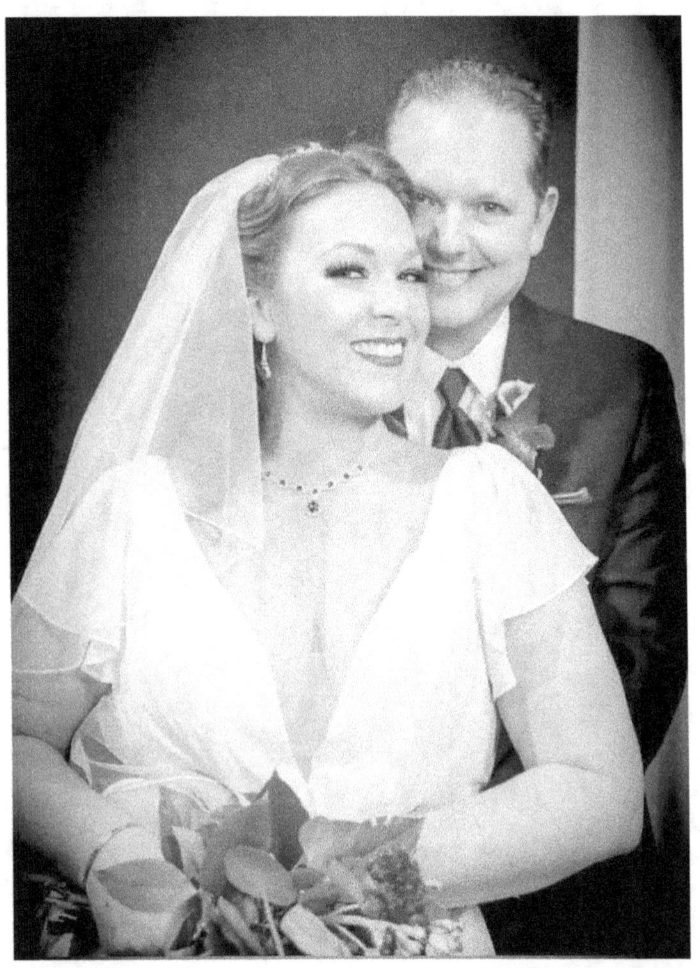

Our wedding, January 26th, 2022

What's on the Menu:

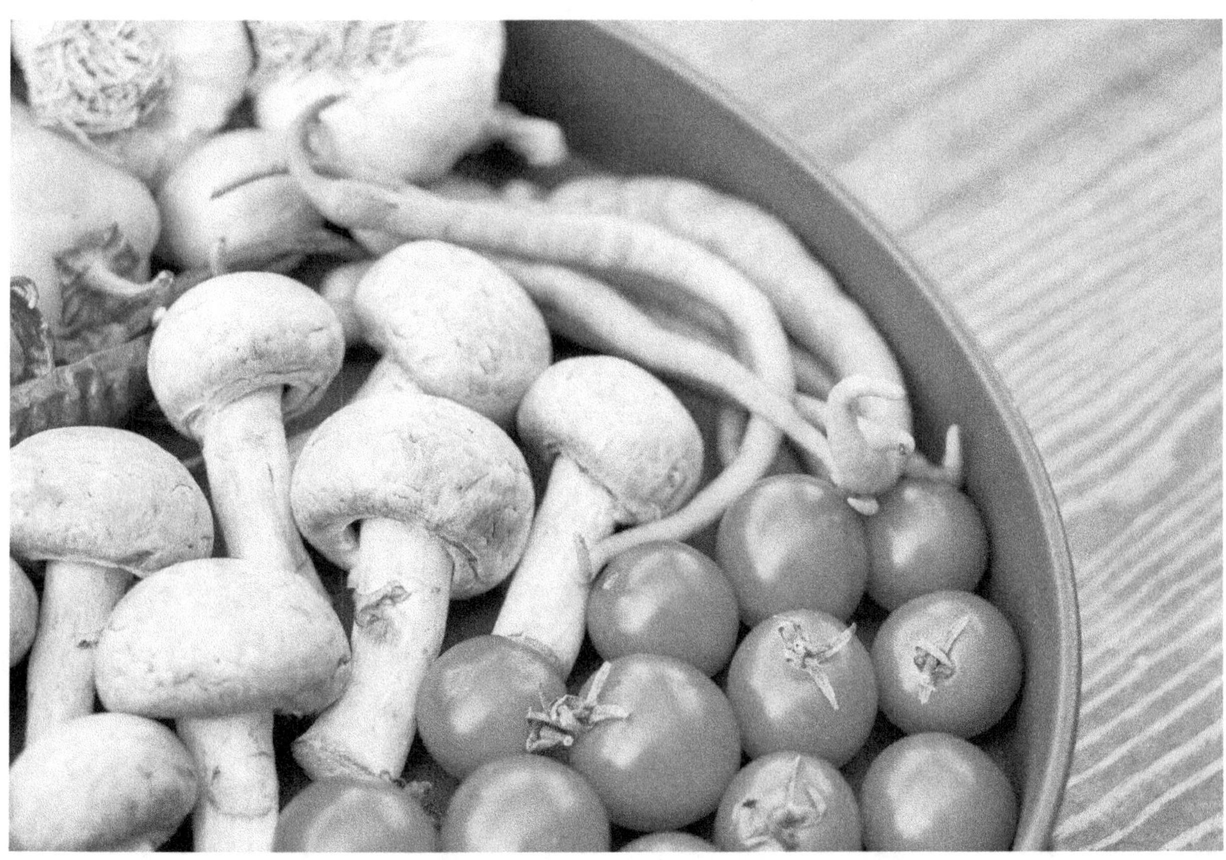

Introduction

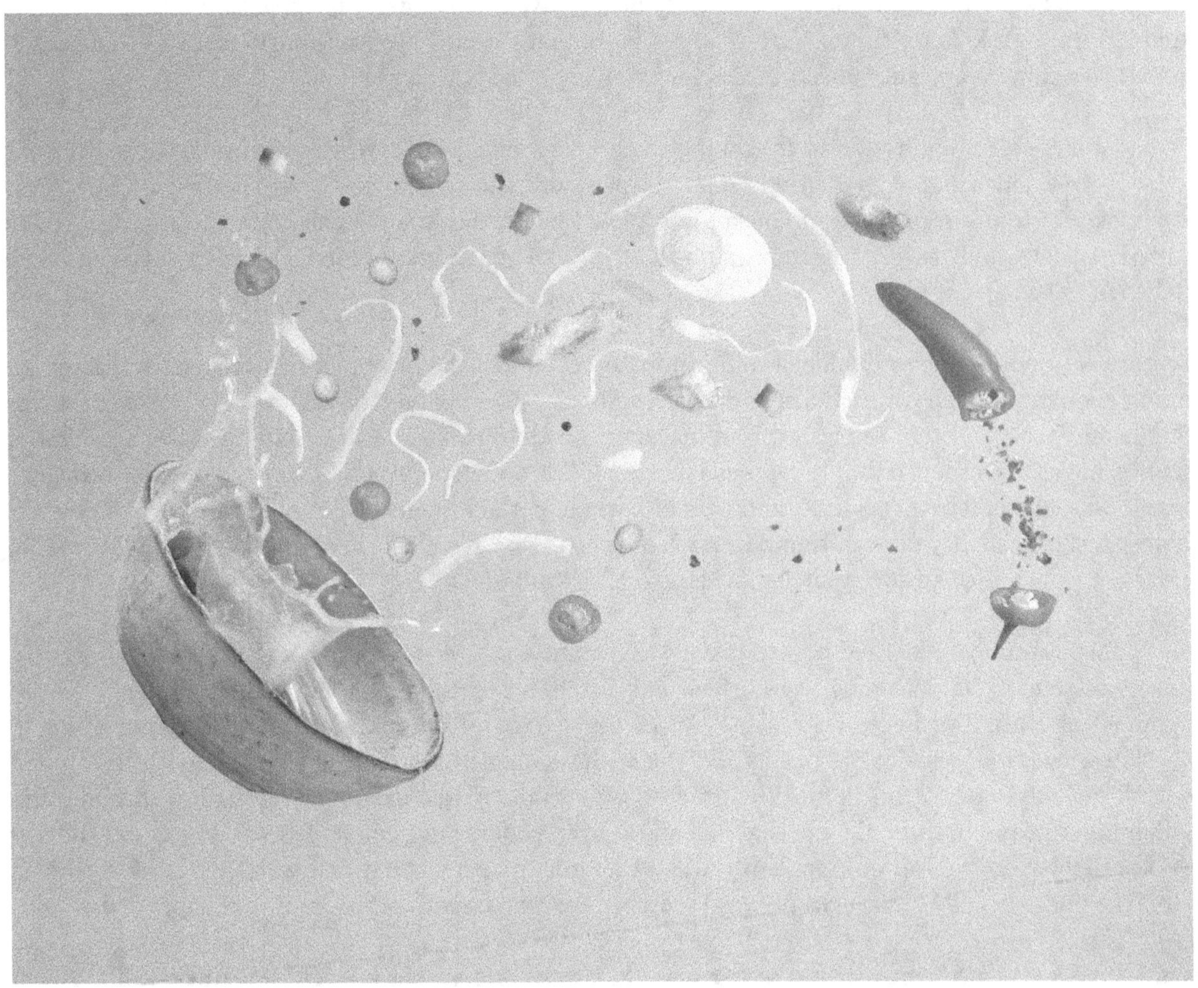

Surviving in the kitchen is more than just learning how to cook without burning off your eyebrows. It's the art of learning more about yourself through patience, combinations, trying new things, and taking time to practice a few things. Just as it is in life, some recipes are quite easy. Others take a bit more work. In the end, the final product is worth it just about every time.

I've often been found making jokes about why and how I learned to cook in my constant effort to put others at ease through humor. As with most jokes, there's usually some truth behind them.

"I learned how to cook out of self defense."

My mother hated cooking and would often complain about it. Still, without passion and a sense of purpose in it, she managed to create some rather tasty meals! Eventually she went to work full time and it was often left up to us kids to "fin for ourselves." At least, that's what I always thought she was saying at the time. It was many years later I discovered she was saying "fend" all along.

We had a large standing freezer in the dining room in my mid-teens. Boy, was it stocked to the brim with frozen entree chicken pot pies. That's one recipe I promise you'll never see in this or any future cookbooks. I simply cannot *stand* chicken pot pies. I spent too many meals trying to dig through the burned crust to find a frozen center waiting patiently. They're gross. First lesson to surviving in the kitchen: *don't eat gross food.*

My mother tried to teach my older brother how to cook when he was in his early teens, but he wasn't patient enough with the instructions, and as a result, she wasn't patient enough with him. One particular disaster he forgot to drain the water from macaroni noodles, so he had man-and-cheese soup. We were rather poor at the time, so that became his meals until it was gone. Another time he tried to brown the meat for lasagne before it was time, and he had a whole pot of lasagne-spice chili to eat. By the time I hit my teens, she was fairly tired of trying to teach anyone to do what she never really enjoyed. If I was going to learn, it would be in an empty kitchen with no one else at home.

One of the first things I learned how to make was peanut butter cookie dough *without* any raw eggs. The dangers of salmonella poisoning were drilled into my brain by then, so I had some rudimentary basics engrained at least. I've never been a big fan of cookies, or of chocolate, so I would often forgo the chocolate chips, *and* usually the baking. I'd freeze the dough in a flat sheet in a sandwich bag, hidden beneath pot pies, and I'd break small chunks off when nobody was looking. Eventually I shoved off my mothers fear of me burning the house down and started cooking eggs at twelve. (To her credit, I'd once left a potholder on the top of a tea kettle when the announcement that Princess Diana's death hit the news. The potholder slid off, caught fire, and scorched the wall before we realized what happened.)

By the time I was a fifteen-year-old teen runaway, I was comfortable enough in a kitchen that I would often cook for the people I was staying with. It was usually pretty simple, but I could at least cook full meals from scratch.

At sixteen I was determined to take a chemistry class because I loved the experience of how chemistry worked in the kitchen. It was fascinating to me! I failed the class. There might be several different reasons for this, not the least of which was my perpetual habit of running away every time the cops dragged me back home, my growing habit of skipping school, my plummeting self esteem, and my growing hatred for school due to the severe bullying at harassment I received, but the fact remains. Chemistry was *not* in my bag of tricks. I started to believe I was stupid. I was buying into what other people were saying about me. I let them define who I was. I allowed my joys and passions to be ground into dust. I played the piano, until my small keyboard was taken away as punishment. I sang in choir, until my parents didn't allow me to take choir anymore. I always loved drawing, but would get in trouble for drawing what I was feeling or trying to express. Slowly I gave up on so many things I loved - except cooking.

Since nobody knew I was occasionally cooking private meals when nobody else was home, I was never met with the same criticism. It took years before I was finally able to cook for someone else, and even then I was simply putting flavors together and seeing what happened. Some things were complete disasters. Others were great successes I never wrote down and are now lost in the cracks of time forever. But my favorites, the ones I continued to make until the process was burned into my memory, are the ones you'll find in this book.

Eight years ago I had the plan to write a cookbook. I'd put on a little weight over the years and wanted to take it off. In a period of four months, I shed fifty pounds. It was through my own cooking, making sure that I ate healthy foods that I prepared for myself. People watched the weight shed like rain off Italian roof tiles and wanted to know what I'd done. Some folks grew concerned about me, fearing I was starving myself. The truth was quite the opposite. I was eating three *large* meals a day! They were filled with lean meats, flavorful vegetables, and even some of my favorite chocolate-less chocolate chip cookie dough. I ate quite well, quite often, and I found great success. But I found myself embroiled in a bitter, ugly divorce and I lost the motivation and the time to write the book. I was working two full time jobs just trying to survive. There were days that the only thing I could manage to do was cook a meal for myself.

Five years ago I had another plan to write a cookbook. Once more I found myself lacking time and energy for most things. I was **still** working two full time jobs and barely covering the cost of my small one bedroom apartment. I was on an extremely tight budget and couldn't afford the nice little extras, like cookie dough or cable tv, or a new shirt. I was surviving on an average of only $2 per day for my food every month. I spent $60 a month on groceries and *nothing* went to waste. You might even find tips to using up some partial items in the recipes in this book - a throwback to those days of near starvation.

In spite of having very little food and successfully surviving anyway, I started to gain weight. It's no secret that a salad might be $9 on the same menu where French fries are only $0.99 but that wasn't the secret to my weight gain. I didn't know why I was continually gaining weight in spite of limited means until only last year, when I discovered I had thyroid disease. A non-functioning thyroid can really screw a person up.

The first two cookbook ideas that I had planned aren't even *close* to what this one turned out to be.

My mother hated cooking. Without passion she managed to create some rather tasty meals. With that knowledge as my basic inspiration and guide, the idea of this book was created. Where she lacked passion, I had it in spades. Where she created some rather tasty meals, and I never got those recipes from her before she was out of my life forever, I wanted to make sure my favorite things that other people like are available to those who want to learn how to cook the way I did. It doesn't take a culinary school to learn how to feed those you love.

Food is important in so many ways. It can make enemies into friends. It can make friends into enemies (I have stories...). It can heal broken hearts, and mend strained relationships. It can show love and compassion when words aren't enough, and provide warmth when there is no other source for it to come. And it can become a part of a family legacy.

I hope you enjoy these recipes, and when you make them, think fondly of the people in your life, be they still living or long gone. Maybe share a meal (or dessert) with a neighbor. Food has a way of unexpectedly changing the world - or at least the perception someone might have of it.

One word of advice before you start - each time you find something you want to make, be sure to read the whole recipe before you start anything. I can't tell you how many of my recipes came about because I didn't do that, and had to improvise along the way!

Quick tips and kitchen tricks!

- **Read the recipe carefully before you start cooking.** This will help you to understand the steps involved and make sure that you have all of the necessary ingredients.
- Gather all of your ingredients and tools before you start cooking. This will help you to stay organized and avoid making a mess.
- Preheat your oven or stovetop before you start cooking. This will help you to cook your food evenly.
- Use a timer. Get several of them if you need to. I have five currently, although I often use the timer function on my phone these days. This simple step will help you to avoid overcooking your food.
- Taste as you go. This will help you to adjust the seasonings to your liking.
- Have fun! Cooking should be enjoyable. If you're not having fun, it will show in your food.
- Don't overcrowd your pan or baking sheet. If you add too much food to a pan or baking sheet, it will steam instead of cook evenly.
- **Don't be afraid to experiment.** Cooking is a great way to be creative and try new things.
- Clean up as you go. This will help you to avoid a big mess at the end of cooking.
- When boiling eggs, start with cold water. Adding eggs to boiling water can cause them to crack. Cover the eggs with water. The eggs should be completely submerged. Add a teaspoon of vinegar or salt to the water. This can help to prevent the eggs from cracking *and* make them easier to peel. If you want to make deviled eggs, cook the eggs for a shorter amount of time. This will make the yolks softer and easier to mash.
- When cooking bacon, use a large skillet. You want enough room for the bacon to cook evenly without crowding. Don't preheat the skillet. Put the bacon in the skillet while it's still cold. This will help to prevent curling the bacon, and the heat should never be above a medium heat. It's a slower method to cooking bacon, but the fat doesn't pop as much and the texture is so much nicer!

Breakfast

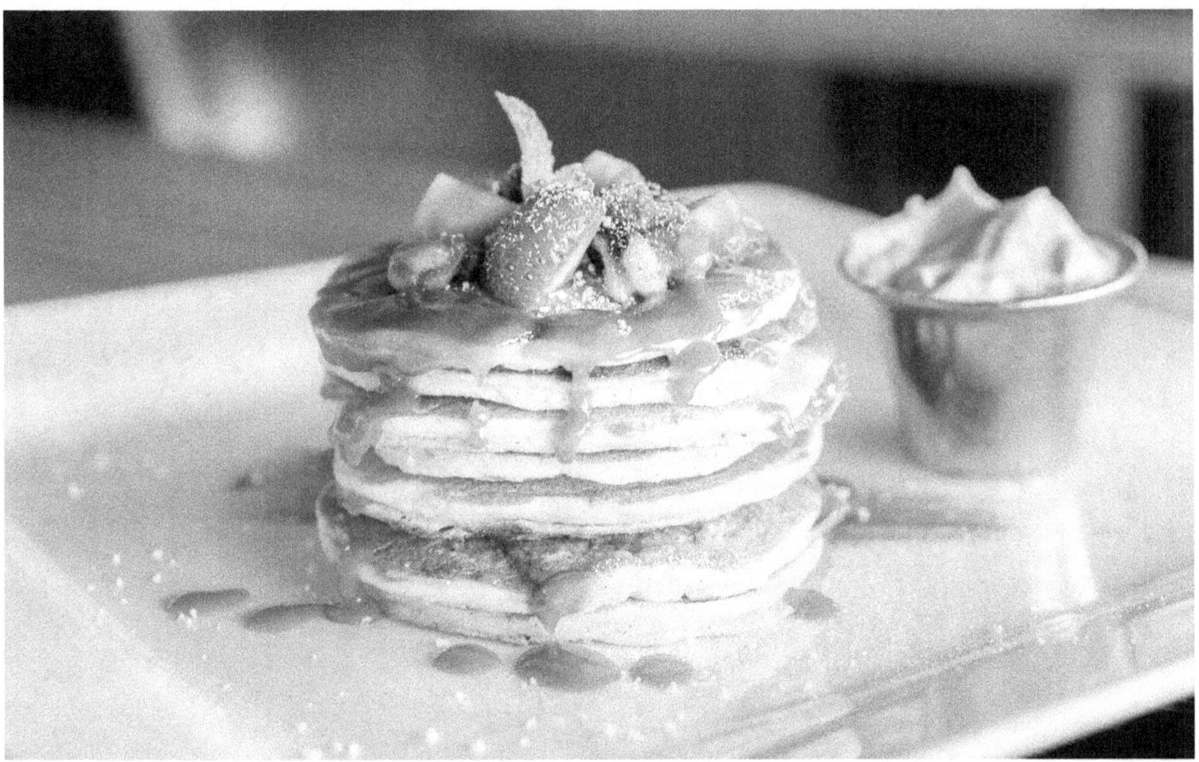

It's long been said that breakfast is the most important meal of the day. For years I struggled with this because I wasn't sure how much I believed in that saying. Breakfast was boring. Usually I was in a hurry to get to work and didn't have the time to spend on making a 45 minute breakfast. Eventually I started finding more recipes that I could either prepare in advance or wouldn't take as long to make in the mornings. Some of them were flavorful enough to make it worth getting up a bit earlier for. I grew up hating breakfast (except on the rare Sundays when my father would make pancakes), but since then I've grown to love it and it's become one of my favorite meals. But when it's both breakfast and dessert? That's when my world comes to life. YUM. Eating healthy is definitely a struggle some days, but thanks to some of my recipes we've been able to find a fairly healthy balance.

Nutty Delicious Granola

There are those days when nothing beats a big bowl of sliced strawberries and bananas on homemade granola with milk or yogurt. To kick up the flavor a bit, you can add some Hershey's cocoa powder (unsweetened) or some coffee flavoring syrup instead of maple syrup. My favorite to use is pumpkin spice because I can be very *basic* at times) or S'mores syrup. DELISH!

Ingredients

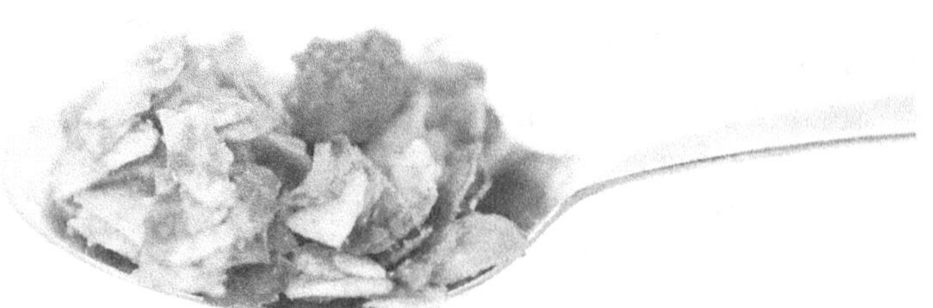

- 4 cups dry rolled oats
- 2 tbs Pepitas
- 2 tbs Sunflower seeds, shelled
- 2 tbs slivered almonds
- 1 tbs chia seeds (white)
- 1 med egg white
- 2 tsp maple syrup
- 2 tsp ground cinnamon
- 1 tsp orange or lemon zest

Directions

1. Preheat the oven to 180°C. Line 2 baking trays with baking paper.
2. Combine oats, pepitas, sunflower seeds, almonds and chia seeds in a large bowl. Whisk the egg white, maple syrup and cinnamon in a small bowl. Add egg white mixture to coat oats mixture and toss to combine. Scatter over lined trays.
3. Bake for 10 minutes, swapping trays and stirring halfway through cooking.
4. Remove from the oven and sprinkle evenly with orange rind. Bake for a further 2 minutes or until granola is lightly golden.
5. Set aside on trays to cool completely.

For a beautiful homemade holiday gift, simply spoon into sterile glass jars, screw the lid on, cover the lid with a square of colorful fabric and tie with a pretty seasonally appropriate ribbon. This goes really well for anything from 4th of July to Christmas.

Best Overnight Oats (with variations)

Ingredients

Base recipe
- ½ cup old fashioned rolled oats
- ½ cup unsweetened almond milk, plus more to thin if desired
- ¼ cup plain fat-free greek yogurt
- 1 pinch salt
- 1 - 3 tsp honey or maple syrup to taste (can substitute sweetener)

Pumpkin
- ⅓ cup canned pumpkin
- ¼ tsp cinnamon
- 1 pinch each nutmeg and cloves
- ⅛ tsp vanilla extract
- 1 Tbsp dried cranberries, for topping
- 1 Tbsp raw unsalted pumpkin seeds , for topping

Chocolate
- 2 - 3 tsp cocoa powder, to taste
- 1 Tbsp creamy peanut butter
- ½ well ripened banana, mashed
- ¼ tsp vanilla extract
- ½ Tbsp mini chocolate chips for topping
- 1 Tbsp shredded toasted coconut, for topping

Berry Chia Seed
- ½ cup fresh berries such as chopped strawberries, whole blueberries or raspberries ,
- ¼ tsp vanilla extract
- 1 ½ tsp chia seeds

Banana Almond Flax
- 1 small ripe banana, mashed
- 1 Tbsp creamy almond butter
- 1 Tbsp ground flax seeds
- 3 drops almond extract

Apple Pie
- ½ cup chopped crisp sweet apples
- ¼ tsp ground cinnamon
- 1 pinch ground nutmeg
- 1 Tbsp chopped pecan for topping

Instructions

1. Add oats, almond milk, yogurt, salt and honey or maple syrup to a 16 oz. jar or bowl. Add mix-ins listed for desired flavor (don't add toppings until the next day). Stir then cover and refrigerate overnight. Thin with more almond milk if desired, add toppings if listed. DONE!

Scrambled Eggs with Smoked Salmon

Ingredients

- ¼ pound sliced smoked salmon
- 12 eggs
- ½ cup heavy cream
- Salt and freshly ground black pepper
- 2 tablespoons butter
- 12 to 15 blades of fresh chives, finely chopped

Directions

1. Reserve 2 slices of salmon for garnish. Chop the remaining salmon into very small pieces.
2. Whisk your eggs and cream together. Add ½ of your chopped chives and season eggs with salt and pepper. Preheat a large nonstick skillet over medium heat.
3. Melt butter in the pan and add eggs, stirring to scramble. When eggs have come together but remain wet, stir in the chopped salmon. Remove the pan from the stove. Garnish the eggs with remaining salmon and chives and serve right out of the warm pan.

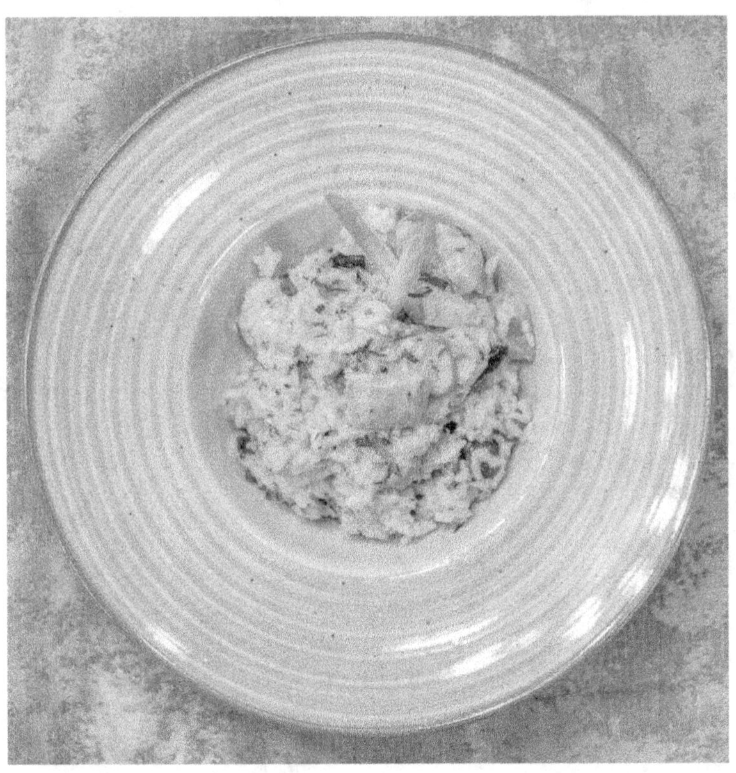

Egg In A Hole Sandwiches

Ingredients

- 6 slices thick-cut peppered bacon
- ¼ cup mayonnaise
- Jalapeño-style hot sauce, as needed
- Kosher salt and freshly ground black pepper
- 4 slices Texas toast
- 4 tablespoons salted butter
- 4 large eggs
- 4 slices pepper jack cheese
- 1 small tomato, sliced
- Green leaf lettuce, for topping

Directions

1. In a large cast-iron skillet over medium heat, cook the bacon until crisp, 12 to 14 minutes. Remove to a plate and set aside. Drain the grease from the skillet but do not clean. When cool enough to handle, tear the bacon slices in half.
2. Meanwhile, mix the mayonnaise and hot sauce to taste in a small bowl. Season with salt and pepper.
3. Using a biscuit cutter or the rim of a glass, cut a hole in the center of each Texas toast slice.
4. Melt 2 tablespoons of the butter in the bacon skillet and add 2 of the Texas toast slices. Toast the bread slightly, 1 to 2 minutes. Crack an egg into the hole in each piece of toast and sprinkle the eggs with salt and pepper. Cook the eggs until set on the bottom, 2 to 3 minutes. Using a spatula, carefully flip the toast with the egg, season the other side and spread with the mayonnaise mixture. Top each with a slice of cheese to slightly melt and cook until the egg is the desired done-ness. Remove to a cutting board and repeat with the remaining butter, toast, eggs, mayo mixture and cheese.
5. To build the sandwiches, divide the bacon between 2 of the egg-in-a-hole toast pieces, on top of the cheese. Top each with some tomato slices and lettuce, then top with a remaining egg-in-a-hole toast piece. Serve immediately or wrap in foil to keep warm.

Egg-Stuffed Bacon and Cheese Muffins

Ingredients

- 6 slices bacon
- 10 large eggs
- Nonstick cooking spray, for the muffin tin
- 1 ⅔ cups all-purpose flour, plus more for dusting the eggs (see Cook's Note)
- 1 ½ teaspoons baking powder
- ¾ teaspoon kosher salt
- ½ teaspoon baking soda
- ¼ teaspoon freshly ground black pepper
- Pinch of granulated sugar
- ½ cup vegetable oil
- ½ cup nonfat plain Greek yogurt
- 4 ounces Irish Cheddar, shredded on the large holes of a box grater (about 1 cup)
- ¼ cup grated Pecorino Romano (about 1 1/2 ounces)
- 4 scallions, thinly sliced (about 1/4 cup)
- Flaky sea salt and hot sauce, for serving

Directions

1. Put the bacon in a large skillet and place over medium heat. Cook, flipping occasionally, until golden brown and crispy, about 8 minutes. Drain on a paper towel-lined plate, then finely chop.
2. Meanwhile, fill a large bowl with lots of ice and water; set aside. Bring a large saucepan of water to a boil over medium-high heat. Gently lower 6 of the eggs into the water with a slotted spoon and cook until soft boiled (the whites have set but the yolks are still runny), 5 minutes (see Cook's Note). Transfer the eggs immediately to the ice water bath to stop the cooking and let sit until completely cool, about 15 minutes. Carefully peel the eggs and reserve.
3. Preheat the oven to 425 degrees F and spray a 6-cup jumbo muffin tin generously with nonstick cooking spray.
4. Whisk the flour, baking powder, kosher salt, baking soda, pepper and sugar in a medium bowl until evenly combined. Whisk the vegetable oil, yogurt and remaining 4 eggs in a large bowl until smooth and combined. Stir the flour mixture into the yogurt mixture until just combined (do not overmix), then gently fold in the Cheddar, Pecorino Romano, scallions and reserved bacon until just combined. Transfer to a piping bag or resealable freezer bag and snip the tip. Put a couple tablespoons of flour in a small bowl.
5. Pipe enough batter into each prepared muffin cup to just cover the bottom and help anchor the soft-boiled eggs. Carefully dust the soft-boiled eggs in the flour, shaking off any excess (this will help the batter to adhere), then place 1 upright in each muffin cup. Pipe the remaining batter around and on top of the eggs, making sure the eggs are completely coated. Use a rubber spatula or offset spatula to help smooth out the tops of each muffin (they should look domed).

6. Bake until the muffin tops are light golden brown, the batter is just cooked through and the eggs inside are soft and jammy, about 16 minutes. Let the muffins sit in the tin for just 5 minutes, then transfer to a wire rack. Enjoy warm, cut in half with a sprinkle of flaky sea salt and a few dashes of hot sauce.

FOR STORING: let the muffins come to room temperature, then refrigerate in an airtight container for up to 5 days.

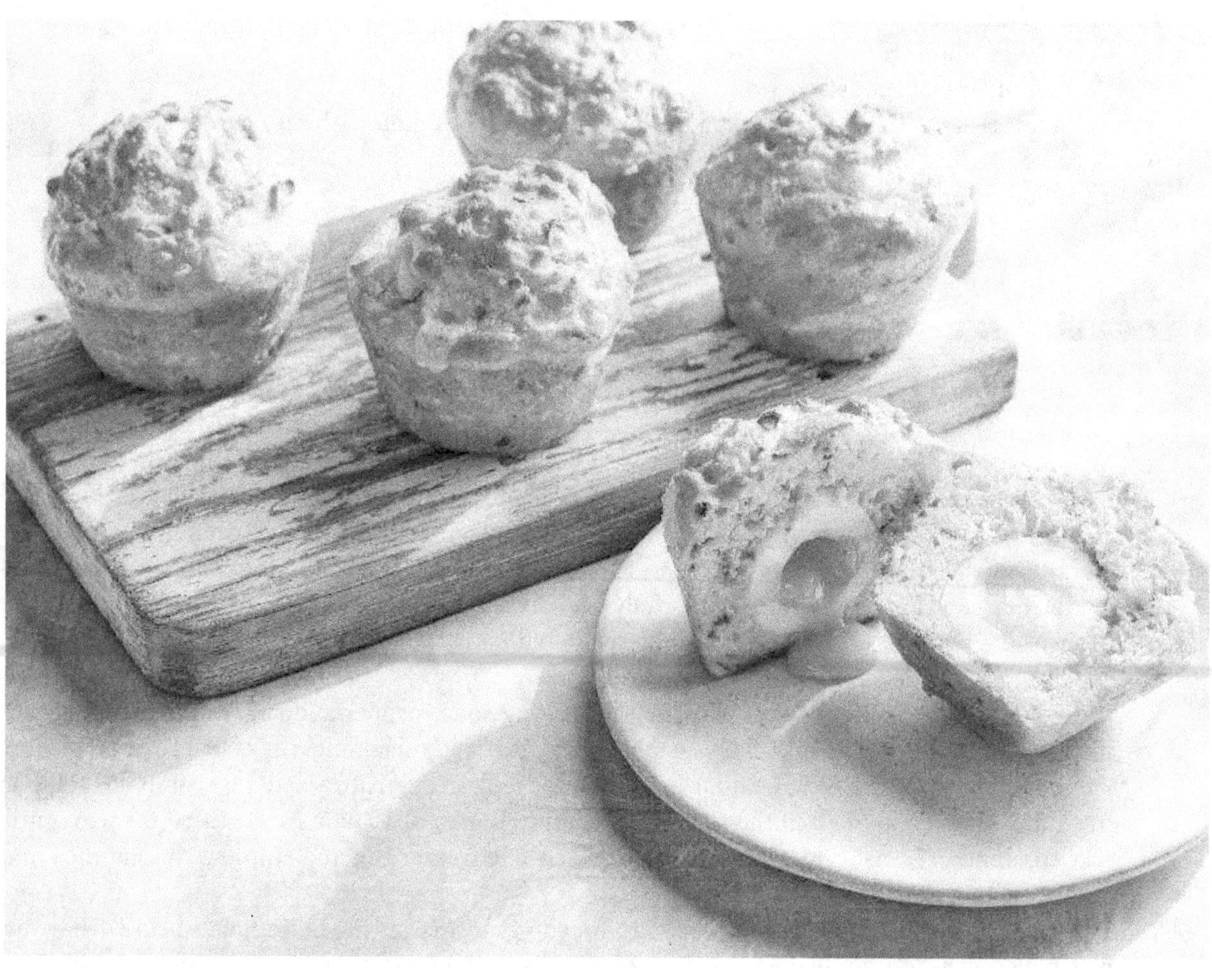

Castroville Omelet

Traveling the coast of California was always a pleasure, and while on a map the little town of Castroville seems like a little spot of nothing, nestled into the heart of the outer layers is a tiny little omelet house that deserves all the credit for this fantastic recipe. Castroville at one time was the Artichoke Capital of the world, which might explain some of the ingredients in this recipe. Though the restaurant appears to be closed now, the flavors live on.

Ingredients

- Non Stick Cooking Spray
- ¼ cup sliced green onions (white portion only), reserve green portion
- 3 cloves garlic, minced
- 1 cup canned artichoke hearts, drained, patted dry
- ½ cup chopped red bell peppers
- 8 pitted Greek kalamata olives, chopped
- ½ teaspoon dried oregano leaves
- ½ teaspoon dried basil leaves
- ¼ teaspoon ground black pepper
- 3 tablespoons grated Parmesan cheese, divided
- 8 eggs, lightly beaten

Directions

1. Spray medium skillet with cooking spray; heat over medium heat. Add white portion of green onions and garlic; cook 1 minute, stirring occasionally. Add artichokes, bell peppers, olives, oregano, basil and black pepper. Cook for 8 minutes, or until vegetables are crisp-tender, stirring occasionally. Remove vegetables from skillet; cover to keep warm.
2. Pour eggs into the same skillet. Allow the eggs to cook as they are *without* moving the skillet or lifting the cooked egg up. Cook until the eggs are almost set on the surface but still look moist.
3. Spoon vegetable mixture over half of omelet; sprinkle with 2 tablespoons cheese. Fold the omelet in half.
4. Slide onto a serving plate. Top omelet with remaining 1 tablespoon cheese and reserved green portion of green onion. Cut into 4 wedges to serve.

Hashbrown Omelet

Ingredients

- 3 Tbsp olive oil
- ¼ cup finely diced green bell peppers
- ¼ cup finely diced canadian bacon
- Salt and fresh ground pepper
- 2 cups frozen shredded hash browns (do not thaw)
- 2 large eggs
- 2 slices cheese
- ¼ cup finely diced Roma tomatoes
- 1 Tbsp thinly sliced scallions
- ½ ripe avocado, thinly sliced

Directions

1. Heat 1 tbsp of the olive oil in a medium sized skillet over medium high heat. Add the bell peppers, canadian bacon, and salt. Do not add the pepper, as it has a tendency to burn at higher temps. Cook, stirring occasionally until the peppers are just tender and the bacon begins to brown in spots. Transfer the veggies to a small bowl and return the skillet to the heat.
2. Add 1 more Tbsp of the olive oil to the same skillet, swirling the pan to evenly coat. Add the shredded hash browns in a single layer and press down with the back of a spatula. Cook, undisturbed, until the bottom is golden brown and crispy, about 10 minutes. Flip the hashbrowns over, add the remaining 1 tbsp of oil around the edge of the skillet, then continue to cook until the other side is golden, about 5 minutes more.
3. Whisk the eggs with a pinch of salt and the black pepper in a small bowl until thoroughly combined.
4. Reduce the heat under the skillet to medium low. Break apart the hashbrowns slightly, then pour the eggs over top in an even layer (sometimes I use a small ladle to get it as even as possible without disturbing the hashbrowns). Cook until the eggs are just set. Lay the cheese over the top evenly. Then sprinkle over the cooked peppers, bacon, tomatoes, and scallions. Continue to cook until the cheese is just melted, about one minute more.
5. Fold the omelet in half, and serve hot with a garnish of cheese, scallions, and a touch of pepper.

Stuffed Acorn Squash

Ingredients

- 2 small uncooked acorn squash, halved lengthwise, seeds removed
- Non stick cooking spray
- ½ tsp salt
- ¼ tsp freshly ground Black pepper
- ¼ tsp Dried oregano
- 4 Eggs
- Fresh spinach leaves
- ½ cup diced Roasted red peppers (packed in water)
- ¼ cup crumbled feta cheese
- 1 tsp fresh minced Dill

Directions

1. Preheat the oven to 425°F. Line a baking sheet with parchment paper.
2. Cut a thin slice off the bottom of each squash half so it sits flat. Place squash halves, cut side up, on prepared pan and coat with cooking spray; sprinkle with salt, pepper, and oregano. Roast until squash is just tender and a paring knife can pierce flesh without much resistance, about 25 minutes.
3. Sprinkle squash halves with more salt and pepper (optional); line the bowl with fresh spinach leaves and crack an egg into each one over the spinach. Evenly divide peppers over top.
4. Return squash to the oven; bake until eggs are set to your liking, about 15 minutes for a still-runny yolk and up to 20 for a set yolk. Sprinkle each with 1 Tbsp feta and some dill. Serve immediately.

Jalapeno Cheddar Grits with Bacon and Eggs

Ingredients

- 2 tablespoons butter
- 2 jalapeno peppers, minced
- 2 cups water
- 2 cups milk
- ½ teaspoon salt
- 1 cup old-fashioned grits
- 1 ½ cups shredded cheddar cheese
- black pepper
- Thick cut bacon
- 4 eggs

Directions

1. Melt butter over medium-high heat in a medium saucepan. Add jalapeno and cook for 2 minutes to soften.
2. Add water, milk, and salt and bring to a boil. Turn heat to low and gradually whisk in the grits. Cover and cook for 15 to 20 minutes, stirring occasionally.
3. While the grits are cooking, set the bacon in a skillet to cook at medium heat. Set the bacon in while the skillet is still cold to prevent curling.
4. With about five minutes remaining for the grits to cook, cook the eggs over medium (solid cooked white, warm liquid yellows) in a separate skillet.
5. When the bacon is done, dice the cooked bacon and mix into the grits mixture. Stir in cheddar cheese and black pepper to taste. Pour the cooked grits into two bowls and serve two eggs over the top.

Sheet Pan Vegetable Frittata

So this recipe is as versatile as it is delicious. I wasn't really sure my husband would like this one the first time I made it since it doesn't have what he considers to be any substantial amount of meat (and eggs don't count to him). I was pleasantly surprised when he not only loved it, but asked for seconds, and wanted to know how difficult it would be to take to work! The next page has a couple of other recipes that use this same veggie frittata for some make-ahead ideas, and the breakfast sandwich has worked out incredibly well for him. There are dozens of other things you can do with this recipe, and have fun!

Ingredients

- Non stick Cooking spray
- 1 ½ cups thin sliced zucchini (about 2 medium)
- 1 ½ cups thin sliced yellow squash (about 2 medium)
- 1 cup halved grape tomatoes
- 1 medium sweet red pepper, cut into thin strips
- ½ cup 2% milk or unsweetened almond milk
- 1 tsp salt
- ½ tsp black pepper
- ½ tsp dried thyme
- 12 large eggs
- ¾ cup shredded sharp cheddar cheese
- ¼ cup chopped chives

Directions

1. Preheat the oven to 400°F. Coat a large (18-by-13-inch) sheet pan with cooking spray. (I tend to also line mine with foil for easy cleanup.)
2. Combine the zucchini, squash, tomatoes, and bell pepper on the prepared pan and spread into an even layer, avoiding overlap as much as possible. Bake at 400°F until the vegetables are crisp-tender, about 15 minutes.
3. Reduce the oven temperature to 350°F. In a large bowl, whisk the milk, salt, black pepper, thyme, and eggs. Fold in the cheese and chives. Pour the eggs over the vegetables on the pan, stirring to redistribute the cheese and chives if necessary.
4. Bake at 350°F until the eggs are set, 15 to 17 minutes. Run a thin knife or offset spatula around the edges of the frittata to loosen it from the pan. Store the frittata in the refrigerator for up to 5 days or freeze for up to 1 month.

Frittata Avocado Toast

Ingredients

- 1 piece oof the Sheet-Pan Veggie Frittata (see prior recipe)
- ½ medium Avocado
- 1 slice Whole wheat bread, toasted
- ⅛ tsp salt

Directions

1. On a microwave-safe plate, microwave the frittata on High until heated through, 45 seconds to 1 minute.
2. Place the warm frittata on the toast. Using a fork, mash the avocado with the salt and place on top of the frittata. Serve immediately.

Frittata breakfast sandwiches

Ingredients

- 1 piece sheet-Pan Veggie Frittata (see previous recipe)
- 1 slice cooked Canadian bacon
- ⅓ cup fresh baby spinach
- 2 thin slices Fresh tomato
- 1 Everything bagel, toasted
- Thin sliced sharp cheddar

Directions

1. On a microwave-safe plate, arrange the frittata and top with the bacon. Microwave on High until the frittata is heated through, 45 seconds to 1 minute.
2. Layer the frittata, bacon, spinach, and tomato on the bottom half of the bagel, top with cheese. Add the top half of the bagel and serve!

Steak, Spinach and Brie Crepes

My husband can't stand mushrooms so I have a little fun improvising with these. Originally the recipe called for blue cheese instead of brie, but I've discovered the soft, nuttiness of brie pairs so beautifully with the flavors of steak and balsamic. Of course you could always use blue cheese instead, now that I've told you the secret. Try both! And let me know which one you like more.

Ingredients

Crepes
- 2 large eggs
- 3/4 cup milk I use 2%
- 1 cup all purpose flour
- 3 tablespoons butter
- 1/4 teaspoon salt
- 1/2 cup water

Filling
- 2 ounce beef tenderloin filets
- freshly crack coarse black pepper
- coarse salt
- 2 tablespoons butter
- 1 clove garlic minced or grated
- 6-12 ounces baby bella mushrooms sliced
- 6 ounces fresh spinach
- 2 tablespoons balsamic vinegar
- salt and pepper to taste
- a pinch of fresh nutmeg
- 4 to 8 ounces brie cheese, cut into small pieces
- fresh parsley for garnish

Balsamic Glaze
- 1/2 cup balsamic vinegar
- 1 teaspoon brown sugar optional

Directions

1. To make the crepes. Add butter to a small saucepan and heat over medium heat. Whisk constantly until brown bits appear on the bottom, about 5-6 minutes, then immediately remove from heat and set aside. Combine all the remaining ingredients in a blender or food processor. Add the browned butter and pulse for 30 seconds or until well combined. Place the crepe batter in the refrigerator for about 30 minutes. This allows the bubbles to subside so the crepes will be less likely to tear during cooking. The batter will keep for up to 48 hours.
2. Heat a 12 inch non-stick pan. Add butter or cooking spray (I like to use cooking spray) to coat. Pour 1/3 cup of batter into the center of the pan and swirl to spread evenly. Cook for 30 seconds

and flip. Cook for another 10 seconds and remove to the cutting board. Lay them out flat so they can cool. Continue until all batter is gone. Makes about 10 crepes.

3. To make the balsamic glaze, add the vinegar and brown sugar (if using) to a small saucepan and bring to a boil. Reduce to a very low simmer and cook for 10-15 minutes, until liquid reduces by about half and is slightly syrupy. Remove from heat, pour the glaze into a bowl or glass to pour, and set aside to cool and thicken.

4. Cook the steak using your preferred method - I like to cook it to medium in a well seasoned cast iron skillet. Once the steaks are cooked, place them on a cutting board. Let them rest 10 minutes before slicing against the grain into 1/4 inch strips.

5. Meanwhile, heat a medium skillet over medium high heat, add 2 tablespoons butter and toss in the mushrooms in a single layer. Don't stir them! Let them sizzle until they have caramelized on the bottom, about 2 minutes. When the bottoms are caramelized, toss them once and add the spinach. Season with salt and pepper, to taste. Continue cooking for about 5 minutes or until the spinach is beginning to wilt. Add the garlic and cook for about 10 seconds. Add the balsamic vinegar, and simmer until the mushrooms have soaked up all remaining vinegar. Remove from the heat, taste and adjust seasonings if needed.

6. To assemble, layer a crepe flat on a plate and sprinkle on the spinach and mushrooms. Add a few slices of steak and a generous sprinkle of brie cheese. Fold the crepe up into triangles or little burritos. Drizzle with the balsamic glaze and sprinkle with fresh parsley.

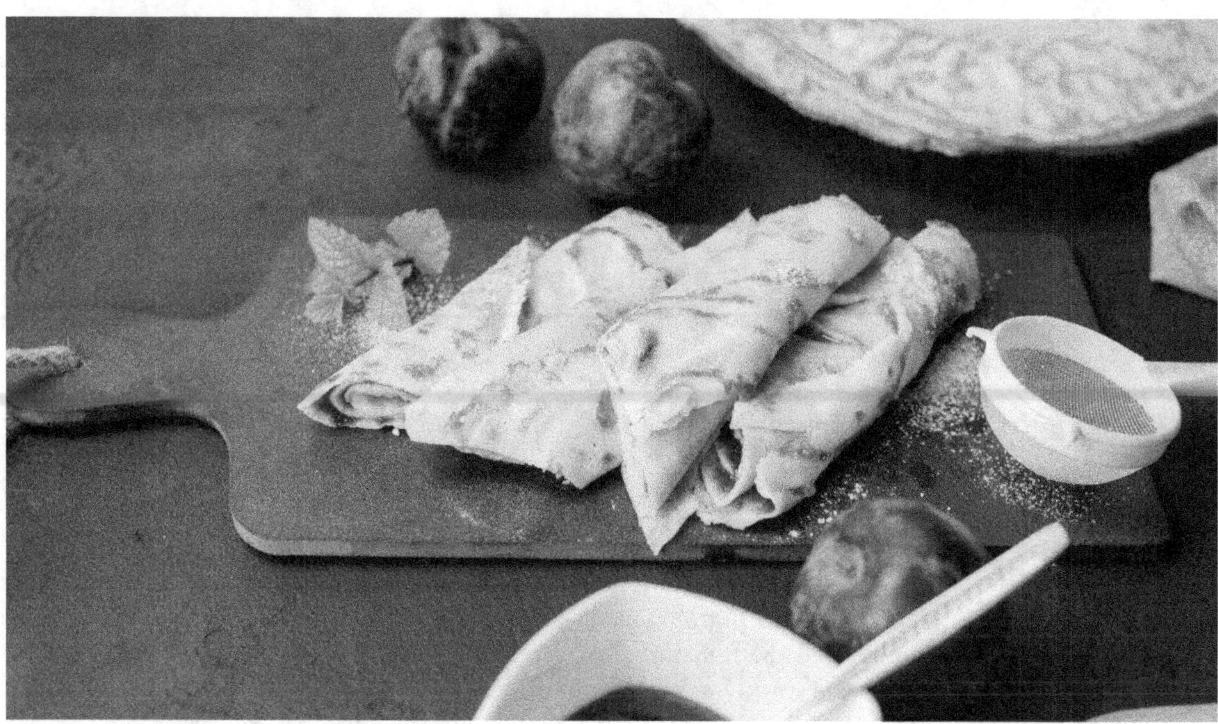

New Orleans French Toast

The first time I ever made this for my husband he was terribly confused. He couldn't understand how someone could make french toast out of french bread! In New Orleans it's known as Pain Purdue instead of French Toast, but I have two different recipes for it, depending on my mood at the time. You'll find the other recipe on the next page, named New Orleans Pain Perdu. You might be surprised to find yet a *third* recipe for french toast in the book, but that one is slightly different.

Ingredients

- 2 large eggs
- 1 cup milk, half and half, coconut milk, or almond milk
- pinch salt
- 1 tablespoon granulated sugar, honey or maple syrup
- 1 teaspoon vanilla extract
- 1 teaspoon ground cinnamon
- 8 slices french bread
- Butter and syrup

Directions

1. Whisk. To save on dishes and cleanup, I whisk together the eggs, milk, sweetener, vanilla extract, and ground cinnamon right into a shallow dish I'll use to dip my bread in.
2. Dip. Once I have whisked the egg mixture together well, I place my bread slice in on one side and then quickly flip it over to the other side since some sandwich bread will absorb the liquid super quickly. You'll want to be sure that you are dipping your bread and not leaving it for any time to soak so that the bread does not absorb too much liquid. Make sure to follow this so your bread does not get too wet. This will prevent your French toast from becoming soggy.
3. Cook. Once both sides of the bread are coated with the liquid, I place them into the skillet with melted butter set over medium heat. They only take a few minutes to cook, about 2 to 3 minutes on each side.
4. Serve. Serve immediately with your syrup of choice. I also love to serve with fruit like fresh berries (I love blackberries, blueberries, strawberries, and raspberries). A dollop of homemade whipped cream is always a good idea!

New Orleans Pain Perdu

Ingredients

- ½ pint fresh strawberries, hulled and sliced
- 2 tablespoons sugar, divided
- 3 tablespoons orange liqueur (like Grand Marnier), divided
- 6 extra-large eggs
- 1½ cups milk or half-and-half
- 2 tablespoons honey
- 1½ teaspoons pure vanilla extract
- 1 teaspoon grated orange zest
- 2 teaspoons kosher salt
- 1 large brioche loaf or french bread
- Unsalted butter
- Vegetable oil
- ½ cup (1½ ounces) sliced blanched almonds, toasted
- Confectioners' sugar, to serve
- Butter and syrup

Directions

1. Combine the sliced strawberries, 1 tablespoon of the sugar, and 1 tablespoon of the orange liqueur in a small bowl and set aside.
2. Preheat the oven to 250°F.
3. In a large bowl, whisk together the eggs, milk, honey, 1 tablespoon of sugar, 2 tablespoons orange liqueur, the vanilla, orange zest, and salt. Slice the bread in ¾ inch slices. Pour the egg mixture into a large shallow plate and soak a few slices of bread for 4 minutes, turning once.
4. Heat 1 tablespoon each of butter and oil in a very large saute pan over medium heat. Take each slice of bread from the egg mixture, dip one side in the toasted almonds, and place in the saute pan, almond side down. (While you're cooking each batch, add more bread to the egg mixture to soak.) Cook for 2 to 3 minutes on each side, until nicely browned.
5. Place the cooked bread on a baking sheet and keep it warm in the oven. Wipe out the pan with a dry paper towel, add more butter and oil, and continue to fry the remaining soaked bread until they're all cooked. Sprinkle it with confectioners' sugar and serve hot with the strawberries, butter, and syrup.

Banana Bread French Toast

I had made banana bread the week before and it was getting old. We'd had an extremely busy week and hadn't made time to devour it the way we normally did, and I needed a way to use it up in a hurry, so I made this one weekend for my husband. It was a massive hit, and since the banana bread I make (see bread section of the book) is a rather heavy bread, there were some leftovers he was able to take to work the following week. He had several people ask what he was eating and many of them asked if they could have the recipe so I've included it here. This one is for Marianna.

Ingredients

- 3 eggs
- 3 tablespoons sweetened condensed milk
- 1 teaspoon vanilla extract
- 2 tablespoons butter
- 1 loaf banana bread (see bread section of the book)
- 1 tablespoon confectioners' sugar for dusting

Directions

1. In a shallow bowl, whisk together the eggs, sweetened condensed milk and vanilla with a fork. Set aside.
2. Melt butter in a large skillet over medium heat. Slice banana bread into 4 thick slices. Dip each slice into the egg mixture, then place in the hot pan.
3. Cook on each side until golden brown, but be careful when turning! The bread can be a bit delicate. Dust with confectioners' sugar just before serving, and smother with fresh strawberries and bananas.

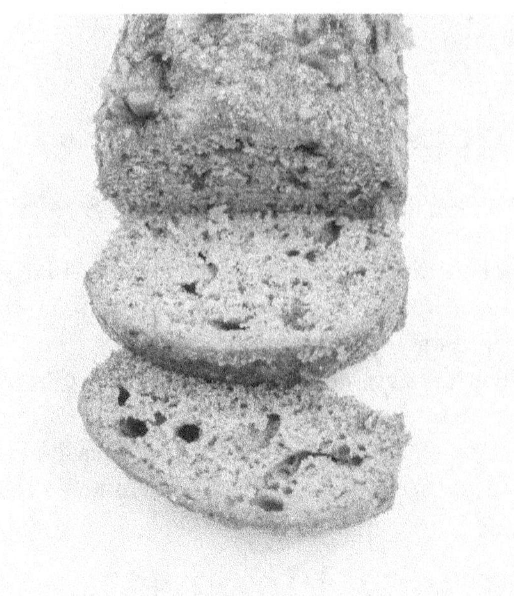

Velvety Herb Luncheon Scrambled Eggs

Ingredients

- 9 large eggs
- ¼ cup milk or cream, plus a splash
- ¼ cup butter
- 1 tablespoon minced fresh marjoram or oregano
- 1 tablespoon minced fresh thyme
- ½ scallion, minced (green only)
- 2 tablespoons freshly grated Parmesan cheese
- Salt and freshly ground black pepper
- Lemon wedges, for serving
- Green Salad, recipe follows
- Green Salad:
- 1 head green, red or butter lettuce, torn into small pieces (5 cups mesclun salad mix)
- Classic Dijon Vinaigrette:
- 1 teaspoon Dijon mustard
- 1 ½ tablespoons red wine vinegar
- ¼ cup olive oil
- Salt and freshly ground black pepper

Directions

1. In a medium bowl, whisk the eggs plus 1/4 cup of milk or cream until no longer stringy, about 1 minute.
2. Over medium-low heat, melt butter in a large nonstick saute pan. Pour the eggs into a pan and using a wooden spoon or rubber spatula, gently stir the eggs and cook over low heat. The eggs will turn creamy with soft curds.
3. When the eggs appear as half cooked, toss in the marjoram, thyme, scallion, Parmesan cheese, salt and pepper, and stir to distribute. Once the eggs are no longer runny, but still very creamy and moist, immediately pour a little splash of milk (1 or 2 teaspoons) on the eggs and stir. Remove the eggs from the heat. Serve immediately with wedges of lemon as garnish and Green Salad.

Classic Dijon Vinaigrette:

4. In a small bowl, whisk together the mustard and the vinegar. Slowly whisk in the olive oil to make an emulsion. Season with salt and pepper.
5. Toss the green salad with the vinaigrette and serve.

Overnight waffles

The story of how I stumbled onto overnight waffles is a bit embarrassing to be perfectly honest with you. It all started out because I wanted to make homemade bread for some guests from out of the country. My hope was to impress them with my cooking and baking skills with a recipe from my favorite cookbook I'd had for many years. I was chatting with them while preparing my ingredients, and by the time I'd dumped them into the bowl and gave it a stir, it hadn't registered in my brain yet that I'd accidentally combined two different recipes into one - a homemade bread recipe, and a waffle recipe that was on the same page next to it. (This is actually why I adamantly left only one recipe per page in this book. Otherwise a cookbook can be extremely difficult to work with when you're dyslexic like I am.) At the time I was rather poor and didn't want to toss out the ingredients, so I was determined to just stick with what I had and figure something out. I still made the bread, but the waffles I accidentally made were THE big hit.

Ingredients

Night Before:
- ½ cup warm water
- 1 tablespoon active-dry yeast
- ½ cup melted butter
- 2 cups whole or 2% milk
- 1 teaspoon salt
- 2 tablespoons sugar (optional)
- 3 cups all-purpose flour

The Next Day:
- 2 large eggs, beaten
- ½ teaspoon baking soda

Directions

1. Combine the yeast and the water in a large mixing bowl and let stand for a few minutes. Stir to make sure the yeast dissolves into the water. Melt the butter over low heat or in the microwave. Combine the butter with the milk, salt, and sugar (if using). Test with your finger to make sure the mixture has cooled to lukewarm, then stir it into the dissolved yeast mixture. Add the flour and stir until a thick, shaggy dough is formed and there is no more visible flour.
2. Cover the bowl with plastic wrap and let it sit on the counter overnight. The batter will double or triple in bulk as it rises.
3. The next morning, beat the eggs together and add them to the batter along with the baking soda. Using a whisk or hand blender, beat the eggs and baking soda into the batter until completely combined.
4. Make the waffles according to your waffle maker's instructions, cooking until the waffles are golden-brown. Cooking time will vary with your waffle maker, but it is typically 4 to 6 minutes.
5. Waffles are best if served immediately, but reheat well in the toaster. Waffles can be frozen for up to 3 months and toasted straight out of the freezer for quick work-morning leftovers.

Best Ever Pancakes

Ingredients

- 1½ cups all-purpose flour
- 2 tablespoons sugar
- 1 teaspoon baking powder
- ½ teaspoon baking soda
- ½ teaspoon salt
- 1 cup buttermilk (can substitute plant based milk)
- 2 large eggs, room temperature
- ¼ cup butter, melted
- 1 teaspoon vanilla extract
- Optional: Mixed fresh berries, whipped cream, maple syrup and butter

Directions

1. In a large bowl, whisk together the first 5 ingredients. In another bowl, whisk all of the remaining ingredients; stir into dry ingredients just until moistened.
2. Preheat the griddle over medium heat. Lightly grease the griddle. Pour batter by ¼ cupfuls onto griddle; cook until bubbles on top begin to pop and bottoms are golden brown. Turn; cook until the second side is golden brown. Serve with toppings as desired.

Best Ever Banana Pancakes

Ingredients

- 1 cup milk
- 1 egg (beaten)
- 2 Tbsp butter (melted)
- 1 tsp vanilla extract
- 1½ cups all purpose flour
- 3 Tbsp dark brown sugar
- 1 Tbsp baking powder
- ½ tsp salt
- 2 small bananas (mashed)
- OPTIONAL
- ½ tsp cinnamon
- bananas (sliced)
- maple syrup
- mini chocolate chips

Directions

1. In a small bowl, whisk together the wet ingredients.
2. In a larger bowl, combine the dry ingredients.
3. Mash 2 small bananas (you'll need 1 cup of mashed bananas total, so adjust according the size of bananas used)
4. Add the wet ingredients to the dry and add the mashed bananas. Fold together gently until just combined.
5. Heat 1 Tbsp butter in a skillet over medium heat.
6. Add pancake batter ½ to ¾ per pancake.
7. Cook until bubbles form and pop, then flip. Cook for another minute or two, until golden brown.
8. Add bananas, syrup and chocolate chips to your pancake stack.

Pancake Bread

Ingredients

- Nonstick cooking spray, for the loaf pan
- Pinch ground cinnamon
- 1 stick plus 1 tablespoon (9 tablespoons) unsalted butter, at room temperature
- 2 cups plus 2 tablespoons all-purpose flour (see Cook's Note)
- 1 cup plus 2 tablespoons packed dark brown sugar
- Kosher salt
- 1 teaspoon baking soda
- 1/2 teaspoon baking powder
- 1 cup sour cream
- 2/3 cup pure maple syrup, plus more for serving
- 2 teaspoons pure vanilla extract
- 2 large eggs

Directions

- Position an oven rack in the center of the oven and preheat to 350°F.
- Thoroughly grease a 9-by-5-inch loaf pan with nonstick spray, then line with parchment, leaving a 2-inch overhang on the 2 long sides of the pan. Grease the parchment with nonstick spray.
- Using the tines of a fork, smash the cinnamon, 1 tablespoon butter, 2 tablespoons flour, 2 tablespoons brown sugar and a pinch of salt together in a small bowl until combined and buttery clumps form. Set aside until ready to bake.
- Whisk together the baking soda, baking powder, remaining 2 cups flour and 1 teaspoon salt in a medium bowl until combined.
- Whisk together the sour cream, maple syrup and vanilla in a small bowl until completely combined and no lumps of sour cream remain.
- Beat the remaining 8 tablespoons butter in a large bowl with an electric mixer on medium-high speed until light and creamy, about 3 minutes. Gradually add the remaining 1 cup brown sugar and beat until light and fluffy, 3 minutes more. Add the eggs one at a time, beating until fully incorporated after each addition; continue to beat until the mixture is light and fluffy, about 1 minute more. Reduce the speed to low.
- Add the dry ingredients in 3 additions, alternating with the sour cream mixture in 2 additions, beginning and ending with the dry ingredients.
- Scrape the batter into the prepared loaf pan and smooth the top. Sprinkle with the reserved cinnamon and butter crumb mixture. Bake until the top is brown and a tester inserted in the center comes out clean, 1 hour to 1 hour 10 minutes. Transfer the pan to a wire rack and let the bread cool in the pan for 30 minutes. Run a paring knife around the sides to loosen and use the parchment overhang to carefully lift the bread out of the pan. Let sit on the rack until cooled, about 1 hour more.

Breakfast Bread Pudding

I don't know how to tell you this, but I might be addicted to this recipe. It's easy, full of flavor, and makes me feel like I'm eating dessert for breakfast. What's not to love? It's not as sweet as a dessert (depending on how much syrup you add), but the 'kapow' of flavor gets to me every single time.

Ingredients

- 5 eggs
- 2 extra egg yolks
- 2 ½ cups half-and-half
- ⅓ cup honey
- 1 ½ teaspoons pure vanilla extract
- 2 teaspoons orange zest (apx2 oranges)
- ½ teaspoon kosher salt
- Brioche loaf
- ½ cup golden raisins
- Maple syrup, to serve

Directions

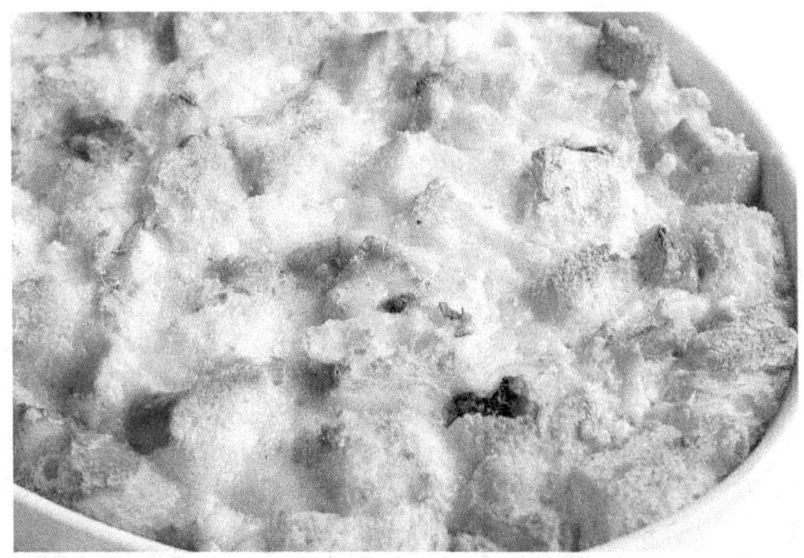

1. Preheat the oven to 350°F.
2. In a medium bowl, whisk together the whole eggs, egg yolks, half-and-half, honey, vanilla, orange zest, and salt. Set aside.
3. Slice the brioche loaf into 6 (1-inch) thick pieces. Lay half brioche slices flat in a 9 by 14 by 2-inch oval baking dish. Spread the raisins on top of the brioche slices, and place the remaining slices on top. Make sure that the raisins are between the layers of brioche or they will burn while baking. Pour the egg mixture over the bread and allow to soak for 15 minutes, pressing down gently.
4. Bake for 55 to 60 minutes or until the pudding puffs up and the custard is set. Remove from the oven and cool slightly before serving.

Banana Caramel Dutch Baby

I know not everyone has a Dutch Oven or a Cast Iron Skillet, but they're incredibly simple to take care of once you do get one, and they can make some of the most amazing meals you've ever had, including this dish, or a juicy New York Strip Steak to die for. I was scared of them for years myself, but my husband had one when we got married and I learned pretty quickly how to use it. This recipe was an instant hit, and of course I've added my own twist to the mix. Just make sure your ingredients are at room temperature before you begin the process or it won't turn out quite the same. (I'm actually typing this recipe as I'm still tasting the lingering flavors of this breakfast and almost wishing I had more.)

Ingredients

- 3 large eggs *at room temperature*
- ½ cup all purpose flour
- ½ cup milk, *at room temperature*
- 1 tsp granulated sugar
- 3 tsp brown sugar
- ½ tsp cinnamon, halved
- Pinch of nutmeg
- 4 Tbsp butter, chopped
- 1 ½ bananas, separated
- 1 cup sliced strawberries

Directions

1. Preheat the oven to 425°F with the 10 inch cast iron skillet inside the oven.
2. In a medium bowl, combine the eggs, flour, milk, granulated sugar, ¼ tsp of cinnamon and the nutmeg with a whisk. Beat until blended.
3. In a separate bowl, stir together ½ of a sliced banana with the brown sugar and remaining cinnamon, being extra careful not to smash the banana.
4. Once the oven is preheated, remove the skillet and add the butter. As soon as the butter has melted (be sure to watch it so it doesn't burn) add the sliced bananas and brown sugar mixture. Spread evenly across the bottom of the skillet quickly.
5. Immediately add the egg mixture over the bananas, then return the pan to the oven and bake for 20 minutes until it's golden brown. Without opening the oven, lower the temperature to 300°F and bake for another five minutes.
6. Once the timer goes off, remove the skillet from the oven and place on a flat surface to cool for two to three minutes. This helps the Dutch Baby to pull away from the sides and bottom of the pan. As it's cooling, prepare the other banana by slicing it as a fresh fruit garnish with the strawberries. Serve with butter and syrup, and watch them gobble it up!

Beef, Pork, Bird, & Beyond

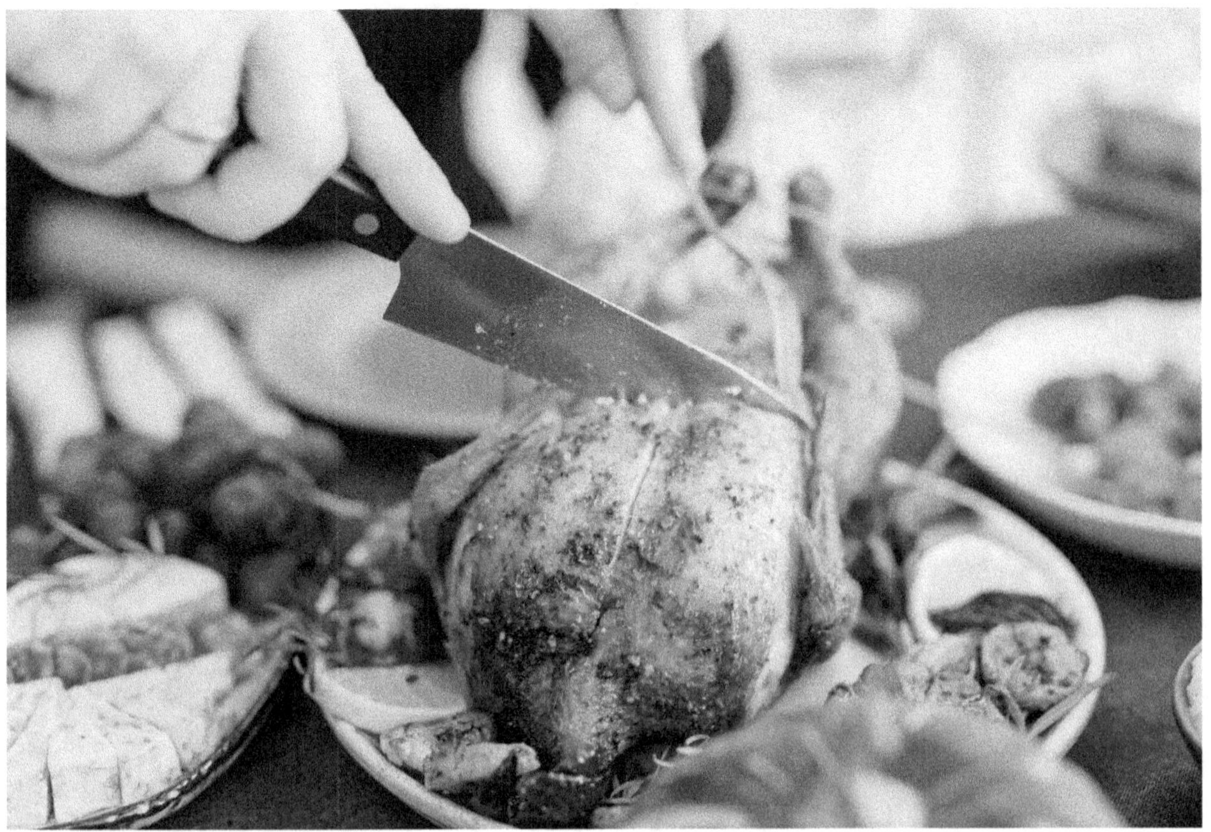

In my own kitchen, this is where the real learning began. Those chicken pot pies got very old very fast. For a while I was convinced that I'd rather starve than ever eat another one of those frozen lava pies. I started with some simple recipes, then expanded on those with things I began to taste in dishes from the restaurants I visited while living in different parts of the country. Some of my favorite flavors came from New Orleans, but others were cultural blends from the melting pot of Los Angeles. Cooking suddenly became an adventure of flavor, and for a while, a futile practice in budgeting. My first attempt at fashioning a cookbook was to be called "Two Dollars a Day" because that's what I had been living on at the time. Due to the rising and falling of inflation, that title wasn't a very practical one. By 2018 I had to extend my budget to a whole $2.25 a day average.

My husband has a joke about "if it doesn't have four legs and a mama, it ain't meat." The first time he told me that I couldn't help but to laugh, but then I realized he was serious. He doesn't consider eggs or chicken to be meat. Still, I thought it was prudent to add Chicken (and a few other things) to this list anyway, because so much of the rest of the *sane* world does. (Just kidding, Honey. Sort of.)

The Best Pork Chops

I spent years being afraid of pork chops! When we ate them in my family growing up they were often dry and hard in the middle, leaving me to believe that pork was just a dry, hard meat. It didn't strike me that they didn't need to be hockey pucks before they were considered to be cooked through! These are so good when served with pork stuffing and roasted brussel sprouts. The rustic flavors combine to create a real 'wow' factor that's worth sharing again and again.

Ingredients

- 2 large eggs
- ½ teaspoon garlic powder
- ½ teaspoon onion powder
- 1 cup wheat breadcrumbs (white breadcrumbs can be substituted)
- ½ tsp salt
- ¼ tsp pepper
- ¼ tsp cayenne (optional)
- 6 thin cut pork chops
- 3 tbsp vegetable oil or olive oil

Directions

1. Preheat the oven to 375° F
2. Whisk eggs, garlic powder, and onion powder together in a shallow bowl. Place breadcrumbs, salt, pepper, and cayenne into a second shallow bowl and mix. Dip pork chops into egg mixture, then press in cracker crumbs to coat. Don't worry about filling every inch of the surface of the pork.
3. Heat oil in a large skillet over medium high heat. Add breaded pork chops and cook until golden brown, 2 to 3 minutes per side.
4. If your skillet is oven safe, transfer the skillet containing pork chops into the oven and bake until no longer pink in the center, about 35 minutes. If your skillet isn't oven safe, transfer the pork chops to a baking sheet (prepared with foil and cooking spray for easy cleanup) and bake for approximately 45 minutes. A thermometer should read 145° internal temperature for the pork chops when they're done.
5. Serve these beauties to family and friends, or just for yourself when you feel like having a delicious pork chop! To mix things up a bit you can add some grated parmesan in with the bread crumbs, too! Try adding some chopped onion and garlic to the oil before cooking the pork chops for added flavor.

Lemon Chicken with Broccoli

Much to my poor husband's chagrin, I have a *lot* of chicken recipes. There was a span of time in my life for about a decade where I wasn't able to eat many meats outside of white meat chicken and non-oily fish. I'd been diagnosed with Crohn's Disease and other meats would cause me to get very sick. Once I learned how to manage my own trauma and move beyond it with research and faith, I beat Crohn's Disease and opened up my cooking experiences once more! But if you see an extraordinary amount of chicken recipes in this book, now you know why.

Ingredients

- 2 Tbsp all purpose flour
- ½ tsp table salt, divided
- ¼ tsp fresh ground black pepper
- 1 lb thin sliced boneless skinless chicken breasts
- 2 tsp olive oil
- 1 ½ cups chicken broth
- 2 tsp minced garlic
- 2 ½ broccoli florets (raw)
- 2 tsp lemon zest (add more if you're like me.)
- 2 Tbsp fresh parsley (optional, but encouraged)
- 1 Tbsp (or more) fresh lemon juice

Directions

1. On a plate or shallow bowl, combine 1 ½ Tbsp flour, ¼ tsp salt, and pepper; add chicken and turn to coat.
2. In a large nonstick skillet, heat the oil over medium-high heat. Add the chicken and cook, turning, until lightly browned and cooked through, about 5 minutes; transfer the chicken to a plate.
3. Put 1 cup of broth and the garlic in the same skillet; bring the mixture to a boil over high heat, scraping up browned bits from the bottom of the pan with a wooden spoon. Add the broccoli; cover and cook for 1 minute.
4. In a small cup, stir remaining 1/2 cup broth, 1/2 Tbsp flour, and 1/4 tsp salt; add this mixture to the skillet and bring it to a simmer over low heat.
5. Cover and cook until the broccoli is crisp-tender and the sauce is slightly thickened, about 1 1/2 minutes. Stir in the chicken and the lemon zest; heat through.
6. Remove the skillet from the heat and stir in the parsley and lemon juice; toss to coat.

Skinny Orange Chicken

Ingredients

- 2 cups all purpose flour
- 2 large eggs, beaten
- 2 cups panko bread crumbs
- 1 lb boneless skinless chicken breasts, cut into chunks
- Salt and pepper to taste
- Juice and zest of 2 oranges
- ⅓ cup low sodium soy sauce
- ¼ cup honey
- 2 cloves garlic, minced
- 2 tsp freshly grated ginger
- 2 Tbsp cornstarch
- 2 cups of cooked rice (look for the sticky rice recipe!)
- Sesame seeds for garnish
- Sliced green onions for garnish

Directions:

1. Preheat oven to 400° F and line a baking sheet with parchment
2. Set up a dredging station with one bowl of flour, one of eggs, and one of panko bread crumbs. Dredge the thicken in each, in that order. Season generously with salt and pepper.
3. Arrange the chicken on the parchment lined baking sheet and bake until no longer pink, about 18 to 20 minutes.
4. Meanwhile: Make the sauce! In a small saucepan over medium heat, combine the juice of two oranges, soy sauce, honey, garlic, ginger, and cornstarch. Whisk until combined and cook until thickened, about 5 minutes.
5. Transfer chicken to a large bowl and toss in the orange sauce.
6. Serve over rice with orange zest, sesame seeds and green onions as a beautiful garnish.

Slow Roasted Rabbit

This might seem like a strange place to talk about cat food, but that's where I'm at right now. What else can I say about this recipe? No, it's not cat food. It's substantially tastier than that, and quite a rich food. So what's the connection to cat food, you ask? I'll tell you. My husband and I make every ounce of the food our cats eat specifically to give them the best shot at a long and healthy life (there's soooo much crap in manufactured cat food it's not even funny). While shopping for ingredients for the cat food one day we came across a section of frozen rabbit. I told him that I'd never made any rabbit and I wanted to give it a shot! That desire surprised the both of us, but the resulting recipe was even more of a surprise. We loved it!

Ingredients

- 1 (3 pound) rabbit, cleaned and cut into pieces
- 1 tablespoon ground black pepper
- 1 ¾ teaspoons salt
- ¼ cup vegetable oil (or bacon grease)
- 1 onion, chopped
- 1 cup water
- ¾ cup bbq sauce
- 3 dashes of liquid smoke
- 1 ½ tablespoons Worcestershire sauce
- ½ cup white wine
- 1 tablespoon paprika
- 1 to 2 cloves garlic, chopped
- Baby potatoes, halved.

Directions

1. Preheat the oven to 350°F (175° C).
2. Season rabbit pieces with pepper and salt.
   Heat vegetable oil in a large skillet over medium-high heat. Add rabbit; cook in hot oil until brown on all sides. Place in a 9x13-inch baking dish.
3. Combine onion, water, ketchup, Worcestershire sauce, sugar, paprika, and garlic in a medium bowl; mix well, then pour over the rabbit. Toss the potatoes in the bowl to lightly coat and add around the rabbit.
4. Bake uncovered in the preheated oven, basting about every 20 minutes, until very tender, about 90 minutes. An instant-read thermometer inserted into the meat nearest the bone should read at least 160°F.
5. Serve piping hot with lots of hearty sides like garlic green beans and mashed potatoes with gravy made from the remaining sauce after the rabbit has cooked! This also pairs very nicely with some crusty sourdough bread.

Chicken Pierre

I once made this for my husband and I for dinner and had some leftovers in the freezer for a quick meal. When we went on a trip to visit his family, he had a young coworker come over to babysit the house and cats. I pulled out the Chicken Pierre leftovers and let him know he could eat them (and a few other items I'd made) and our house sitter talked about the Chicken Pierre for *months* after that! Now whenever I make it, I make extra so my husband can take some to work for his coworker, too.

This dish has been a favorite of mine for many years now. It's been a hit every time I've ever made it, and it's versatile enough to be as spicy as anyone can handle. It's got a great mingling of flavors and pairs beautifully with some rustic mashed potatoes to soak up more of the tomato based sauce, and you can never go wrong with some prosciutto wrapped asparagus on the side, either. This is a rather traditional version of the recipe, but if you were to exclude the flour coating on the chicken, you can put the rest of the ingredients in a crockpot on high for 4 hours to have an almost identical meal.

Ingredients

- 6 skinless, boneless chicken breast halves
- ¼ cup all-purpose flour
- ½ teaspoon salt
- 1 pinch ground black pepper
- 3 tablespoons butter
- 1 (14.5 ounce) can stewed tomatoes, with liquid
- ½ cup water
- 2 tablespoons brown sugar
- 2 tablespoons distilled white vinegar
- 2 tablespoons Worcestershire sauce
- 1 teaspoon salt
- 2 teaspoons chili powder
- 1 teaspoon mustard powder
- ½ teaspoon celery seed
- 1 clove garlic, minced
- ⅛ teaspoon hot pepper sauce

Directions

1. In a shallow dish or bowl, combine flour, ½ teaspoon salt and ground black pepper. Coat chicken breasts with flour mixture. Melt butter in a large skillet over medium heat, and brown chicken on all sides. Remove from the skillet, and drain on paper towels.
2. In the same skillet, combine the tomatoes, water, brown sugar, vinegar and Worcestershire sauce. Season with salt, chili powder, mustard, celery seed, garlic and hot pepper sauce. Bring to a boil; reduce heat, and return chicken to skillet. Cover, and simmer for 35 to 40 minutes, or until chicken is tender, no longer pink and juices run clear.

Enchilada Skillet Meal

Ingredients

- 1 pound extra lean ground turkey
- 1 teaspoon ground cumin divided
- 1 teaspoon dried oregano divided
- ½ teaspoon kosher salt divided
- ¼ teaspoon ground pepper
- 3 teaspoons olive oil divided
- ½ yellow onion chopped
- 1 red bell pepper diced
- 3 garlic cloves minced
- 2 ½ cups green enchilada sauce
- ¾ cup salsa
- 1 (4 oz.) can diced green chiles
- 1 (14 oz.) can black beans drained & rinsed
- ¾ cup fresh or frozen corn kernels
- ¾ cup cooked brown rice
- 4 corn tortillas cut into 1 1/2-inch strips
- ¾ cup grated Pepper Jack cheese
- 3 tablespoons minced cilantro

Directions

1. Heat a large nonstick skillet over medium-high heat. Lightly coat with cooking spray. Add the ground turkey, ½ teaspoon cumin, ½ teaspoon oregano, ¼ teaspoon salt and pepper and cook, breaking up with a wooden spoon, until browned. Transfer to a bowl.
2. Reduce the heat to medium and add 2 teaspoons olive oil to the skillet. Add the onion and cook, stirring occasionally, until the onion is tender and starting to brown, 3 to 4 minutes.
3. Add the remaining 1 teaspoon olive oil and stir in the red bell pepper. Cook for 1 minute. Stir in the garlic, remaining ½ teaspoon cumin, remaining ½ teaspoon oregano and ¼ teaspoon salt. Cook for 1 minute.
4. Add the enchilada sauce, salsa, green chiles, black beans, corn, rice and cook ground turkey to the skillet. Increase heat and bring the mixture to a boil. Reduce the heat and simmer until the sauce has thickened slightly, about 10 minutes.
5. Stir in the corn tortillas, then sprinkle the cheese over the mixture. Cover the skillet for a minute to allow the cheese to melt.
6. Garnish with cilantro. Serve.

Key West Chicken

When I first came across this recipe I instantly had visions of citrus lime chicken, and it surprised me that the lime flavor wasn't very strong at all! You can always increase the lime to give it more of that citrus flavor, but regardless of what's done to it, this recipe is delicious. Alternatively, this chicken can also be air fried or baked with vegetables on the same tray

Ingredients

- 3 Tbsp soy sauce
- 1 Tbsp honey
- 1 Tbsp vegetable oil
- 1 ½ tsp lime juice (fresh)
- 1 tsp garlic, chopped
- 4 skinless, boneless chicken breast halves.

Directions

1. Using a shallow bowl or container, add vegetable oil, honey, soy sauce, garlic, and lime juice. Stir to mix well.
2. Place the chicken in the marinade. Coat well. Cover with plastic wrap, place in the refrigerator for a minimum of 30 minutes.
3. Heat outdoor grill at high heat.
4. Prepare the grill by lightly oiling the grill grate to prevent sticking.
5. Remove chicken from the refrigerator and discard the marinade.
6. Grill the chicken for approximately 6-8 mins. per side or until chicken is fully cooked and the juices run clear. Serve with grilled veggie skewers, baked potato, roasted broccoli, or corn on the cob for a fantastic side.

Best Chicken Enchiladas

By now you might be wondering why so many of the recipes start with the word "Best" in front of them. That's because these were the best of the collection of similar recipes I had and I only wanted to share my most favorite ones in this book. It took some kitchen experiments to figure out which were the best, and the criteria was complex. I had to judge them by the ease of creation, the simplicity of ingredients, the complex flavor combinations, and 'mouth feel.' It's a thing.

Ingredients

- 1 (10 ounce) can enchilada sauce, divided
- 4 ounces Cream Cheese, cubed
- 1 ½ cups salsa
- 2 cups shredded chicken
- 1 (15 ounce) can pinto beans, rinsed and drained
- 1 (4 ounce) can chopped green chilies
- 8 of the 10 inch flour tortillas
- 1 cup shredded Mexican blend cheese
- Optional: shredded lettuce, chopped tomato, fresh cilantro, diced onions, sour cream, black olives, Sliced avocado, guacamole, etc.

Directions

1. Preheat the oven to 350°F.
2. Spoon ½ cup enchilada sauce into a greased 13" x 9" baking dish. In a large saucepan, cook and stir the cream cheese and salsa over medium heat for 2-3 minutes or until blended. Stir in the chicken, beans, and chilies.
3. Place about 6 tablespoons of chicken mixture down the center of each tortilla. Roll up and place the enchiladas seam side down over sauce. Top with remaining enchilada sauce; sprinkle with cheese. (I also like to add a light sprinkling of sliced black olives.)
4. Cover and bake for 25-30 minutes or until the cheese has melted and the enchiladas are heated through. Serve with lettuce, tomato, sour cream and olives if desired.

Air Fryer Rotisserie Cornish Hen (or baked)

This has been a recipe in the making for a few years now. The first time I made this I didn't have an air fryer or rotisserie, and instead had to bake it in the oven the old fashioned way. If you don't have an air fryer rotisserie, you can do the same and it still comes out AMAZING.

If you're going to bake this in the oven, whatever part of the bird you want to be the juiciest (the breast or the thigh) just make sure you set the bird that side down in the roasting pan. You can also take a center slice from the lemon to lay on the top of the bird for a bit of a caramelized citrus flavor at the end of roasting. Bake it in the oven at 350° for 1 hour 15 minutes. If desired, every 10 or 15 minutes of roasting, brush additional butter or oil over the skin of the Cornish hens for added flavor and crispiness. Of course it is important not to overcook it, and make sure that the internal temperature at the thickest part reaches 165° before serving.

Ingredients

- 1-2 small Cornish Hen(s), thawed
- Honey
- Cayenne Pepper
- Juice of one lemon
- Remaining lemon, quartered
- Garlic powder
- Onion powder

Directions

1. Preheat your Air Fryer on the rotisserie setting to 350°F.
2. Place the quartered, juiced lemon inside the cavity of the bird.
3. Slide the rotisserie bar through the cavity of the bird and secure it in place. Truss the legs with kitchen twine.
4. In a small bowl mix the honey, cayenne pepper and lemon juice together. Brush the honey mixture over the skin of the bird. Sprinkle the entire bird with garlic and onion powders.
5. Place the rotisserie bar into the grooves within the air fryer and set for 2 hours.
6. The bird is done when the thickest part of the meat (usually the thigh) reaches 165°F.

Air Fryer Boneless Pork Chops (or baked)

Again, if you don't have an air fryer, there are alternatives! Instead of preheating an air fryer that you don't have, preheat your oven to 350° and prepare a pan for the chops with a little spray oil. Prepare them exactly the same way, and then bake them for 20 to 30 minutes, until the chops reach 150° F at the center point. Turning them half way through will help with the crispness on both sides. These go incredibly well with brussel sprouts and pork stuffing.

Ingredients

- 4 boneless center cut pork chops, about ½ inch thick
- 1 teaspoon olive oil
- 1 teaspoon garlic powder
- 1 teaspoon onion powder
- 1 teaspoon smoked paprika
- 1 teaspoon salt
- ½ teaspoon cracked pepper

Directions

- Preheat the air fryer to 380° for 5 minutes.
- While the air fryer preheats, drizzle the pork chops with the oil.
- Stir together the garlic powder, onion powder, smoked paprika, salt, and pepper in a small bowl.
- Sprinkle evenly over the pork chops. Rub to coat both sides with the seasoning.
- Place the pork chops in the air fryer and cook for 9-11 minutes or until the pork chops reach 150° internally. Time may vary depending on the thickness of pork chops and the air fryer used.
- Let pork chops rest 5 minutes before serving.

Lemon Chicken with Broccoli

Ingredients

- 2 Tbsp All-purpose flour
- ½ tsp divided,   Table salt
- ¼ tsp fresh ground Black pepper
- 12 oz thin sliced Uncooked boneless skinless chicken breasts
- 2 tsp Olive oil
- 1 ½ cups Fat-free reduced sodium chicken broth
- 2 tsp Minced Garlic
- 2 ½ cups raw broccoli florets
- 2 tsp (or more) Lemon Zest
- 2 Tbsp Fresh parsley, chopped
- 1 Tbsp (or more) Fresh lemon juice

Directions

1. On a plate, combine 1 ½ Tbsp flour, ¼ tsp salt, and pepper; add chicken and turn to coat.
2. In a large nonstick skillet, heat the oil over medium-high heat. Add the chicken and cook, turning, until lightly browned and cooked through, about 5 minutes; transfer the chicken to a plate.
3. Put 1 cup of broth and the garlic in the same skillet; bring the mixture to a boil over high heat, scraping up browned bits from the bottom of the pan with a wooden spoon. Add the broccoli; cover and cook for 1 minute.
4. In a small cup, stir remaining ½ cup broth, ½ Tbsp flour, and ¼ tsp salt; add this mixture to the skillet and bring it to a simmer over low heat.
5. Cover and cook until the broccoli is crisp-tender and the sauce is slightly thickened, about 1 ½ minutes. Stir in the chicken and the lemon zest; heat through.
6. Remove the skillet from the heat and stir in the parsley and lemon juice; toss to coat. Serve over rice, pasta, or by itself.

Shish Tawook

This traditional Lebanese dish is one of my rarely made favorite meals. To make all of the things I like to pair it with (tomato rice, spicy lemon potatoes, garlic sauce, etc) it takes some time and care. This was my favorite thing to order at one particular Los Angeles restaurant and when I moved to Denver I wasn't able to find it available so I had to learn how to make it myself. It was a learning process, figuring out some of the flavors and processes to create them, but I'll never regret the time I spent figuring it out. Shortly after I finalized this recipe, a friend of mine took me to a Denver restaurant that had this exact dish, and once again I stopped making it with any kind of frequency. This recipe is super simple and completely worth ANY effort, but it's the rest of the recipes (you'll find them in the book) that seem to take so much time. (Dedicated to Mark Scopel for showing me that Israeli restaurant in Denver that had Shish Tawook on the menu. I still miss you every day, my friend.)

Ingredients

- 24 ounces boneless, skinless chicken breasts, cubed
- ¼ cup lemon juice
- 2 tablespoons extra virgin olive oil
- 3 cloves garlic (minced)
- 1 ½ teaspoons salt
- ½ teaspoon pepper

Directions

1. In a medium bowl, whisk together lemon juice, olive oil, garlic, salt, and pepper. Toss with chicken cubes and marinate overnight.
2. Preheat the oven to 350°F and spray a baking sheet with cooking spray.
3. Spread chicken in a single layer and bake until golden brown and cooked through, about 20 minutes.

Chakhokhbili (Georgian Chicken with Herbs)

You mean you can't pronounce that word? Not surprising, most Americans can't. I had a friend who grew up in Georgia (not the State) who laughed at me every time I tried. Marco was the one who told me the basics for this recipe, and somehow he knew how to tell me in a way that I wouldn't forget it. He had been a scientist for NASA in the 1970's and 1980's so he was a pretty smart fella anyway. But when Marco retired he opened his own restaurant in San Diego and loved to charm the ladies from his wheelchair. That was how we met! Every time I make this, I think of him (though his grandmother's recipe will always be better than mine.) This goes extremely well with the Lebanese tomato rice recipe, too!

In loving memory of Marco and the fabulous Kafe Sobaka Pomegranate of San Diego, CA. (Now closed)

Ingredients

- 2 ½ lb. chicken breasts with skin & bone, halved
- Salt and pepper to taste
- 4 tbsp olive oil
- 1 large onion (diced)
- 2 more tbsp olive oil
- 1 red bell pepper
- 3.5 lb fresh tomatoes, diced
- 1 cup red cooking wine
- 1-2 jalapeños sliced
- 1 small chili pepper
- 2 tsp fenugreek seeds
- 2 tsp coriander seeds
- 2 dried bay leaves
- 6 to 7 saffron strands (optional)
- ½ cup fresh parsley, chopped
- ½ cup fresh basil, chopped
- 2-3 garlic cloves, pressed

Directions

1. Season the chicken with salt and pepper.
2. In a large heavy bottomed pot, heat 4 tbsp olive oil over high heat until it's smoking hot. Add the seasoned chicken and brown on both sides. Remove the chicken and set aside.
3. In the same skillet add an additional 2 tbsp olive oil and bring the heat to medium high. Add the diced onion and cook for about 2 minutes. Then add in the diced bell pepper. Cook for an additional 3 minutes.

4. Add in the chopped tomatoes and red wine. (If you do not have in season tomatoes use pre diced tomatoes, preferably Pomi or San Marzano brand). Cover the pot with a lid and cook over medium heat for 10 minutes.

5. Add the chicken back into the pot by nestling it into the tomato mixture and season with salt. Start with 1 tsp. You may add more later according to your liking. Place the lid back over the pot and cook the chicken for about 30 more minutes.

6. Use a spice grinder to grind the fenugreek, coriander, bay leaves and saffron into a powder. Add this to the pot with the sliced jalapeños, chili pepper, chopped cilantro, and pressed garlic. Bring to a boil and remove from heat. Serve hot over seasoned rice or cheese bread. This dish can also be served alone as a Georgian chicken stew.

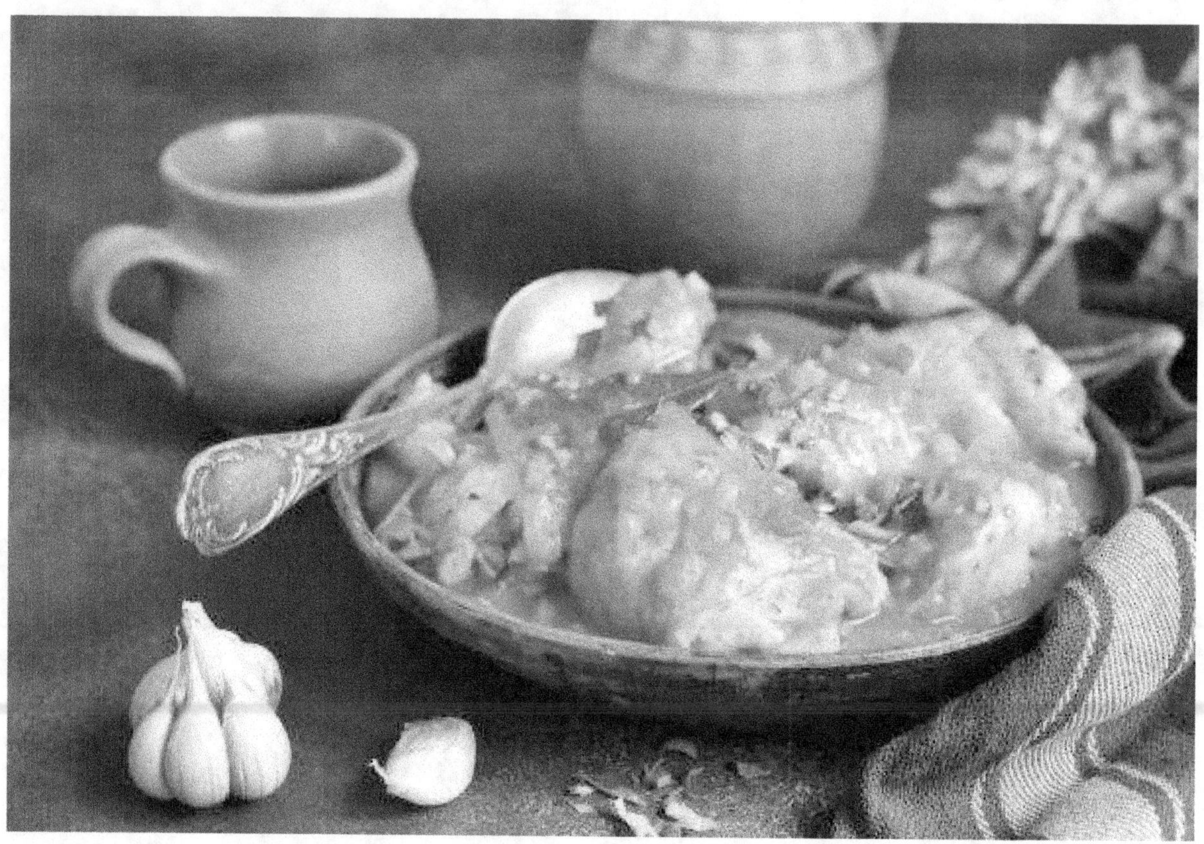

Skinny Orange Chicken

I followed a couple different diet programs in the past, one which worked extremely well and supplied me with some fantastic flavorful recipe ideas that genuinely did help me to eat healthier and lose weight! This is one of those amazing recipes, but there are many sprinkled throughout the book.

Ingredients

- 2 c. all-purpose flour
- 2 large Eggs, beaten
- 2 c. panko bread crumbs
- 1 lb. boneless skinless chicken breasts, cut into chunks
- kosher salt
- Freshly ground black pepper
- Juice and zest of 2 oranges
- 1/3 c. low-sodium soy sauce
- 1/4 c. honey
- 2 cloves garlic, minced
- 2 tsp. freshly grated ginger
- 2 tbsp. cornstarch
- 2 c. cooked jasmine rice
- Sesame seeds, for garnish
- Sliced green onions, for garnish

Directions

1. Preheat the oven to 400°F and line a baking sheet with parchment.
2. Set up a dredging station with one bowl of flour, one of eggs, and one of panko. Dredge the chicken in flour, then coat in eggs and cover in panko. Season generously with salt and pepper.
3. Arrange chicken on a parchment-lined baking sheet and bake until no longer pink, 18 to 20 minutes.
4. Meanwhile, make sauce: In a small saucepan over medium heat, combine orange juice, soy sauce, honey, garlic, ginger, and cornstarch. Whisk until combined and cook until thickened, about 5 minutes.
5. Transfer chicken to a large bowl and toss in orange sauce.
6. Serve over sticky rice (see recipe listed in the Side Items section) with orange zest, sesame seeds, and green onions.

Hand Rolled Lasagna

Make this dish at your own risk. In my own experience, this dish destroyed a budding friendship, but launched a romance.

Ingredients

- 9 lasagna noodles
- 2 lbs super lean ground turkey or beef
- 1 medium onion, diced
- 3 garlic cloves, minced
- 2 cans (one 28 oz, one 15 oz) crushed tomatoes
- 2 cans (6 oz each) tomato paste
- ⅔ cup water
- 2 tbsp sugar
- 3 tbsp plus ¼ cup minced fresh parsley, divided
- 2 tsp dried basil
- ¾ tsp fennel seed
- ¾ tsp salt, divided
- ¼ tsp coarsely ground pepper
- 1 large egg, lightly beaten
- 1 carton (15 oz) Ricotta cheese
- 4 cups shredded part-skim mozzarella cheese
- ¾ cup grated parmesan cheese

Directions

1. Preheat oven to 375°F
2. Line a casserole dish (9x9) with foil and spray with non-stick cooking spray.
3. Cook noodles according to package directions and drain.
4. Cook the ground turkey or beef and onion over medium heat until meat is no longer pink, breaking the meat into crumbles. Add garlic and cook for one minute.
5. Stir in tomatoes, tomato paste, water, sugar, 3 tbsp parsley, basil, fennel, ½ tsp salt and pepper. Bring to a boil. Reduce heat, simmer, uncovered for 30 minutes, stirring occasionally.
6. In a small bowl, mix the egg, ricotta cheese, and remaining parsley and salt. Combine the two bowls a little at a time, mixing the hot into the cold ingredients to avoid cooking the egg.
7. Add a thin layer of spaghetti sauce to the bottom of the casserole dish.
8. Spread 2 to 3 tbsp of the mixture into the end of a noodle and roll gently in your hand, spreading the mix evenly throughout as you roll. Set this roll into the dish lined and primed casserole dish, near the corner, to keep the roll upright and intact. Repeat this process with the remaining lasagna noodles, filling the casserole dish.
9. Top the rolls with a spoonful of the filling mixture to fill up any open space. Sprinkle it with mozzarella cheese, and then parmesan cheese.

10. Bake these rolls in the sauce lined casserole dish, covered, for 25 minutes. Bake uncovered for 25 minutes longer or until bubbly. Top with more mozzarella and let it melt. Let stand for about five minutes before serving.

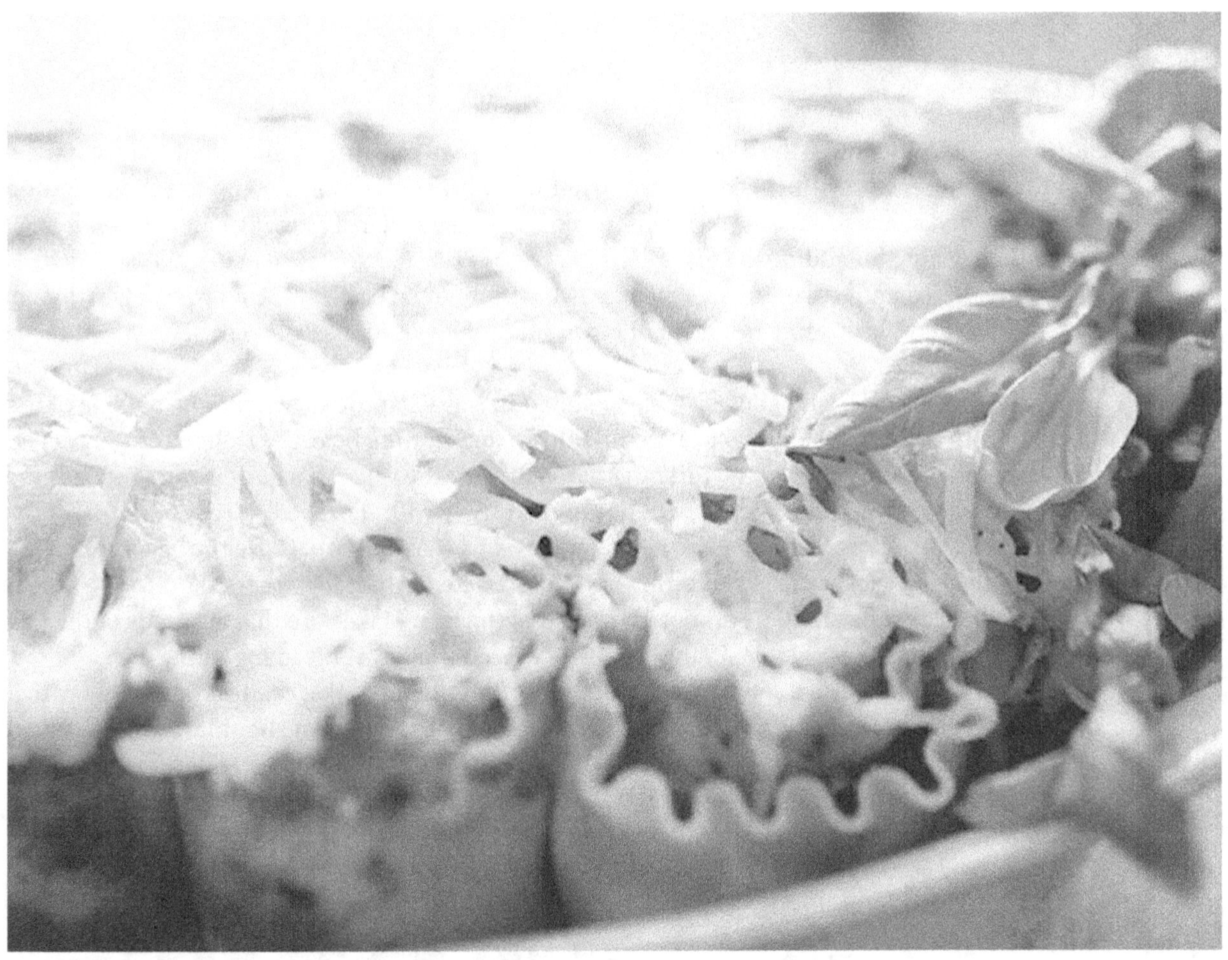

Thanksgiving Turkey

What's a cookbook without at least ONE holiday recipe? But don't look now - I also have a killer ham recipe that you're bound to love if you like ham even a little.

Ingredients

- 1 teaspoon dried basil
- 1 teaspoon garlic powder
- 1 teaspoon dried sage
- 1 teaspoon dried thyme
- 1 teaspoon onion powder
- 1/2 teaspoon freshly ground black pepper
- 1 tablespoon kosher salt
- 1 recipe turkey gravy (next page)

Directions

1. Arrange a rack in the lower third of the oven to ensure that your turkey has plenty of clearance, then heat to 350°F. Spray the inside of your oven bag with cooking spray. Add the flour, twist to close briefly, and shake to coat the bag with the flour. Set the bag in a roasting pan and roll it back to ready the opening for adding the turkey.
2. Combine the herbs and seasoning in a small bowl. Combine the basil, garlic powder, sage, thyme, onion powder, and black pepper in a small bowl. Place the salt in a second small bowl. Set these aside.
3. Remove the turkey's neck and giblets, or save for another use. Pat the cavity and the outside of the turkey dry with paper towels and place breast-side up on a cutting board or rimmed baking sheet. Season the outside and cavity of the turkey generously with the salt — it's okay if you don't use the full amount called for here. Season the exterior of the turkey with the dried spice rub.
4. Place the turkey breast-side up in the roasting bag inside a roasting pan. Close the bag tightly with either the included closure (for some this is an oven safe zip-tie; for others it's a twist tie). If you've lost the closure, simply tie a knot in the end of the bag. Make sure that any ends of the bag are tucked inside the roasting pan. Using scissors, cut 6 (1/2-inch) vents in top of the bag.
5. Roast the turkey undisturbed for 2 to 2 1/2 hours (for a 15lb bird). You can test the turkey with a probe thermometer inserted into one of the bag's vents — the thigh meat should reach an internal temperature of at least 175°F and the breast 180°F.
6. Remove the turkey from the oven and rest, sealed in the bag, for 15 minutes. Use caution when cutting open the bag, as some steam can remain in the bag.
7. Carve the turkey as desired. Serve with turkey gravy (see next page)

Turkey Gravy

Ingredients

- Pan drippings from Thanksgiving Turkey
- 1/4 cup unsalted butter
- 1/4 cup all-purpose flour
- 2 teaspoons chopped fresh thyme
- 1 tablespoon chopped fresh parsley leaves
- Kosher salt and freshly ground black pepper, to taste

Directions

1. Strain pan drippings through a fine-mesh sieve; discard solids and reserve 2 1/2 cups pan drippings; set aside.
2. Melt butter in a medium saucepan over medium heat. Whisk in flour and thyme until lightly browned, about 1 minute.
3. Gradually whisk in reserved pan drippings. Bring to a boil; reduce heat and simmer, whisking constantly, until thickened, about 5-10 minutes. Stir in parsley; season with salt and pepper, to taste. Serve warm.

Holiday Ham

Every single time I see this recipe I chuckle to myself. There was an original television show for a while that I loved, and in one particular episode the sister of the main character is tasked with preparing food for guests. What she comes up with is nothing more than exactly what she calls it - hot ham water. It's a great episode, a horrible recipe, and nothing at all like you'll find below. My husband told me that this was the best ham he thought he'd ever had in his life - exactly the opposite of hot ham water.

Ingredients

- 1 ready-to-eat ham, bone in, no water added (about 7 or 8 pounds for a half a ham)
- 1 ½ cups water or chicken stock
- ¼ cup white wine

Glaze:

- ½ cup Dijon mustard
- ¼ cup brown sugar
- 2 tablespoons dark rum
- 2 tablespoons apple cider vinegar

Directions

1. Preheat the oven to only 300° degrees. Remove any tough skin. Score fat in a diamond pattern with a sharp knife, being careful not to cut into the meat of the ham. Add the 1 ½ cups water or chicken stock and ¼ cup white wine to the bottom of a roasting pan.
2. Place ham, fattier side up, in the roasting pan and roast on a middle rack of the oven. A good roasting guideline is about 15 minutes per pound with the final internal temperature at about 140°F.
3. While the ham is roasting, mix together all the ingredients for the glaze. About halfway through the roasting time, increase the temperature to 350° and begin brushing the ham with the glaze, repeating about every 15 minutes. If the sugar starts to burn the bottom of the pan, add more chicken stock or water.
4. When the ham is finished, remove to a cutting board and let rest for 15 minutes before carving. If you'd like, deglaze the pan with a little white wine and add the remaining stock of water. Boil in a saucepan to reduce it into a gravy substitute sauce.

Skip!

This one has a fun story associated with it, though it came to me second-hand. It was a cold day in 1953 when my grandfather and grandmother were driving home from a family event. My grandfather had been a picky eater so he didn't eat much that evening and his stomach was growling. My grandmother didn't have the same restrictions and had eaten plenty. My grandfather kept asking what they would have for dinner once they arrived home, and my grandmother had no intention of cooking with a full stomach. She jokingly said they would just skip. When they got home, my grandfather's stomach won out and she finally gave in. What she came up with was a mixture of sauteed onions and potatoes with ground beef all cooked together in a single skillet.When she set the plate before him, and after he gave it a good dose of ketchup zigzagged over the top, he dug in. "I never heard of Skip before, but we might need to have this more often. This is good!" (Of course I added my own touch to it.)

Ingredients

- 3 tablespoons extra-virgin olive oil, divided
- 1 pound 90% lean ground beef
- 2 teaspoons ground cumin
- ¾ teaspoon salt
- ¼ teaspoon ground pepper
- 3 medium Yukon Gold potatoes, diced (½ inch)
- 1 medium yellow onion, chopped
- 1 yellow bell pepper, diced (½ inch)
- 1 Poblano pepper, diced (½ inch)
- 2 cloves garlic, minced
- 1 bunch kale, stemmed and roughly chopped
- 2 plum tomatoes, cored and diced (1/2-inch)
- 1 scallion, thinly sliced crosswise (optional)

Directions

1. Heat 1 tablespoon of oil in a large cast-iron skillet over medium-high heat. Add beef, cumin, salt and pepper; cook, stirring often to break up the meat, until evenly browned, about 6 minutes. Using a slotted spoon, transfer the beef to a paper-towel-lined plate; do not wipe out the pan. Add 1 tablespoon of oil to the drippings in the pan. Add potatoes; cook, stirring occasionally, until the potatoes begin to caramelize and are tender, about 20 minutes. Transfer the potatoes to the plate with the beef.
2. Heat the remaining 1 tablespoon oil in the skillet over medium heat. Add onion, bell pepper and poblano; cook, stirring occasionally, until tender, about 6 minutes. Add garlic; cook, stirring often, until aromatic, about 1 minute. Add kale and tomatoes; cook, stirring often, until the kale is wilted and the tomatoes are heated through, about 3 minutes. Stir in the beef and potatoes. Sprinkle with scallions, if desired.

Gorgeous Pork Loin

Ingredients

- 3 cloves garlic, minced
- 1 tablespoon dried rosemary
- salt and pepper to taste
- 2 pounds boneless pork loin roast
- ¼ cup olive oil
- ½ cup white wine

Directions

1. Preheat the oven to 350° F. Crush garlic with rosemary, salt, and pepper in a mortar and pestle to make a paste.
2. Pierce meat with a sharp knife in several places and press garlic paste into the openings. Rub pork loin with the remaining garlic mixture and olive oil. Set into an oven-safe pan.
3. Place pork loin into the preheated oven, turning and basting with pan liquids every 30 minutes. Cook until the pork is no longer pink in the center, 90 minutes to 2 hours. An instant-read thermometer inserted into the center should read 145° F . Remove roast to a platter and keep warm.
4. Place the pan onto the stove over medium-high heat and pour wine into it. Heat wine and stir to loosen browned bits from the bottom of the pan. Simmer for 3 to 5 minutes. Slice pork loin and serve with pan juices.

NOTE: The National Pork Board recommends the following cook times for roasting pork loin at 350°

- New York Pork Roast (2 pounds): 26-28 minutes per pound
- New York Pork Roast (3-5 pounds): 20-25 minutes per pound
- Sirloin Pork Roast (2 pounds): 26-28 minutes per pound
- Sirloin Pork Roast (3-5 pounds): 20-25 minutes per pound
- Pork Crown Roast: 12-15 minutes per pound
- Rack of Pork: 25-40 minutes per pound

Medium-Rare: 145-150° F
Medium: 150-155° F
Medium-Well: 155-160° F
Well: 160° F

Amazing Turkey Burgers

Ingredients

- 1 pound lean ground turkey
- ½ teaspoon garlic powder
- ½ teaspoon onion powder
- 3 Tablespoons sriracha
- 1 teaspoon Worcestershire sauce
- ¾ teaspoon salt
- ½ teaspoon freshly ground pepper
- ¼ cup Feta cheese (reduced fat)
- ½ medium onion, finely diced.
- ⅓ cup bread crumbs
- 1 egg
- 4 buns
- 1 tablespoon canola oil , or use pan spray

For serving:
- Condiments: ketchup, mustard, mayonnaise, BBQ sauce
- Toppings: lettuce, tomato, onion, pickles, avocado, bacon, cheese, etc.

Directions

1. Mix together the turkey, garlic powder, onion powder, sriracha, Worcestershire sauce, salt and pepper, egg, feta, onion, and breadcrumbs. Using a fork, mix together—try not to mix it too much.
2. Shape into 4 patties about ½ inch thick.
3. Use your thumb to make a depression in the center of each patty. If grilling, place the patties on a parchment lined plate and freeze for 20 minutes.
4. Cooking options:
5. Skillet: Heat the canola oil in a nonstick griddle or large nonstick frying pan over medium-high heat. (Or spray generously with non-stick cooking spray). Once hot, cook the patties for 4-5 minutes on each side.
6. Grill: Freeze the patties for 20 minutes before grilling (this will help the hold their shape.) Grill for a few minutes on each side, until cooked through.
7. Oven: Bake at 375 F for 25-30 minutes. Then sear on a hot pan for 2 minutes on each side.
8. Serve on buns, with the condiments of your choice.

NOTE: If you want to melt a slice of cheese onto the burger, Provolone and Pepper Jack both work wonderfully. Just add them for the last few minutes of the cook time and watch the magic happen.

Coconut Chicken

You'll see more notes about pairing this with other island themed dishes if you look at the Hawaiian roasted vegetables (in "side dishes") or mango salsa (in "Snacks and Appetizers"). These flavors all compliment one another beautifully and will make you wonder why you haven't been cooking like this all your life. Fairly healthy and simple, these dishes will bring the flavor of the islands to your own kitchen table no matter where you live.

Ingredients

- 4 boneless, skinless chicken breasts
- ½ cup flour
- 1 tsp salt
- ½ tsp black pepper
- 2 large eggs
- ½ tsp cayenne pepper
- 1 ½ cups *unsweetened* shredded coconut
- 1 cup panko breadcrumbs (I prefer wheat)
- 4 tbsp coconut oil

Directions

1. Preheat the oven to 350°F
2. In a shallow bowl, combine the flour, salt, and pepper. In a second shallow bowl, whisk the eggs and cayenne pepper. In a third shallow bowl, combine the shredded coconut and panko breadcrumbs.
3. First, dredge each chicken breast in flour. Then dip the floured chicken into the egg wash, letting the excess drip off before moving on. Next, dredge the egg washed chicken breast in the coconut-panko mixture, pressing lightly to make sure the coconut sticks.
4. In a large skillet, heat the coconut oil over medium *low* heat. Saute the chicken 1 to 2 minutes per side until the coconut is golden brown. Place the chicken on a rack over a foil lined baking tray. Place the baking tray in the oven and bake for 10 minutes until the chicken is cooked through the rest of the way. Test with a thermometer to make sure the internal temp of the chicken is at least 170°. Keep warm until ready to serve.

Instant Pot Pineapple Chicken

I admit it, I jumped on the instant pot craze when that was happening a few years ago now. But I also have to admit that it's one of the best investments I could've made on nights when I'm busy and haven't had a chance to prepare for making a nice dinner. I can take frozen ingredients to a full dinner in less than 30 minutes. To me, that's worth every penny.

Ingredients

- 4 frozen chicken breasts (separated)
- ⅓ cup pineapple juice
- ¼ cup pineapple chunks
- ¼ cup onion pieces (about the same size as the pineapple)
- ⅓ cup soy sauce
- ⅓ cup brown sugar
- 1 Tbsp ground ginger
- 2 tsp garlic powder
- Salt and pepper to taste

Directions

1. Add all of the ingredients to the pressure cooker, starting with the chicken breasts. Set the pressure cooker to 10 minutes on high pressure and turn the valve to seal in the steam. It will take the instant pot longer to reach pressure because the chicken is frozen, but it shouldn't be longer than 12 minutes.
2. Once the cook time has elapsed, let the pressure release naturally for 5 minutes, and then do a quick release.
3. Remove the chicken from the liquid and let it rest for 5 to 10 minutes before serving.

This recipe also pairs incredibly well with the Quick Sticky Rice recipe from the side dishes, and that Mango salsa in the appetizer's section.

Lemon Garlic Skillet Chicken

This recipe is so beautifully paired with a nice parmesan risotto. The delicate flavors bring to mind the coasts of California when I find myself missing the flavors of the place I called home for fourteen years. There are very few things I'll ever truly miss about California, but the variety of food is definitely a big one for me. The food in Colorado is great too! I mean, we have restaurants here that specialize in wild game. You'd never find that in Los Angeles at an affordable price without having to have it flown in yourself. But the delicate french infusion foods I gravitated to on a chilly night in Los Angeles aren't as easily accessible out here. So I had to change that for myself.

Ingredients

- 2 Tbsp butter
- 3 skinless, boneless chicken breasts
- 1 ½ tsp salt
- 1 ½ tsp ground black pepper
- 2 tbsp garlic powder
- 1 lemon, juiced

Directions

1. Melt the butter in a skillet over medium high heat.
2. Season the chicken with the salt and pepper, then place the chicken in the melted butter. Cook the chicken, carefully flipping frequently, until browned. This will take about five minutes.
3. Sprinkle 1 tbsp of garlic powder over the chicken pieces, then flip and repeat with the second side. Cook each side for 2 minutes.
4. Pour the lemon juice over each side of the chicken and cook until no longer pink in the center, about 5 to 10 minutes more. Test with an instant read thermometer to make sure the internal temperature is 170° before serving.

Spectacular Broiled Chicken Thighs

The first time I ever made this dish it was before I was married and I had a male roommate who ate like a bird. It would take a lot to get that horrible roommate to exit his room and interact with any sense of human decency, but this one accomplished it. Not only did he come out to see what I was making, but he asked if he could try it, then requested seconds. It was rare he ever wanted a second taste, much less a second helping of any dish I made. This pairs really well with a baked potato for more rustic flavors.

Ingredients

- 1 tbsp olive oil
- 2 tsp garlic powder
- 2 tsp chili powder
- 1 tsp ground cumin
- 1 tsp smoked paprika
- 1 tsp paprika (not smoked)
- ¼ to ½ tsp cayenne pepper, to taste
- 2 tsp dried oregano
- 1 ½ tsp black pepper
- 1 tsp salt
- 3 lbs boneless skinless chicken thighs

For honey vinegar glaze:

- 6 tbsp honey
- 2 tsp + 2 tbsp apple cider vinegar, divided.

Directions

1. Preheat oven to broil
2. Place an oven rack about 6 inches from the top of the oven.
3. Combine the garlic powder, chili powder, paprika, cumin, oregano, pepper, salt, and olive oil together in a bowl and whisk until combined. Toss the chicken with the spice mix to coat evenly.
4. Prepare the glaze by combining the honey with 2 tsp of the vinegar in a small bowl and stir well.
5. Arrange the chicken thighs by putting a wire rack over a large baking tray and arrange the chicken on the wire rack. Broil the chicken for five minutes on each side (for a total of 10 minutes). Remove the chicken from the oven and brush half of the glaze on the chicken. Broil for one minute. Remove the chicken from the oven and turn over, brush the chicken with the remaining honey mixture and broil for 1 to 2 minutes more, until the chicken is nicely browned. Remove the chicken from the oven and sprinkle it with the remaining 2 Tbsp of vinegar.
6. Let the cooked chicken rest for 5 minutes before serving. Sprinkle with fresh cilantro if desired.

Saffron Risotto with Lemon Chicken

Ingredients

- 8 oz yellow onion
- Grated zest and juice of one lemon
- Small handful of fresh parsley
- 1 oz blanched almonds
- ½ tsp dried thyme
- 1 clove garlic, minced
- 2 tbsp olive oil
- Salt and fresh ground black pepper to taste
- 4 chicken breasts *with* skin
- 4 Tbsp butter
- Small pinch of saffron (not safflower)
- 8 oz risotto rice
- 4 oz white wine
- 5 oz hot chicken or vegetable stock
- 4 tbsp fresh parmesan cheese
- Fresh thyme sprigs

Directions

1. Preheat the oven to 400°F.
2. Finely chop the onion and set aside.
3. In a food processor, blend the zest, parsley, almonds, thyme, and garlic for a few seconds. Slowly add the oil and process until combined. Season with the salt and pepper.
4. Spread this mixture *under* the chicken skin.
5. Place in a roasting tin. Brush with 2 Tbsp melted butter. Pour the lemon juice over the chicken. Cook at 400° F for 25 minutes, basting occasionally.
6. Melt the remaining butter in a pan. Fry the onion until soft. Stir in the uncooked rice and saffron.
7. Add the wine and hot stock a little at a time, allowing the rice to absorb the liquid after each addition. This will take about 25 to 30 minutes.
8. Once the risotto rice is tender, remove from the heat and stir in the parmesan. Serve with the chicken, pouring over any juices from the roasting pan. Garnish with the fresh thyme!

Seafood

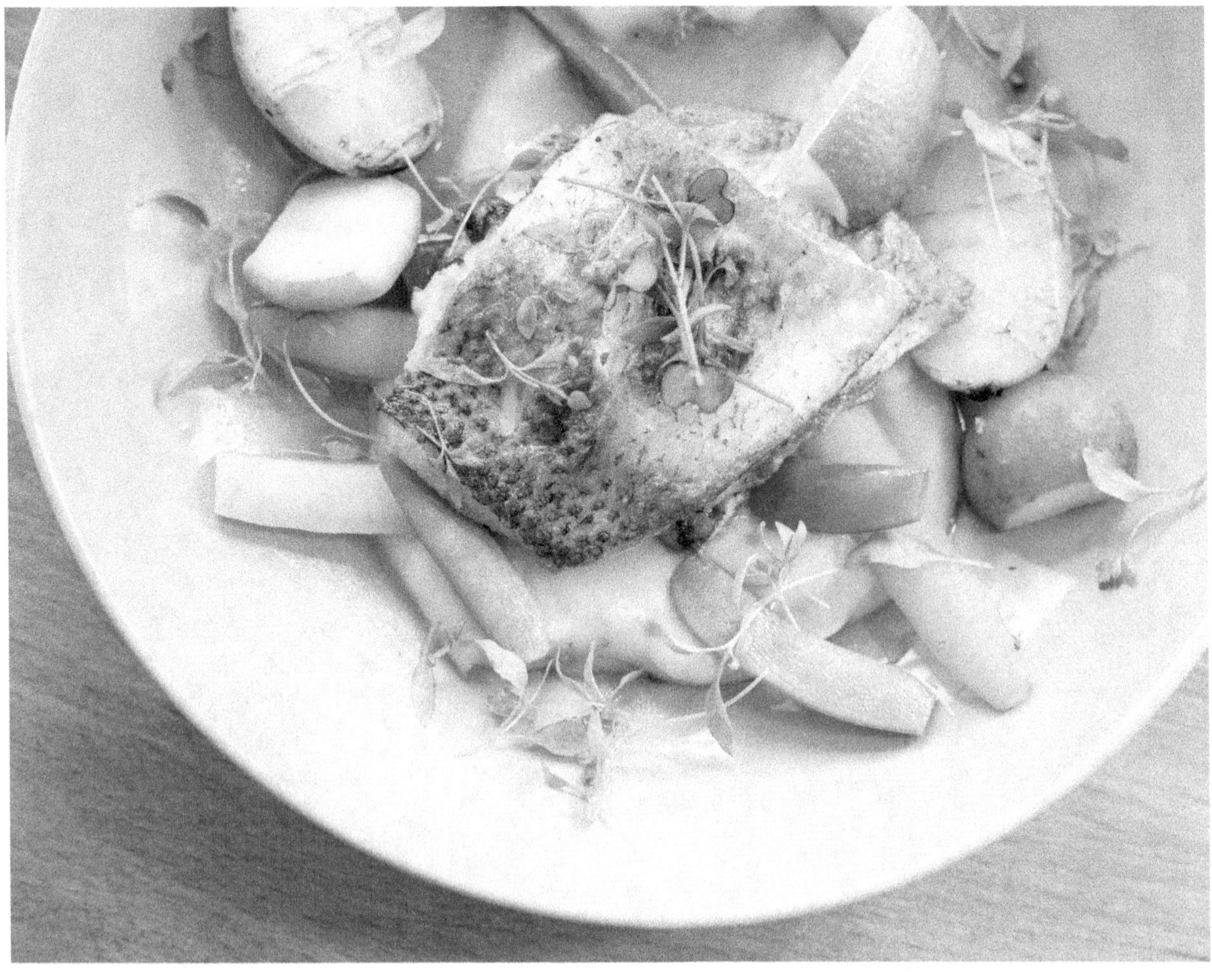

I had been cooking for many years before I could afford fresh seafood, even when I was living in Los Angeles. Seafood also intimidated me. Not that I was scared of fish, or of the little legs on shrimp, but the horror stories I grew up with, My mother had me convinced that unless it was canned fish, there was no possible way someone could cook it successfully in their home to where it both tasted good and was safe to consume. When I learned the truth, I started going out of my way to research seafood recipes, finding what flavors paired best with it, and learning all I could about their multitude of textures. It was both delicious and rewarding.

Stuffed Mediterranean Swordfish Steaks

I discovered this recipe when a former roommate came home with some swordfish and gave me the challenge of creating something magical out of it. At first I was scared. I had no idea how to cook swordfish, or even if I liked it! I'd never tasted swordfish before. After doing a bit of research on flavors that pair well with it, I came up with this recipe and it's been a hit every time I've ever served it. This can also be cooked on an open grill in the summer! If you enjoy wine, it's fabulous with a dry Chardonnay. I love serving this over some baked asparagus for a delightfully beautiful plate.

Ingredients

- 2x 8 oz swordfish steaks (about 2 inches thick)
- 2 tbsp olive oil, divided
- 1 tbsp fresh lemon juice
- 2 cups fresh spinach, rinsed, dried and torn into bite size pieces
- 1 tsp additional olive oil
- 1 clove garlic, minced
- ¼ cup crumbled feta (I prefer fat free or reduced fat if available)
- 2 tbsp salted butter, split.

Directions

1. Preheat oven to 400° F. (If your skillets aren't oven safe, preheat a roasting pan in the oven at the same time).
2. Cut a slit in the swordfish steaks to create a pocket that is open on one side only.
3. In a cup, mix together 2 tablespoons of olive oil and lemon juice. Lay the fish in the lemon oil and let it rest for five to ten minutes per side.
4. In a medium sized skillet, heat 1 tbsp olive oil over medium heat. Cook spinach in the skillet until wilted, toss with the leftover lemon juice and olive oil mixture. Remove from heat, and stuff the spinach into the pockets cut in the steaks. Retain a little spinach for a garnish. Place feta over the spinach inside the pocket. Retain a little feta for a garnish.
5. Place the swordfish in the skillet and cook until browned, 2 to 3 minutes. Turn the swordfish over and brown for 2 minutes.
6. If your skillet is oven safe, transfer the skillet to the oven and roast until just cooked through, about 8 to 10 minutes or until desired doneness. If your skillet isn't oven safe, use the preheated roasting pan. For easy cleanup, line the pan with foil and spray with cooking spray.
7. Add 1 tbsp salted butter to the top of each swordfish steak and let it melt before serving. Top with remaining spinach and feta before serving.

White Wine Yellowfin Tuna Steaks

These are fabulous served with hearty sides like a baked potato and asparagus, or just a salad. They're extremely versatile and well worth the minimal effort required to make them.

Ingredients

- ¼ cup(s) sherry or white wine
- 2 Tbsp low sodium soy sauce
- 1 Tbsp fresh lime juice
- 2 tsp olive oil
- 1 ½ lbs uncooked tuna
- ¼ tsp salt
- ½ tsp pepper

Directions

1. Combine the first 3 ingredients in a small bowl, stirring well with a whisk. Set aside.
2. Heat oil in a large nonstick skillet over medium-high heat. Sprinkle steaks with salt and pepper; add steaks to pan. Cook 4 minutes on each side until steaks are medium-rare or desired degree of doneness.
3. Transfer steaks to a serving dish, and keep warm. Pour sherry mixture into the pan. Cook for 1 to 1 ½ minutes or until reduced to 2 tablespoons, stirring to deglaze pan. Pour over steaks. Serve!

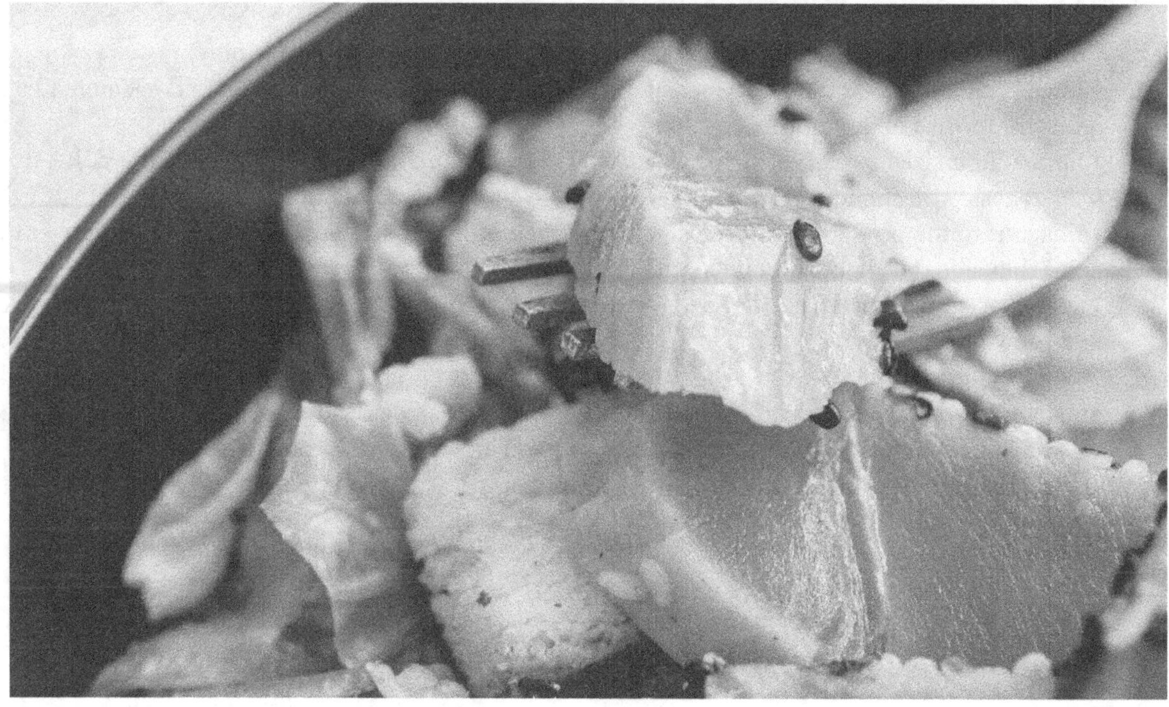

Gorgeous Tuna Steaks

These tuna steaks go soooo well sliced over a fresh salad with the sauce as a salad dressing, or served with a baked potato and asparagus. They're extremely versatile and well worth the minimal effort required to make them. The first time I ever cooked these for my husband he asked if I'd be willing to cook them again for company. That's a pretty big compliment.

Ingredients

- 2 ahi tuna (yellowfin tuna) steaks, about 4 oz. each, 1" thick
- 2 tablespoons soy sauce
- 1 tablespoon toasted sesame oil see notes
- 1 tablespoon honey see notes
- 1/2 teaspoon kosher salt
- 1/4 teaspoon black pepper to taste
- 1/4 teaspoon cayenne pepper (optional)
- 1 tablespoon canola oil or olive oil
- green onions, toasted sesame seeds, and lime wedges for serving (optional)

Instructions

1. Pat the ahi tuna steaks dry with a paper towel. Place on a plate or inside a plastic bag.
2. Mix the soy sauce, toasted sesame oil, honey, kosher salt (leave out if marinating for more than a couple hours), pepper, and cayenne pepper until honey is fully dissolved. Pour over the ahi tuna steaks and turn over to coat completely.
   *Optional: allow to marinate for at least 10 minutes, or up to overnight in the refrigerator.
   *Optional: Reserve a spoonful or two of the marinade before coating the fish for drizzling on top after you've cooked it.
3. Heat a medium skillet, preferably non-stick or a well-seasoned cast iron skillet, on medium-high to high until very hot (or medium medium-high for nonstick).
4. Add the oil to the hot pan. Sear the tuna for 1 - 1½ minutes on each side for medium rare (2 -2½ minutes for medium-well to well, 30 seconds for very rare - this will vary based on thickness of the tuna steaks.
5. Remove to a cutting board and allow to rest for at least 3 minutes. Slice into 1/2 inch slices and serve garnished with green onions, toasted sesame seeds, and a squeeze of fresh lime juice, if desired.

Smoked Trout with Roasted Radishes and Fennel-Stone Fruit Salad

Ingredients

- 12 ounces small to medium radishes, trimmed (and halved, if needed)
- 1 tablespoon olive oil
- ¼ teaspoon black pepper
- 1 teaspoon kosher salt, divided
- .50 cup sour cream
- 2 teaspoons grated lemon zest
- ¼ cup almond oil
- 3.50 tablespoons wildflower honey
- 1.50 tablespoons aged sherry vinegar
- 3 cups thinly sliced fennel, plus fennel fronds for garnish
- 2 cups thinly sliced unpeeled under ripe stone fruit (such as peaches or apricots
- 2 cups (8-ounce) packages hot-smoked trout filets (such as Ducktrap River of Maine), skin discarded
- Flaky sea salt, for garnish
- Toasted baguette slices, for serving

Directions

1. Preheat the oven to 450°F. Toss together radishes, olive oil, pepper, and 1/4 teaspoon kosher salt on a rimmed baking sheet; arrange any halved radishes cut sides down. Roast in a preheated oven until the radishes are tender and lightly browned, about 15 minutes. Let cool for 5 minutes.
2. While radishes cool, stir together sour cream and lemon zest in a small bowl. Whisk together almond oil, honey, vinegar, and 1/2 teaspoon kosher salt in a separate small bowl until creamy; reserve 1/4 cup vinaigrette for drizzling. Combine sliced fennel, stone fruit, remaining vinaigrette, and remaining 1/4 teaspoon kosher salt in a large bowl; toss to coat.
3. Spread 2 tablespoons of sour cream mixture along one side of each of 4 plates to form a semicircle. Decoratively pile fennel mixture and radishes on sour cream mixture. Gently break each trout filet in half crosswise, and place alongside fennel mixture. Garnish fennel mixture with fennel fronds and sea salt. Drizzle reserved 1/4 cup vinaigrette evenly over trout. Serve alongside toasted baguette slices.

Shrimp and Grits

The first time I ever had Shrimp and Grits it was in a hotel restaurant in Tulsa, Oklahoma. I was about to start my in-the-sky testing as a trained flight attendant. I'd gone through all the classes on the ground, and this would be an anxiety riddled few days for the new girl. So what did I do? I went hunting for some good comfort food the night before. The shrimp at this restaurant were some of the largest I'd ever seen in my life, but I've been able to modify it for the normal sized shrimp that we usually get in the grocery stores instead of the ones that are larger than a lobster. This dish might seem labor intensive, but I can promise you that if you like shrimp, it's worth every minute spent making it.

Ingredients

For the Grits
- ¾ cup grits (uncooked)
- ¼ teaspoon salt
- 6 oz cheddar cheese (grated)
- 3 Tbsp butter

For the Shrimp
- 4 Tbsp butter
- ¾ cup chopped onion
- ½ cup chopped green bell pepper
- 2 garlic cloves, minced
- 1 14.5 oz can of fire roasted diced tomatoes
- ½ teaspoon dried thyme
- 1 Tbsp flour
- ½ tsp smoked paprika
- 1 tsp Cayenne pepper
- ½ to 1 cup shrimp stock (see right)
- 1 Tbsp tomato paste
- ⅓ cup heavy cream
- 2 tsp Worcestershire sauce
- 1 lb medium to large raw shrimp, shells reserved!
- 2 dashes hot sauce (Tabasco preferred)
- Salt to taste
- 2 Tbsp chopped fresh parsley

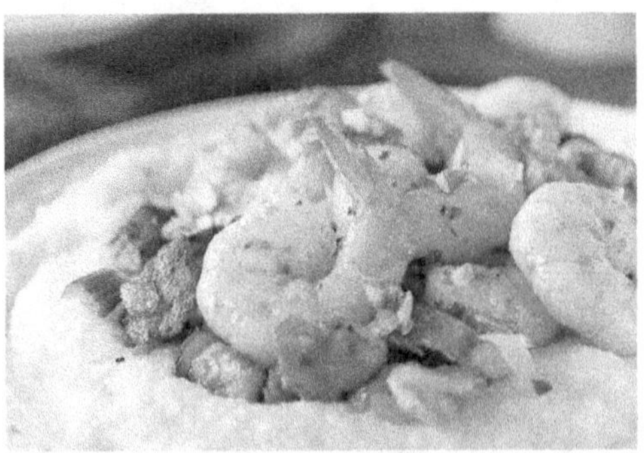

Shrimp stock:

To make the shrimp stock, combine the shrimp shells and 2 cups of water. Boil these until the liquid is reduced by ½ and strain the shells out.

Directions

1. For the grits: bring 3 ½ cups of water to a boil and stir in the grits. Reduce heat to low, cover and cook for 15 to 20 minutes, until the grits are tender and the liquid has been absorbed. Remove from the heat, add the salt, cheese, and butter. Stir until melted. Keep warm.
2. For the shrimp: melt the butter in a large skillet over medium heat and sauté the onion, pepper,

and garlic until softened (about 5 minutes).

3. Add the can of tomatoes with their juice and the thyme. Bring to a simmer. Cook for 3 to 4 minutes.
4. Sprinkle with the flour and stir well. Add the smoked paprika, cayenne pepper, and ½ cup of the shrimp stock and cook for 3 minutes more.
5. Add the tomato paste and stir until blended. Add the cream, worcestershire and hot sauce.
6. Add the shrimp and more shrimp stock if needed to create a spoonable sauce that generously coats the shrimp as they cook. Heat through until shrimp are cooked completely, being careful not to let it come to a boil. Taste for salt.
7. Place a portion of the grits in the center of each plate and spoon shrimp over or around it. Sprinkle the final dish with the fresh parsley before serving.

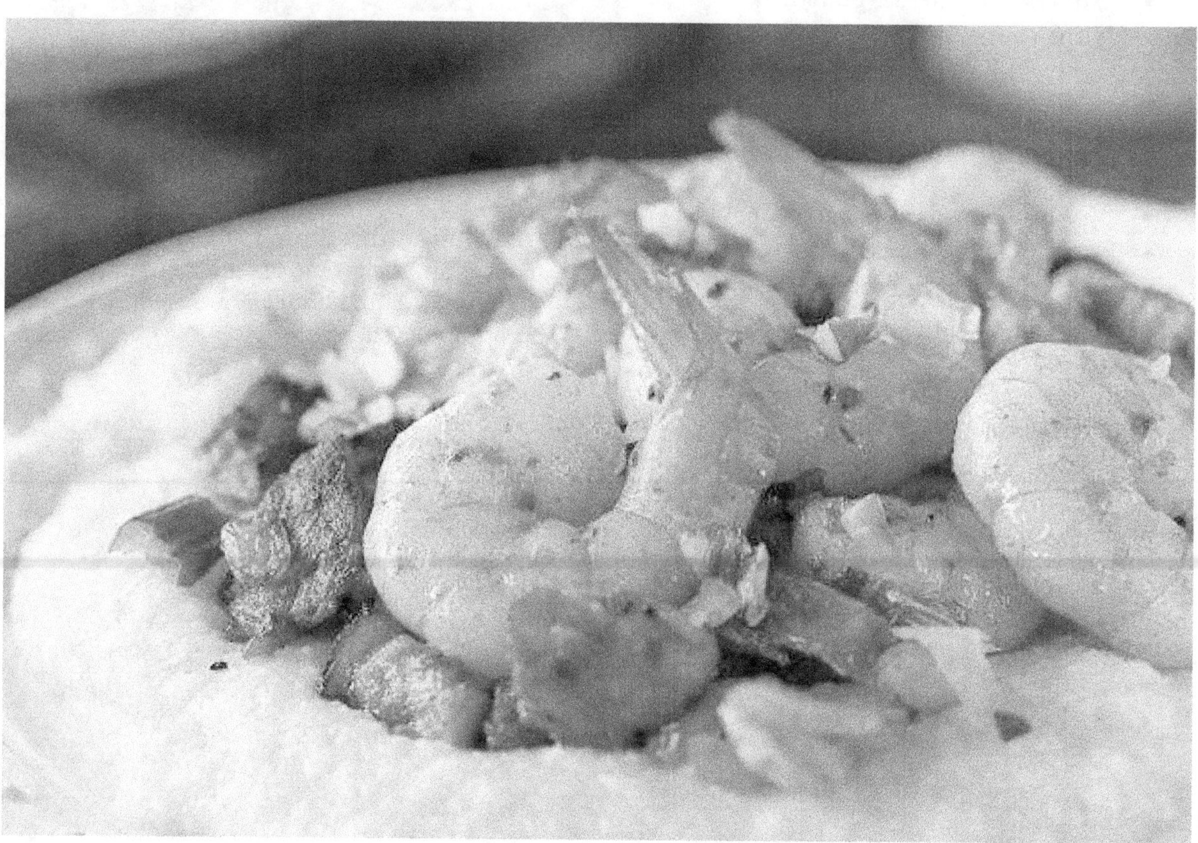

Oven Fried Catfish

This was originally a diet program recipe that I'd found and made changes to. It's incredibly lean and healthy while still packed with flavor and adventure. If your family likes catfish, they're sure to like this fantastic meal. It goes incredibly well with hush puppies and fries, but also with collard greens and a baked potato. This was originally a 'challenge' meal for me. A roommate brought home some catfish and challenged me to make it edible. Little did he know I loved catfish. I'd just never cooked it before!

Ingredients

- yellow cornmeal
- ½ cup(s) smoked paprika
- 1 tsp dried thyme
- 1 tsp table salt
- 1 tsp celery seed
- ½ tsp onion powder
- ½ tsp garlic powder
- ½ tsp black pepper
- ½ tsp cayenne pepper
- ½ pinch, freshly ground
- ½ cup fat free skim milk or unsweetened almond milk
- cooking spray
- 1 lb catfish filet(s) separated into 4 pieces
- Lemon wedges

Directions

1. Preheat the oven to 425°F. Mix cornmeal, paprika, thyme, salt, celery seeds, onion powder, garlic powder, black pepper and cayenne pepper together in a shallow bowl. Pour milk into another shallow bowl.
2. Coat a large nonstick baking sheet with cooking spray. Dredge filets first in milk, then in cornmeal mixture, coating both sides and pressing cornmeal mixture gently to adhere. Place coated filets on a baking sheet and lightly spray each with cooking spray.
3. Bake until cooked through, about 15 minutes. Let stand at room temperature 2 minutes before serving. Serve with lemon wedge.

Super Easy Skinny Tilapia

Ingredients

- 4 tilapia filets (about 6 ounces each)
- 1 tablespoon butter, melted
- 3 tablespoons fresh lemon juice
- 1-1/2 teaspoons garlic powder
- 1/8 teaspoon salt
- 2 tablespoons capers, drained
- 1/2 teaspoon dried oregano
- 1/8 teaspoon paprika

Directions

1. Place tilapia filets in an ungreased 9x13-inch baking dish.
2. In a small bowl, combine the butter, lemon juice, garlic powder and salt. Pour evenly over the filets. Sprinkle capers, oregano and paprika over tilapia filets.
3. Bake, uncovered, at 425°F for 10-15 minutes, or until the fish filets flake easily with a fork.

Broiled Salmon with Lentils

Ingredients

- ¾ cup lentils
- ½ small onion, chopped
- 2 Tbsp red wine vinegar
- 1 tbsp olive oil
- 1 tbsp dijon mustard
- 1 clove garlic, minced
- ⅓ cup chopped fresh parsley
- Chopped celery leaves
- Coarse salt and ground pepper
- 4 skinless salmon filets (6 oz each)
- Nonstick cooking spray

Directions

1. Heat the oven broiler.
2. Combine lentils and 2 ½ cups of water in a medium saucepan. Bring to a boil, reduce heat and simmer, covered, about 5 minutes. Add onion and celery, cover and continue to cook until the lentils and vegetables are tender, about 15 to 25 minutes more. Drain, reserving cooking liquid. Transfer the lentil and vegetables to a medium bowl.
3. Meanwhile, season the salmon with salt and pepper. Coat a baking sheet with cooking spray. Arrange the salmon on the sheet. Broil until opaque throughout, about 8 to 10 minutes.
4. In another bowl, whisk 2 tbsp of the reserved cooking liquid with the red wine vinegar, olive oil. Mustard, garlic, celery leaves and parsley. Season with salt and pepper. Toss half of this dressing with the lentil and vegetable mixture.
5. Spoon the lentils on to plates, top with the salmon, flaking it into large pieces if desired. Drizzle with the remaining homemade red wine vinegar dressing.

Citrus Baked Salmon with Fingerling Potatoes

Ingredients

- 1 lb fingerling potatoes, halved
- 2 tablespoons olive oil
- 3 shallots, cut into thick wedges
- 1 1/2 cups kumquats, halved (or sub 2 tangerines, mandarins, or Meyer lemons, thinly sliced)
- generous pinch salt and pepper
- 1 lb wild salmon – skinless, and portioned into 4, 4-ounce pieces
- a few thyme sprigs

Citrus Marinade:

- 2 tablespoons olive oil
- 1 tablespoon honey
- 2 garlic cloves, finely minced (use a garlic press)
- zest from one orange, divided
- juice from one orange, divided
- 1 teaspoon kosher salt
- 1/2 teaspoon cracked pepper
- 1/4 teaspoon cayenne

Garnish: additional thyme sprigs, squeeze of orange

Directions

1. Preheat oven to 425°F (you will turn this down later in recipe)
2. Place potatoes, shallots, and citrus on a parchment-lined baking sheet and drizzle with olive oil and sprinkle with salt and pepper. Toss to coat well and spread out. Bake for 20-25 minutes, or until potatoes are fork-tender.
3. While the potatoes are roasting, make the citrus marinade. Stir the olive oil, honey, garlic, 1/2 of the orange zest, 2 tablespoons of the orange juice, salt, pepper and cayenne in a small bowl. Place the salmon in a shallow bowl and pour the marinade over top, turning salmon to coat all sides. Leave on the counter.
4. When the potatoes are fork-tender, lower heat to 375°F. Give them a quick toss and nestle the salmon in between the potatoes, drizzling any remaining marinade over the salmon filets. Scatter with a few thyme sprigs and bake until salmon is cooked to desired doneness (8-12 minutes, depending on thickness or the filets). If you have a broiler in your oven, broiling the salmon for the last few minutes adds a beautiful color. Garnish with remaining orange zest, thyme and a squeeze of orange juice to taste.

Spaghetti Vongole

There was a chapter in my life where I pursued a job at a local Italian steakhouse in Eagle Rock California to the point that they grew tired of my appearing unannounced to ask for work. Eventually they hired me to be a hostess one busy night, and immediately had to transition into being a server when an unexpected table of 32 guests came in. Over the next year I became very familiar with the menu and fell in love with several dishes. This and the hand rolled lasagne are my own takes on these classic dishes still served at Colombo's Italian Steakhouse in Eagle Rock, California today. My memories of working there and the friends I worked with in 2004 are among my favorites from that decade.

Ingredients

- 1 lb spaghetti
- Salt
- ¼ cup extra virgin olive oil
- 4 cloves garlic, minced
- ½ tsp crushed red pepper
- 2 dozen littleneck clams (scrubbed clean)
- ¼ cup water
- ¼ cup finely chopped fresh parsley
- Freshly ground black pepper

Directions

1. In a large pot of boiling salted water, cook the spaghetti until just al dente according to the manufacturer's recommendation and then drain the spaghetti noodles well.
2. In a large, deep skillet, heat the olive oil. Add the minced garlic and crushed red pepper. Cook over medium high heat, stirring occasionally, until the garlic is lightly browned, about 1 ½ minutes. Add the clams and water, cover and simmer until the clams open and are just cooked through, between five to eight minutes. Discard any clams that don't open.
3. Add the spaghetti and the chopped parsley to the clams in the skillet and season with pepper. Toss over medium high heat just until the spaghetti absorbs some of the juices, about 1 minute. Transfer the spaghetti and clams to shallow bowls and serve while piping hot.

Carolina Fish, Shrimp, and Okra Stew

Ingredients

- 1 lb raw medium shrimp, peeled and deveined (save the shells!)
- 3 cups water
- 1 ½ lbs skinless catfish or cod filets, cut crosswise into 1 inch strips
- 1 tsp salt, plus more to taste
- 2 tablespoons olive oil, plus more for drizzling
- 2 tbsp all purpose flour
- 1 large white onion, chopped
- 1 large red bell pepper, chopped
- 2 medium celery stalks, chopped
- 3 medium garlic cloves, chopped
- 1 14.5 oz can diced tomatoes with juice
- 2 cups frozen sliced okra (or 8 ounces fresh steamed, cut into ½ in pieces)
- 2 tbsp Worcestershire sauce
- 2 tsp chopped fresh thyme
- 2 bay leaves
- 2 tsp Creole seasoning
- ½ tsp black pepper, plus more to taste
- ½ tsp cayenne pepper
- Cooked rice
- Thinly sliced scallions for garnish

Directions

1. Combine shrimp shells and 3 cups of water in a medium saucepan. Bring to a simmer over medium heat. Remove from heat and let it stand for 15 minutes. Pur mixture through a strainer into a bowl and discard the shells. Set this 'shrimp stock' aside.
2. Toss together catfish pieces and salt in a large bowl. Cover and chill until ready to use, up to 1 hour.
3. Heat oil in a large dutch oven over medium heat. Add flour, cook while whisking constantly, until smooth and lightly browned, about 1 minute. Add the onion, bell pepper, celery and garlic. Cook, stirring often and scrubbing the bottom of the dutch oven to prevent it from burning to the bottom. When the veggies are soft, stir in the shrimp stock, tomatoes with juices, okra, Worcestershire, thyme, bay leaves, Creole seasoning, and black pepper.Bring to a simmer over medium high heat. Reduce heat to medium low. Cover and simmer until okra is almost tender, about 15 minutes.
4. Stir in catfish and shrimp. Reduce heat to low. Cover and cook until catfish and shrimp are cooked through, about five to eight minutes. Remove and discard the bay leaves. Season to taste with salt and pepper. Serve with rice. Garnish each plate with scallions and drizzle with olive oil.

Teriyaki Salmon

Ingredients

- 2 salmon filets, 6 oz each
- ½ tsp black pepper
- 2 cloves garlic, minced
- ½ tsp fresh ground ginger
- 2 tbsp soy sauce
- 2 tbsp brown sugar
- 1 tbsp sriracha
- 1 tbsp apple cider vinegar
- ½ cup water
- ½ tsp cornstarch
- Green onions, sliced

Directions

1. Preheat oven to 400°F
2. Spray a large baking pan or baking sheet with non-stick spray. Line with foil and then spray for easier cleanup. Season the salmon filets with pepper and set aside.
3. In a medium mixing bowl, whisk together the garlic, ginger, soy sauce, brown sugar, sriracha, apple cider vinegar, water, and cornstarch. Pour this mixture into a large resealable bag along with the salmon filets. Allow this to sit and marinade for twenty to thirty minutes in the fridge.
4. After the salmon has rested for the desired length of time, remove from the fridge and place the salmon on the baking dish. Bake for fifteen minutes or until flaky. Bake times might vary depending on the thickness of salmon filets and elevation factors.
5. While the salmon is baking, transfer the leftover marinade to a small saucepan. Place on medium heath, bring to a boil, then reduce the heat to a simmer and cook, stirring occasionally until thickened. Remove from heat and set aside.
6. Take salmon out of the oven when it's done. Plate the fish and drizzle the teriyaki sauce over top or serve on the side in a dipping dish. Top with green onions and serve with rice and broccoli as healthy sides.

Shrimp and Feta Skillet

Ingredients

- 2 cans (14.5 each) diced tomatoes with basil, oregano and garlic - undrained
- 2 tsp garlic powder
- 2 tsp dried basil
- Pinch of cayenne pepper
- Red pepper flakes
- 1 ¼ lbs uncooked shrimp, peeled and deveined
- 1 cup crumbled low fat or fat free feta cheese
- Crusty whole grain bread
- Rice or quinoa, cooked

Directions

1. In a large skillet, combine tomatoes, garlic powder, cayenne, and basil. Bring to a boil.
2. Reduce heat, add red pepper flakes.
3. Simmer, uncovered, for four to six minutes or until slightly thickened.
4. Add shrimp, cook and stir for three to four minutes or until shrimp turn pink. Sprinkle feta over shrimp. Serve with crusty bread and rice or quinoa

Tuna melt

Ingredients

- 16 ounces tuna fish, drained
- ¼ cup mayonnaise
- ¼ cup celery, finely chopped
- ¼ cup red onion, finely chopped
- 1 tablespoon dijon mustard
- 2 tablespoons parsley, chopped
- salt and pepper, to taste
- 16 slices bread
- 8 slices cheddar cheese, more if you want a layer on the bottom
- tomato, sliced
- ¼ cup butter, softened

Instructions

1. In a medium sized bowl combine the tuna, mayonnaise, celery, red onion, dijon mustard, parsley, salt and pepper.
2. Butter one side of each slice of bread. Put the butter side down and add the cheese on the unbuttered side. Add the tuna mixture on top. Top with tomato and additional cheese.

Skillet Method

Preheat a skillet to medium heat. Add the sandwich on the skillet and heat for about 2-3 minutes until the cheese starts to melt and it is golden brown. Flip to the other side and cook until the cheese is fully melted and the sandwich is golden brown.

Broiler Method

Preheat a broiler. Spread the bread butter side up and toast for a couple of minutes. Top with cheese, tuna mixture and Broil for 2-3 minutes until cheese is melted.

Seared Scallops with Saffron Risotto

There was this little French bistro in Redondo Beach, California that I loved. You'd never know it was there if you weren't a local or if someone didn't tell you. It was rather unassuming with its strip mall location nestled next to a mailbox store, down the way from the local liquor and smoke stop. The owner was a feisty french woman who loved to take control whenever she could. Her name was Aimee, and her food was even more fabulous than her over-the-top colored glasses and delicate scarves she would tie around her petite neck. The world lost a hidden treasure when Aimee's Bistro closed many years ago, but the love of french cuisine that she introduced me to will live on as long as I have any memory at all.

Ingredients:

- Fresh Scallops
- 3 tbsp Butter
- 1 recipe Lemon Beurre Blanc (see next page)
- ½ cup Arborio Rice
- 5 cups Chicken Stock (Warmed)
- 1 ¼ cup Dry White Wine (Chardonnay)
- 1 cup Fresh Grated Parmesan
- 1 Small Shallot (Minced)
- 3 Cloves of Garlic (Minced)
- 5 strands authentic Saffron
- Salt and Pepper to taste

Directions:

1. Heat a large frying pan over medium heat, when the pan is hot add 2 tablespoons of butter and allow to melt.
2. Add in the minced shallot and sweat down until translucent then add in garlic. Cook garlic for 1 minute then add in the Arborio rice. Stir rice until it is fully coated in the butter and lightly toasted then add in 1 cup of white wine.
3. When wine has started to evaporate add in a small amount (approximately ½ cup) of chicken stock. Constantly stir the rice until the liquid disappears, then add in additional stock. Add in the saffron with the second round of stock.
4. Continue this process alternating between additions of stock and stirring until it evaporates until the rice is cooked. This will take about 45 minutes.
5. When the risotto has about 10 minutes left to cook, start a frying pan over medium high heat. Once the pan has warmed to the correct temperature, add 1 Tbsp of butter. Don't add the butter prematurely. Patience is key with this delicious recipe.
6. Pat the scallops dry and lightly season each side with salt and pepper. Evenly place in the pan and cook for 2-3 minutes per side. Be careful not to overcook scallops because they will turn rubbery.
7. Remove from the pan and allow to rest. As they rest, start your Beurre blanc (see next page) sauce.

8. When the sauce is finished, finish the risotto by adding in the ¼ cup of remaining white wine, cook this out until wine evaporates, about 1 minute, then add in the parmesan. Adjust seasoning with salt and pepper.
9. Plate scallops then top with hot Beurre blanc sauce, add risotto and top with fresh grated parmesan.

Lemon Beurre Blanc

Ingredients

- 2 Lemons, juiced
- ¾ cup Dry White Wine
- 12 tbsp *cold* butter, cubed
- 3 Sprigs Fresh Thyme
- 1 Shallot, minced

Directions

1. Start sauce by bringing the wine, juice from two lemons, shallot and thyme leaves to a boil. Let this boil for 5 minutes, then turn down the heat to a simmer.
2. With the sauce over low heat, start slowly adding butter 1 small piece at a time and constantly whisk each cube before adding the next one in. Each cube should take about 2 to 3 minutes to incorporate. This delicate sauce will get rich and creamy from the butter.

Shrimp Jambalaya

Ingredients

- 2 pounds shrimp in the shell
- 2 tablespoons corn, peanut or vegetable oil
- 2 tablespoons flour
- 1 cup finely chopped onion
- 1 cup finely chopped green onions or scallions
- 1 cup finely chopped green pepper
- 1 cup finely chopped celery
- 1 tablespoon finely minced garlic
- 1 cup cooked ham cut into ½-inch cubes
- 2 cups crushed tomatoes
- ½ teaspoon dried thyme
- 1 teaspoon dried oregano
- 1 cup uncooked long-grain rice
- Salt and freshly ground pepper to taste
- 5 cups shrimp stock (see Shrimp and Grits recipe) or water
- ½ cup finely chopped green onion or scallions, optional, for garnish

Directions

1. Peel and devein the shrimp. (Prepare the shrimp stock by combining the shrimp shells and 2 cups of water. Boil these until the liquid is reduced by ½ and strain the shells out.)
2. Heat the oil in a kettle or large saucepan with a heavy bottom over medium heat. Add the flour, and cook, stirring constantly, until lightly browned. Be careful not to burn the flour.
3. Add the onion, green onions, green pepper, celery and garlic. Cook, stirring, until wilted.
4. Add ham and stir. Add the tomatoes, thyme and oregano, and bring to a boil.
5. Stir in the uncooked rice. Add salt, pepper and shrimp broth.
6. Reduce heat to medium-low, and simmer, uncovered, about 25 minutes; add the shrimp and stir.
7. Cook about 10 minutes longer or until it has thickened, but is still slightly soupy. Serve in bowls with chopped green onions on the side as an optional garnish.

Linguini Vongole of Colombo's

You might start to notice that there are a number of recipes in this book that came from my time in Los Angeles. That's no coincidence. Having lived there for fourteen years throughout my 20's and 30's was one of the next experiences I could've had as someone who loves food. One of my favorite places was Colombo's Italian Steakhouse in Eagle Rock, California. I worked there as a server for some time and tried practically everything on the menu. I never exactly 'stole' the recipes from the restaurant, and theirs will always be better than my own, but I did the best I could once I moved away and couldn't go there for my favorites anymore. This is one of those recipes - not exactly stolen, but a close approximation.

Ingredients

- 1 pound dry linguine
- ¼ cup extra-virgin olive oil, plus more for serving
- 4 garlic cloves, thinly sliced or slivered
- ¼ teaspoon red pepper flakes
- 2 pounds littleneck or Manila clams, scrubbed and rinsed well
- ¾ cup dry white wine (think of getting a Pinot Grigio for this one)
- 1 lemon, juiced
- 3 tablespoons unsalted butter
- Sea salt and freshly ground black pepper to taste
- 2 handfuls fresh flat-leaf parsley, finely chopped

Directions

Prepare the sauce while the pasta is cooking to make sure that the linguine noodles will be hot and ready when the sauce is finished.

1. Bring a large pot of salted water to a boil, add the pasta and cook for 8 to 10 minutes or until tender yet firm, aka "al dente." Drain the pasta well.
2. Meanwhile, heat the olive oil over medium flame in a deep saute pan with a lid. Add the garlic and red pepper flakes; saute for 2 minutes. Add the clams, wine, and lemon juice. Cover and cook, shaking the pan periodically, until all the clams are opened, about 7 minutes. Discard any that have not opened (because this means they're bad. *Do not be tempted to eat them!*
3. Crank the flame up to medium-high heat. Add the hot, drained linguine to the pan; add the butter and season with salt and pepper. Toss the pasta with the clams so it's nicely coated. Toss in the chopped parsley. Drizzle with a nice dose of olive oil before serving alongside some nice french bread to soak up the sauce with.

Tuna Cakes Like Mom's

This is one of those things my husband will likely *never* try. I guess there's some trauma in his childhood regarding either tuna cakes or salmon patties, I'm not sure which. I know better than to go there with him. But this was a recipe my mother excelled at! I loved tuna cake night when I was a child. I wasn't a big fan of tuna fish sandwiches after a while, but these little things just never went out of style. Maybe one of these days I'll be able to talk my husband into trying them. After all, he hated meatloaf when we met, too. I changed his mind with the turkey sriracha meatloaf the first time I ever made it.

Ingredients

- 3 5-ounce cans tuna
- 2 tablespoons fresh parsley, minced
- 1 green onion, finely minced
- ½ teaspoon garlic powder
- ½ teaspoon kosher salt
- ¾ cup plain panko or coarse breadcrumbs
- 2 tablespoons mustard
- 2 tablespoons mayonnaise
- 2 eggs
- 2 tablespoons olive oil, for cooking

Directions

1. Drain the tuna and flake it into small pieces with a fork, smashing up any big chunks. In a medium bowl, mix it with the parsley, green onion, garlic powder, kosher salt, panko, Dijon mustard, mayonnaise, and eggs. You can also add some Old Bay seasoning if you like. It works well!
2. Form the dough into 8 patties using a ⅓ cup measuring cup to portion it out, then pat it into a patty with your hands. Refrigerate the patties for 15 minutes to firm up the texture (or up to 24 hours to prep ahead).
3. When ready to cook, heat 1 tablespoon of olive oil in a skillet over medium high heat. Add the patties and cook for about 4 to 5 minutes until lightly browned, then gently flip them with a spatula and cook about 3 to 4 minutes more until lightly browned on the other side. Repeat with the next batch, adjusting the heat because the pan will be hotter on the second batch (much like pancakes!).
4. Serve immediately, with a sauce (like remoulade, tartar sauce, artichoke dip, etc). We always had these with cornbread and mixed vegetables. The veggies were boring, but Mom's cornbread was pretty stellar, too.

Ceviche from Hernandez's Mom

I had a decade-long severe *need* to learn how to make this recipe. Let me roll this back a bit. Once upon a time I was the Director of Security for a few different properties in Los Angeles. My staff had been accustomed to leadership that didn't fulfill them or care about them. With required monthly training, I wanted to show to my staff that I genuinely did care about their happiness on the job. I started turning our monthly training meetings into potlucks, and often made some of the recipes from this very book (like the hand rolled lasagna) to take with me to the meetings. Sometimes I spent days in preparation, and the food was always appreciated. One of my employees, Robert Hernandez, was a young father without much time on his hands, so he would ask his mother to make some ceviche for us. The first time it was because he thought it would be his way to get *out* of having to participate in the future, but it backfired. We all loved it and begged for it from then on.

Ingredients

- 1 pound skinless snapper, bass, or halibut filet, sushi-grade
- ⅔ cup fresh lime juice
- 1 teaspoon lime zest
- ⅓ cup rice vinegar
- 1 large red onion
- 1 small (or ½ large) cucumber
- ½ large red bell pepper
- 1 jalapeño pepper, seeded
- 1 avocado
- ¼ cup chopped cilantro
- ¼ cup olive oil
- ½ teaspoon salt
- ¼ teaspoon black pepper
- Fresh lime wedges for serving

Directions

1. Cut the fish into very small cubes (about ¼-inch).Put the fish into a non-reactive container, such as a glass bowl. Combine the fish with lime juice, lime zest, and rice vinegar, and stir gently. Cover the bowl and put it into the refrigerator for 2 to 3 hours, stirring approximately every 30 minutes.
2. Finely dice the onion, cucumber, peppers, and avocado. Mix all of the vegetables, except the avocado, with the chopped cilantro.
3. Drain the fish and stir it into the mixed vegetables. Stir the olive oil, salt, and pepper into the ceviche. Fold in the avocado and season the ceviche with additional salt and pepper if necessary. Garnish with lime wedges

Breads

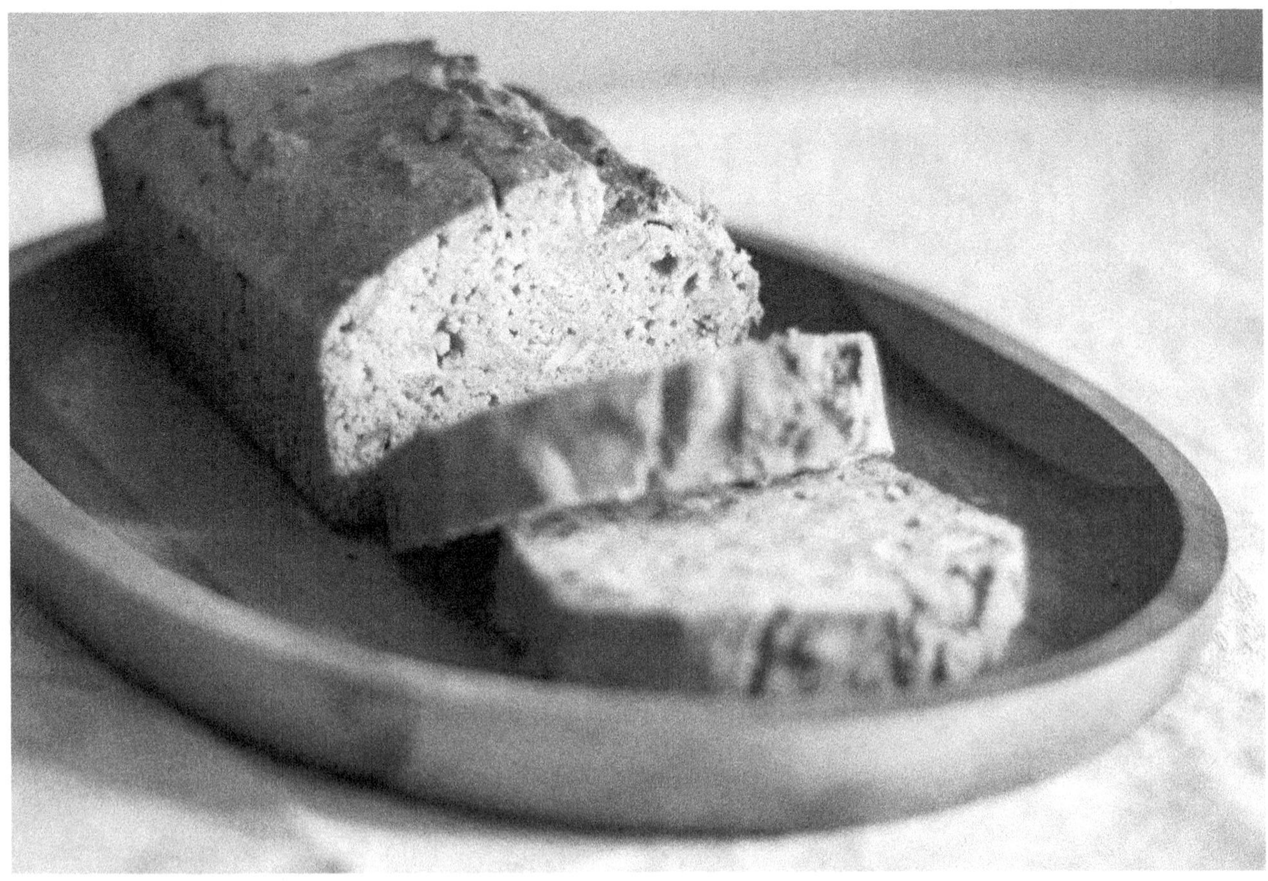

I've never known a kitchen challenge like the one I was faced with when I moved to Colorado. At a mile high elevation, baking bread changed into a completely different and fairly confusing monster with two heads and a forked tail. Once I finally got the basics down, I started to apply what I'd learned to my favorite recipes and things started turning out the way they were supposed to. It just took seemingly forever to get there. For the benefit of this book I'll include the classic recipe I use at sea level, and what I did to make that same recipe work at Denver's elevation. You might be surprised at how simple it really is.

Homemade Bread

Ingredients

- 3 cups all-purpose flour
- 1 teaspoon salt
- 1 teaspoon sugar
- 1 package active dry yeast
- 1 ½ cups warm water (105°F to 115°F)
- 2 tablespoons butter, softened

Instructions

1. In a large bowl, combine 2 cups of the flour, the salt, sugar, and yeast. (For high-altitude baking, add 2 tbsp of additional flour)
2. In a small bowl, combine the warm water and butter.
3. Add the water mixture to the flour mixture and stir until a dough forms.
4. Turn the dough out onto a lightly floured surface and knead for 5-10 minutes, until the dough is smooth and elastic.
5. Place the dough in a greased bowl, cover with plastic wrap, and let rise in a warm place for 1 hour, or until doubled in size.
6. Punch down the dough (once, not repeatedly) and divide it in half.
7. Shape each half into a loaf and place in greased 9x5-inch loaf pans.
8. Cover the pans with plastic wrap and let rise in a warm place for 30 minutes, or until doubled in size.
9. Preheat the oven to 375°F.
10. Bake the loaves for 30-35 minutes, or until golden brown.
11. Remove the loaves from the oven and let cool on a wire rack before slicing and serving.

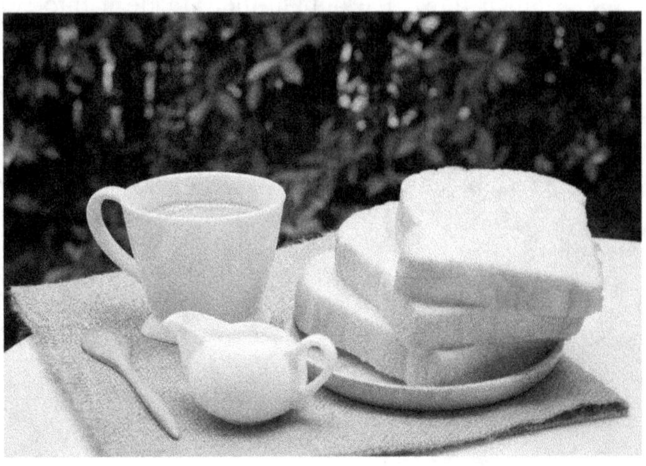

Great Depression Bread

People who know me even a little know that I have a great love of history. Recently I wrote a book called "The Road We Left Behind" primarily set in the 1930's and based on my grandmother's true story. It should come as no surprise to see that there's a historical recipe in this book. If you look hard enough, there might be more than just one or two. When I make this bread, I imagine my grandmother preparing this in her little apartment where she lived over top of the dry cleaners.

Ingredients (makes 2 loaves)

- 4 1/2 C. all-purpose flour
- 1 1/2 tsp. salt
- 1 1/2 Tbsp. yeast
- 1 1/2 C. warm water
- 1 Tbsp. olive oil

Directions

1. In a bowl, stir together flour and salt. Make a small hole in the middle of the flour mixture and pour in the yeast in the hole.
2. Pour warm water in the hole with the yeast and mix with your finger to dissolve.
3. Continue mixing/kneading until there is no more loose flour in the bowl (or until you have a dough ball). If you need to add a little more warm water than the 1 ½ C., then go ahead and do it just a little bit at a time until you have enough.
4. Remove the dough ball from the bowl. Wash and dry the bowl, then spread the olive oil on the bottom and sides of the bowl.
5. Place the dough ball back into the oiled bowl. Flip the dough over once. Cover the top of the bowl with a dish cloth and place the bowl in a warm area.
6. Wait about 1 hour for the dough to rise.
7. Punch down the dough, then divide it into two sections (shaped somewhat like a mini loaf of french bread).
8. Place each section on a lightly floured cookie sheet or in a bread pan. Cover with a cloth and let rise about 1/2 hour more. Preheat the oven to 350°F while it rests.
9. Remove cloth and cook on the center rack in the oven at 350° F for about 30 minutes.
10. Fresh bread is most enjoyed when it's still warm with a pat of butter on it. YUM.

Homemade French Bread

Ingredients

- 2 cups warm water , about 105°F
- 1 Tablespoon active dry yeast
- 2 ½ teaspoons granulated sugar
- 5 cups (650 g) all-purpose flour , more as needed
- 2 ½ teaspoons table salt or fine sea salt
- 1 teaspoon olive oil
- Melted salted butter, optional

Directions

1. In a small bowl, combine the warm water, yeast, and sugar. Let sit for 5 minutes, or until it begins to foam.
2. In a stand mixer fitted with a paddle attachment or in a large mixing bowl, stir together 2 cups of flour and salt. Stir in the yeast mixture on medium-low speed or by hand. Knead in 1/2 cup of the remaining flour in increments until the dough is smooth but not sticky (depending on climate you could use more or less than 5 cups). Add more flour as needed.
3. Rub the olive oil around the dough ball, cover the bowl with a towel and let rest 15 to 30 minutes. If you have more time, let it rise up to 1 hour.
4. Turn the dough onto a well-floured surface and divide it in half. Set one half aside. Roll the other half into a rectangle (about 15 inches). Starting from the long side, roll the dough into a cylinder.
5. Turn both ends in and pinch the seams closed. Round the edges and place onto a baking sheet. Repeat with the second dough ball. Make three diagonal cuts across the top of each loaf. Cover loaves lightly with a towel. Let rise 30 to 60 minutes (the longer the better, if you have the time).
6. Preheat the oven to 400°F. Line a baking sheet with a silicone mat or parchment paper. Bake for 17 to 23 minutes, or until the tops are golden brown. When you knock on it, it should sound hollow. If it's browning too fast, lightly cover with foil and lower the temperature to 375°F.
7. Brush the top with melted butter, if desired. Slice and serve while warm.

Sourdough bread

Ingredients for Sourdough Starter

- 2 teaspoons (10 g) sourdough starter
- 3 tablespoons (25 g) all-purpose flour
- 5 teaspoons (25 g) water
- Dough Ingredients
- ¼ cup (50 g) active sourdough starter (100% hydration)
- 1 ⅓ cups + 2 tablespoons (350 g) water
- 2 teaspoons (10 g) fine sea salt
- 4 cups + 2 tablespoons (500 g) bread flour

Directions

Feed your Sourdough Starter

1. 12 hours before you plan to mix the dough, add the ingredients to make ¼ cup (50 g) of active sourdough starter to a clean jar. Stir until combined, loosely cover the jar and let the starter rise at room temperature.
2. (The ingredients will create a total of 60 g active starter but some of it will stick to the sides of the jar during the transfer, so we are making a little more than needed.)
3. The sourdough starter is ready to use when it has doubled in size and there are plenty of bubbles on the surface and sides of the jar.

Make the bread

1. Transfer 50 g of the active starter and 350 g water into a large mixing bowl. Stir to distribute the starter evenly. Add 500 g bread flour and 10 g sea salt to the bowl and use a stiff spatula or your hands to work the ingredients together until it forms a shaggy mass and there are no dry bits of flour left in the bowl.
2. Cover the bowl and let the dough rest for one hour at room temperature.
3. Stretch and Fold: Wet your hand with a little water to prevent sticking. Pick up the dough on one side and stretch it up and over itself. Turn the bowl a quarter turn and repeat this step until you have turned the bowl a full circle. The dough should form into a tight ball.
4. Cover the bowl and let the dough rest for 30 minutes.
5. Repeat the stretch and fold process one more time to help build volume in the final loaf.
6. Bulk Fermentation: Cover the bowl and let the dough rise for 7-10 hours on your kitchen counter. The dough will have risen by about 50-75%, not doubled, when it is ready to shape.
7. (If the dough has doubled in size and/or is hard to shape, it may be over-proofed. Reduce the rising time on your next bake.)
8. Shape and Second Rise: Turn the dough out onto a lightly floured surface. Shape the dough into a ball by pulling 4 sides of the dough into the middle of itself. Turn the dough over so that it is seam-side down.
9. Use your hands to gently cup the dough, pulling and twisting towards yourself until it forms a

tight skin on the outside.

10. Center the dough onto a piece of parchment paper, seam-side down. Use the parchment paper like a sling to lift the dough up and transfer it into a medium-sized bowl.

11. Cover the bowl with a tea towel and let the dough rest at room temperature for 1-2 hours.

12. Use your thumb to make an indentation in the dough about a ½ inch deep. If the indentation quickly springs back all the way, or almost all the way, it's under-proofed and still needs more time to rise.

13. 30 minutes or so before the dough is ready to bake, preheat your oven to 450°F with the empty dutch oven inside.

14. Using long silicone gloves, carefully remove the hot dutch oven and take the lid off.

15. Score the top of the dough with a razor or a sharp knife. Once again, use the parchment paper as a sling to lift the dough up and transfer it into the dutch oven.

16. Place the lid on the dutch oven, return it to the oven and bake for 20 minutes. Remove the lid and bake for an additional 25-30 minutes or until the crust is golden brown. (The internal temperature of the bread should be around 205-210°F using a digital food thermometer.)

17. Cool: Transfer the baked bread to a cooling rack for 1-2 hours before slicing. The bread will continue to cook inside during this time. If you slice into it too soon, it will result in a gummy loaf.

18. Store: Keep the bread at room temperature, in a bread bag, wrapped in a kitchen towel or beeswax wrap. You can also store the bread, cut-side down, on a cutting board with a cake-stand top covering the bread. Do not refrigerate.

19. Freeze full loaves or individual slices wrapped tightly in plastic wrap and inserted into a freezer-safe container for up to 3 months.

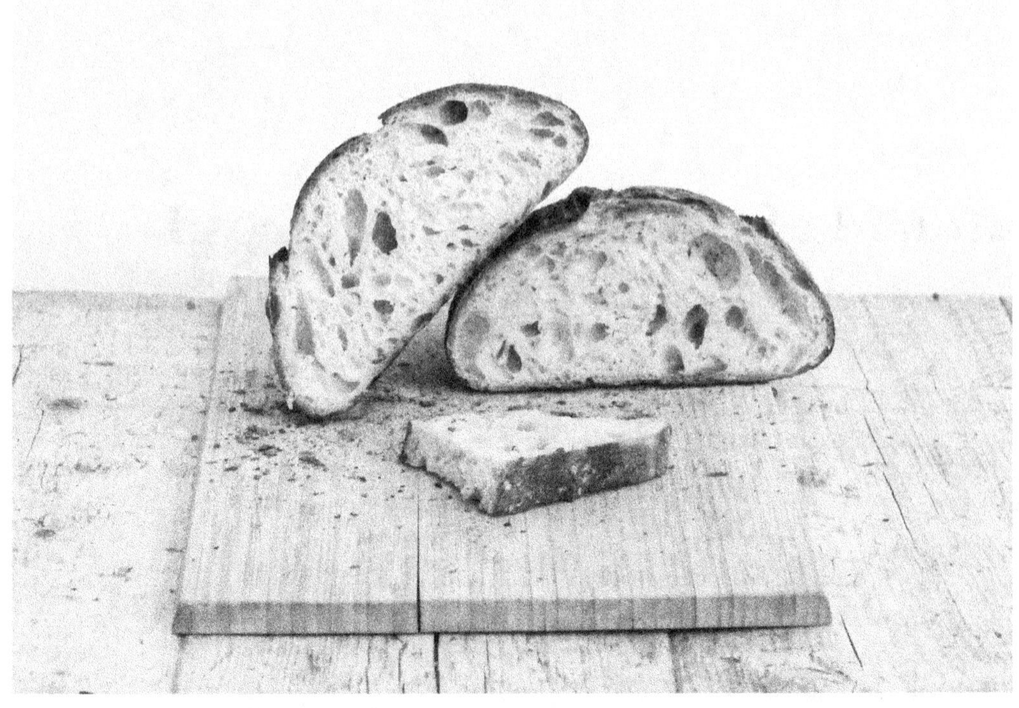

EASY Garlic Bread (with premade bread)

Ingredients

- 1 large loaf French or Italian bread
- 1/2 cup butter, softened
- 2 heaping teaspoons minced garlic (about 2 large cloves)
- 2 teaspoons Italian seasoning*
- 1/4 cup grated Parmesan cheese

Directions

1. Preheat the oven to 375 degrees.
2. In a small mixing bowl, thoroughly mix the butter, garlic, Italian seasoning, and Parmesan cheese.
3. Slice the French bread in half horizontally. Spread each cut side liberally with the garlic butter mixture. Lay each half cut side up on a large rimmed baking sheet.
4. Bake at 375 degrees for 10 minutes. Then broil on high 2-3 minutes, until the outside edges of the bread are toasty and the top is starting to brown. Let cool for a minute, then cut into 1-inch slices. Serve immediately.

Scratch Made Cheesy Garlic Bread

Ingredients

- For the bread dough
- Flour :260 g or 2 cups (loosely packed)
- Milk :160ml or ½ cup +2 ½ tbsp
- Salt :3/4 tsp
- Yeast :1 tsp
- Sugar :19 g or 1 ½ tbsp
- Oil :2 tbsp or 30 ml
- For the topping
- Mozzarella cheese:175g
- Minced Garlic:2 tsp
- Finely chopped Herbs:2 tsp

- Butter:2 tbsp or 30 g
- A pinch of salt

Directions

1. Prepare the bread dough Into a bowl,add all our ingredients together and mix them to form a shaggy mass of dough.
2. Add the milk,sugar,yeast,salt ,butter and flour and mix them together.
3. Transfer the dough onto a clean work surface and knead the dough until the dough become soft and elastic.
4. Only a well kneaded dough can produce soft and fluffy garlic bread .
5. It will be so much easier if you are using a stand mixer to prepare the dough.
6. In a stand mixer, just knead the dough for around 8 minutes using the dough hook attachment.
7. Once we get a soft and elastic dough, let the dough sit and rest for 10 minutes.
8. This will give some time for the dough to rest and this will make it easy for us to roll and shape the dough.
9. After 10 minutes, just roll and shape the dough into a rectangular sheet.
10. Place it on a parchment lined baking sheet.
11. Make square pattern on top of the dough using a sharp knife.Leave 1/8 inch space towards the edge.
12. Take care not to make many small squares..It may look pretty.But we need to add cheese slice in every crease and may end up adding double the amount of cheese and our bread may not turn out as a healthy bread.
13. Spread the top with garlic butter.
14. Insert pieces of mozzarella cheese to fill the creases.
15. Cover the baking tray with a plastic film.
16. Let the dough sit and rise for 30 minutes or until the dough really puff up.
17. Bake at 350° F for 32-35 minutes.
18. The baking time may vary according to the size of the baking tray.The deeper tray will take longer and shallow pan takes shorter time.
19. If the top turns golden brown early, cover the top with aluminum foil and bake properly for 32-35 minutes

Zucchini Bread

Ingredients

- 2 cups all-purpose flour
- 1 teaspoon baking soda
- 1 teaspoon salt
- 1 teaspoon ground cinnamon
- ½ cup sugar
- ½ cup vegetable oil
- 2 eggs
- 1 teaspoon vanilla extract
- 1 cup grated zucchini
- ½ cup chopped walnuts (optional)

Directions

1. Preheat the oven to 350°F. Grease and flour a 9x5 inch loaf pan.
2. In a large bowl, combine flour, baking soda, salt, and cinnamon.
3. In a separate bowl, cream together sugar and oil until light and fluffy. Beat in eggs one at a time, then stir in vanilla.
4. Gradually add dry ingredients to wet ingredients, mixing until just combined. Stir in zucchini and walnuts, if desired.
5. Pour batter into the prepared pan and bake for 50-60 minutes, or until a toothpick inserted into the center comes out clean. Cool in pan for 10 minutes before removing to a wire rack to cool completely.

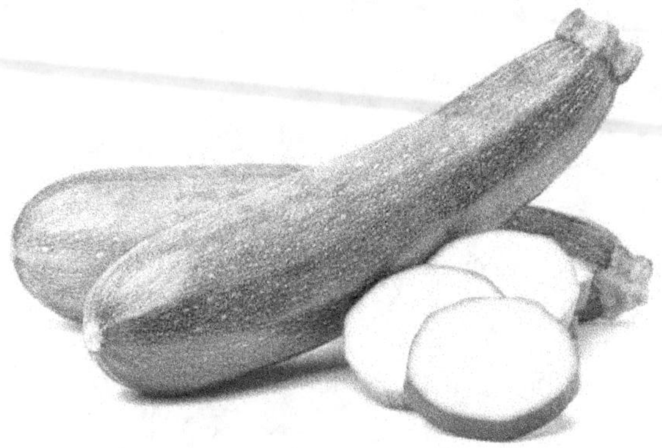

Pumpkin bread

Ingredients

- 2 cups all-purpose flour, spooned into measuring cup and leveled-off
- ½ teaspoon salt
- 1 teaspoon baking soda
- ½ teaspoon baking powder
- 1 teaspoon ground cloves
- 1 teaspoon ground cinnamon
- 1 teaspoon ground nutmeg
- 1½ sticks (¾ cup) unsalted butter, softened
- 2 cups sugar
- 2 large eggs
- 1 (15-oz) can 100% pure pumpkin (I use Libby's)

Directions

1. Preheat the oven to 325°F and set an oven rack in the middle position. Generously grease two 8 x 4-inch loaf pans with butter and dust with flour (alternatively, use a baking spray with flour in it, such as Pam with Flour or Baker's Joy).
2. In a medium bowl, combine the flour, salt, baking soda, baking powder, cloves, cinnamon, and nutmeg. Whisk until well combined; set aside.
3. In a large bowl of an electric mixer, beat the butter and sugar on medium speed until just blended. Add the eggs one at a time, beating well after each addition. Continue beating until very light and fluffy, a few minutes. Beat in the pumpkin. The mixture might look grainy and curdled at this point -- that's okay.
4. Add the flour mixture and mix on low speed until combined.
5. Turn the batter into the prepared pans, dividing evenly, and bake for 65 – 75 minutes, or until a cake tester inserted into the center comes out clean. Let the loaves cool in the pans for about 10 minutes, then turn out onto a wire rack to cool completely.
6. Fresh out of the oven,the loaves have a deliciously crisp crust. If they last beyond a day, you can toast individual slices to get the same fresh-baked effect.
7. Freezer-Friendly Instructions: The bread can be frozen for up to 3 months. After it is completely cooled, wrap it securely in aluminum foil, freezer wrap or place in a freezer bag. Thaw overnight in the refrigerator before serving.

Banana bread
Biscuits
Hamburger buns
Fresh rolls
Potato rolls
Cheddar biscuits
Pancake bread
Shortcut Bagels (2 ingredients)
Hashbrown Omelette
Blueberry Scones
Pumpkin scones

Soups, Chilis & Stews

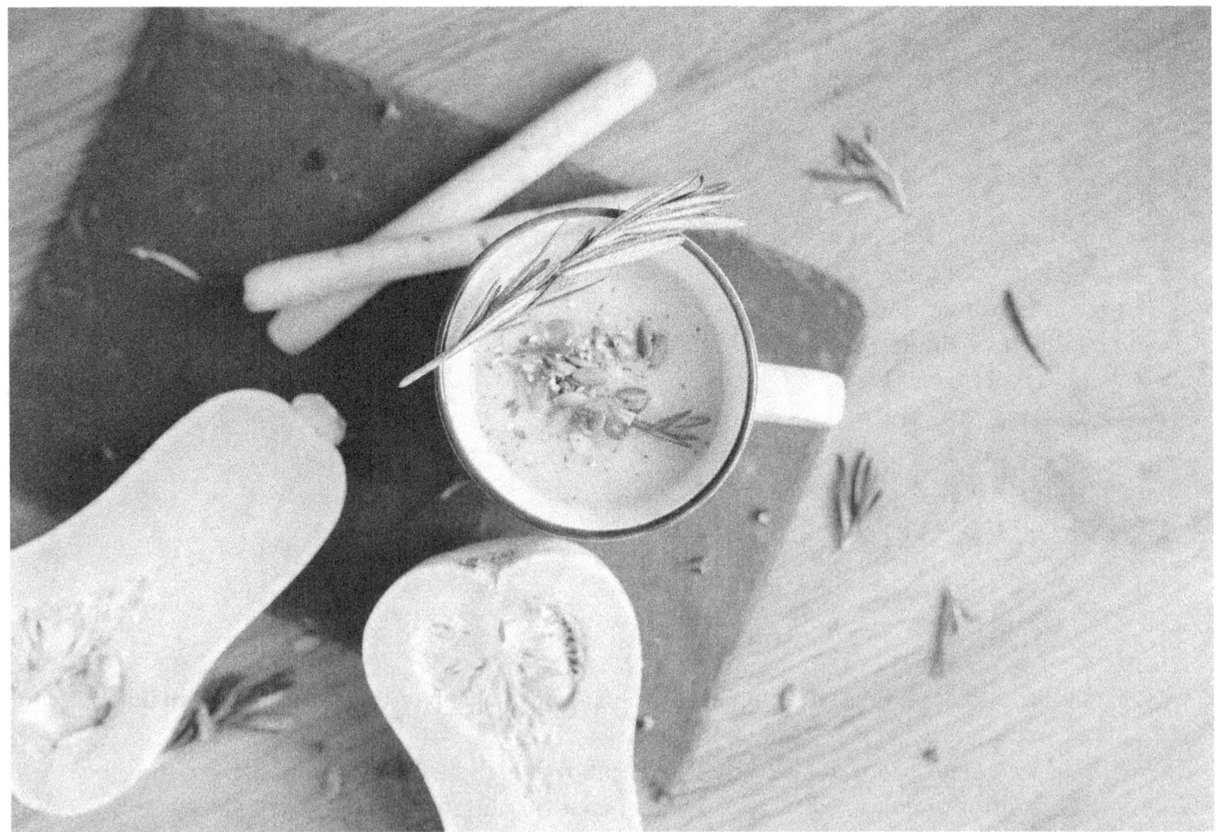

Oh, my fondness for soups... where do I begin? I don't really care for canned soups. I suppose I had too many of those growing up as a kid. That familiar old red label chicken noodle soup is fine when I'm sick, but if I have actually functioning taste buds, I want something with a robust and hearty flavor! Some of these are thick and hearty enough to be considered the entire meal, while others pair so beautifully with a grilled cheese and tomato sandwich, or as an appetizer before a meal of steak and potatoes. My personal favorite, Borscht, can be made either vegan or filled with ground lamb to change it from a side dish to the main course. The winter squash soup (pictured above) is a gorgeous companion to cornish game hen with stuffing.

Cream of Broccoli Soup

To change this one completely, add some low fat Cheddar cheese (to taste) and create a fabulous broccoli cheddar soup that will keep your family or guests guessing what 5 Star resort you purchased it from.

Ingredients

- 2 lbs raw broccoli, stems and florets chopped (tough ends removed)
- 1 medium yellow onion, chopped
- 1 medium clove of garlic, minced
- 4 cups fat free chicken or vegetable broth
- 1 cup evaporated milk
- ½ tsp hot pepper sauce
- ¼ tsp table salt
- ¼ tsp black pepper
- Fresh chives (optional)

Directions

1. Combine onion and garlic in a 2-quart saucepan with 1/4 cup of water. Simmer until onion is soft, about 10 minutes; spoon vegetables into a large pot.
2. Add broccoli and broth to pot; bring to a boil over high heat. Once soup boils, reduce heat and simmer until broccoli is soft but still green, about 8 minutes. Do not cover pot while broccoli is cooking or it will turn gray.
3. Remove soup from heat; puree until smooth in batches in a blender (be careful not to splatter hot liquid) or puree in a pot using an immersion blender. Add evaporated milk and hot pepper sauce to soup; season to taste with salt and pepper. Yields about 1 ¾ cups per serving.
4. Note: Fresh chives brighten the flavor of cream soups. Sprinkle 1 teaspoon of minced chives over each serving. Or, if available, garnish each bowl with 1 chive blossom.

Tomato basil soup

Ingredients

- 2½ pounds roma tomatoes, halved
- ¼ cup extra-virgin olive oil, divided
- 1 medium yellow onion, chopped
- ⅓ cup chopped carrots
- 4 garlic cloves, chopped
- 3 cups vegetable broth
- 1 tablespoon balsamic vinegar
- 1 teaspoon thyme leaves
- 1 loose-packed cup basil leaves, more for garnish
- Sea salt and freshly ground black pepper

Directions

1. Preheat the oven to 350°F and line a large baking sheet with parchment paper. Place the tomatoes cut-side up on the baking sheet, drizzle with 2 tablespoons of the olive oil, and sprinkle with salt and pepper. Roast for 1 hour or until the edges just start to shrivel and the insides are still juicy.
2. Heat the remaining 2 tablespoons of olive oil in a large pot over medium heat. Add the onions, carrots, garlic, and ½ teaspoon salt and cook until soft, about 8 minutes. Stir in the tomatoes, vegetable broth, vinegar, and thyme leaves and simmer for 20 minutes.
3. Let cool slightly and pour the soup into a blender, working in batches if necessary. Blend until smooth. Add the basil and pulse until combined.
4. Garnish the soup with basil leaves and serve with crusty bread.

Pizza Soup

Ingredients

- ½ cup chopped onions
- ½ red pepper, diced
- ½ green pepper, diced
- 2 garlic cloves
- 1 pound 99% fat free ground beef or turkey
- 1 ½ tsp italian seasoning
- Salt and pepper to taste
- ½ cup pepperoni, sliced in half
- 2 cups marinara sauce
- 14.5 oz can fire roasted tomatoes
- 2 to 3 cups beef or chicken broth
- Shredded parmesan cheese
- Fresh basil and croutons for garnish

Directions

1. Set a dutch oven or large pot over medium high heat and brown the ground beef with the onions, bell peppers, and garlic. If using a fattier beef, drain the grease off before continuing.
2. Add the italian seasoning, salt, and pepper.
3. Next, add the pepperoni, marinara sauce, fire roasted tomatoes, and 2 cups of the broth to the pot. Stir to combine. If the soup looks too thin add the remaining cup of broth.
4. Bring the pot to a boil and reduce to a simmer. Place the lid on the pod and simmer for 15 to 20 minutes until the broth has thickened.
5. Remove the soup from the heat and ladle into bowls, top with shredded cheese, fresh basil, and croutons.

You can also top this soup with diced tomatoes, diced red onion, crumbled bacon, sour cream, or tortilla strips. If the soup needs to be thicker, add a half teaspoon of corn flour.

Slow Cooker Tortellini Soup

Ingredients

- 1 lb ground italian sausage
- 24 oz jar of marinara or spaghetti sauce (or homemade sauce)
- 4 cups chicken broth
- 8 hz cream cheese
- 8 oz sliced fresh mushrooms
- 16 oz frozen cheese tortellini
- 2 oz fresh spinach leaves
- 1 lb cooked, shredded chicken breast

Directions

1. In a small saute pan, brown and crumble the sausage until it's cooked through. Place the cooked sausage into the slow cooker.
2. Add the sauce, chicken broth, cream cheese, and mushrooms to the slow cooker. Don't stir or soften the cream cheese - it will do its thing.
3. Cover and cook on low for 6 hours, or on high for 2 to 3 hours.
4. 20 minutes before serving, turn heat to high (if cooked on low). Stir in the shredded chicken breast, spinach, and tortellini. Cover and cook for the remaining time, or until tender and hot. Top with parmesan cheese when serving.

Loaded Baked Potato Soup

Ingredients

- 6 tablespoons unsalted butter
- ⅓ cup all purpose flour
- 4 cups whole milk (can sub for soy, oat, or almond milk)
- 4 cups peeled and cubed Russet potatoes (about 3 to 4)
- 3 green onions
- 1 cup diced or crumbled cooked bacon (plus more for garnish)
- 1 ½ cups shredded sharp cheddar cheese
- ⅓ cup sour cream
- ¼ tsp salt
- ¼ tsp fresh ground black pepper

Directions

1. Melt butter in a soup pot or dutch oven over medium high heat. Slowly add flour while whisking constantly. Continue whisking over heat for one minute. Gradually add milk while continuing to whisk constantly for 2 minutes.
2. Add potatoes and green onions and stir well to combine. Bring to a boil and reduce heat to maintain a simmer. Simmer uncovered for 25 minutes, until potatoes are tender, stirring frequently. Add the bacon, cheese, sour cream, salt, and pepper. Stir until combined and the cheese is melted.
3. Serve hot garnished with bacon, green onions, and cheese on top.

Cauliflower Leek Soup

Ingredients

- 3 tbsp. extra-virgin olive oil
- 2 leeks, cleaned and white and light green parts thinly sliced
- 5 cloves garlic, minced
- 1 russet potato, peeled and chopped
- 1 large head cauliflower, cut into florets
- Kosher salt
- Freshly ground black pepper
- 2 cups low-sodium chicken broth
- Shredded cheddar cheese, for garnish
- Chopped chives, for garnish
- Crumbled bacon, for garnish

Directions

1. In a large pot over medium heat, heat the olive oil. Add leeks and cook until tender, about 10 to 15 minutes. Add garlic and cook until fragrant, 1 minute more.
2. Add potato and cauliflower to pot and season with salt and pepper. Stir. Add broth, bring to a boil, then reduce heat and simmer, covered, until potatoes and cauliflower are tender, about 20 minutes.
3. Remove from heat. Using an immersion blender, blend mixture until smooth. You can also blend this in a blender, but that does require letting the soup cool completely first and reheating it to consume. It's definitely best when hot.
4. Season with salt and pepper to taste, then ladle into bowls and garnish with cheddar cheese, chives, and bacon before serving.

Borscht

I hated beets. I thought they were some of the most disgusting things on the face of the earth. But to my credit, I'd only ever had pickled beets on the side of a salad I really wasn't interested in eating in the first place. The first time I ever tried Borscht it was in a Russian restaurant on a first date down in San Diego, California. The date didn't pan out, but I'd been introduced to Russian food and the rest is history. I never found that original restaurant from the date again, but I did discover Kafe Sobaka Pomegranate and became a loyal customer until I moved away and Marco closed the doors. Now I'm forced to make my own Borscht because there just isn't enough of an Eastern European population in Denver to find the *good* stuff.

Ingredients

- 1 lb ground lamb
- 2 tablespoons olive oil
- 4 red beets peeled and ½ inch diced (approx 1 ½ pounds)
- 2 carrots ½ inch diced
- 1 large russet potato peeled and ½ inch diced
- ½ small green cabbage shaved
- 2 cloves garlic minced
- 4 cups vegetable broth
- 4 cups beef broth
- 2 tablespoons dill fresh, minced
- 2 tablespoons lemon juice fresh
- 1 teaspoon lemon zest
- 1 bay leaf
- salt and pepper to taste
- sour cream (optional) for serving

Directions

1. Add olive oil to a soup pot and set over medium-high heat. When the oil is hot add in the beets, carrots, potatoes, and cabbage. Stir to combine. Add in the ground lamb.
2. Cook for 10 minutes to slightly soften the vegetables and brown the lamb.
3. Add in the garlic and saute for 30 seconds or until fragrant.
4. Pour in the beef and the vegetable broth and add the bay leaf. Simmer for 30-45 minutes or until the beets and carrots are tender.
5. Discard the bay leaf. Stir in the fresh dill, lemon juice, and lemon zest. Taste and season with the desired amount of salt and black pepper.
6. Serve with a dollop of sour cream on top.

Side dishes

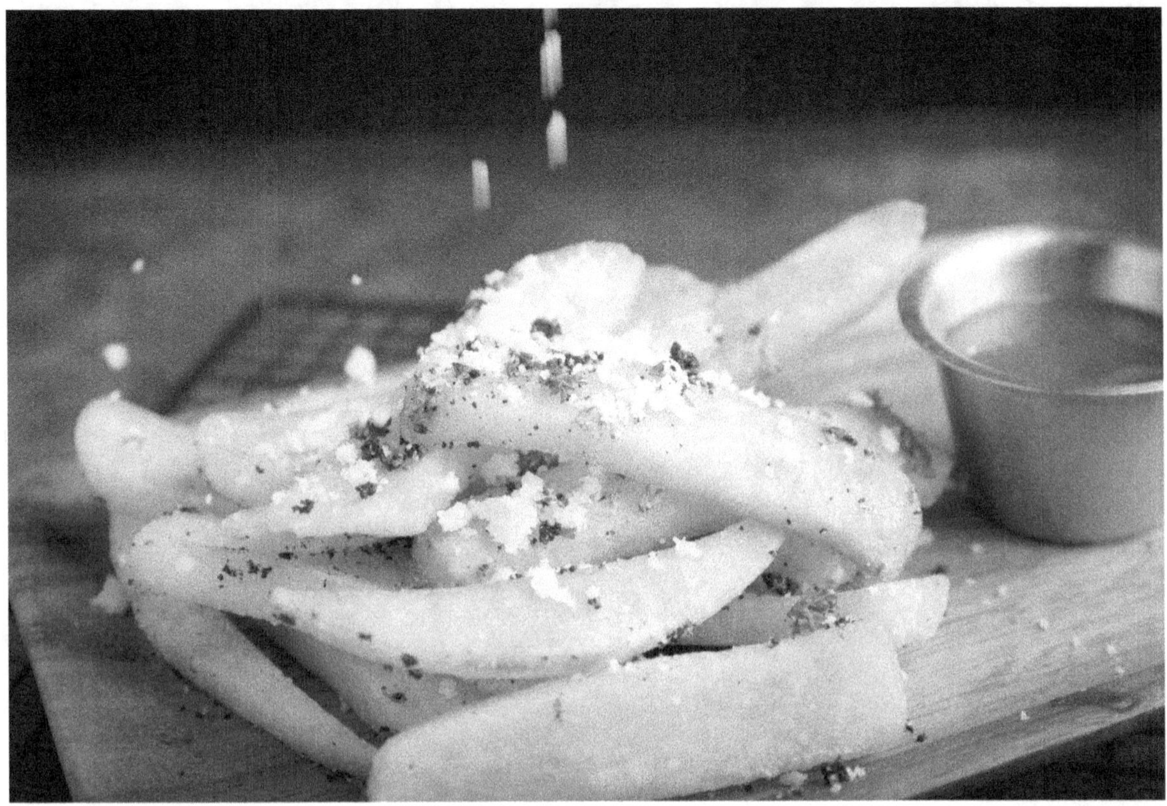

What's a main course without some beautiful little side dishes to go with it? Most of the time I try to have a pair of sides to go with some main dish, but occasionally the side dish takes center stage and everything else fades off into the background. Sometimes there's only one side dish answer to a beautiful main course. As an example, the bleu cheese burgers go so insanely well with the bleu cheese fries that it would be hard to pair anything else with them at all. The traditional burger and fries is an american staple, but the bleu cheese versions of these two bring forth a flavor combination that finally convinced my husband that bleu cheese really is an amazing food.

Ratatouille

Since the first time I saw that charming little rat in Paris cooking a mysterious dish for a food critic, I knew I wanted to try this magical dish called Ratatouille. I researched for the longest time trying to figure out what would be the most beautiful presentation while also providing the best flavor combination. This dish won my heart.

Ingredients

- 2 Tbsp olive oil, divided
- 2 cloves garlic, minced
- 1 cup finely diced white onion
- 1 15 oz can crushed tomatoes
- 2 medium zucchinis
- 2 medium yellow squash
- 1 medium eggplant
- 5 medium roma tomatoes
- 1 tsp Herbs de Provence (Or you can substitute ¼ tsp rosemary, ¼ tsp oregano, ¼ tsp thyme)
- 1 Tbsp fresh basil, chopped
- ½ tsp salt
- ¼ tsp crushed red pepper flakes
- ¼ tsp black pepper

Directions

1. Preheat oven to 350°F
2. Heat 1 tablespoon of the oil in a large saute pan over medium heat, then add onion. Cook until onion softens, about 5 minutes, then add garlic, saute for 30 seconds. Add the crushed tomatoes. Let gently simmer, uncovered, until tomatoes have the texture of a thick paste, about 10 minutes.
3. While tomatoes simmer, thinly slice the unpeeled zucchini, eggplant, and tomatoes into ⅛ inch thick slices (easiest with a mandolin slicer).
4. Remove tomato mixture from heat and stir in seasonings.
5. Spread tomato mixture into the bottom of a large casserole dish or tart pan. Working from the outer edge, layer veggies on top of the sauce in an alternating pattern (ex: eggplant – tomato – zucchini – repeat). You may not use all the veggies, depending on the size of your pan.
6. Brush veggies with remaining olive oil and bake for 1 hour, or until veggies are tender. If the top begins to brown too quickly, cover with aluminum foil.

Lebanese Tomato Rice

This dish pairs so perfectly when served with the Shish Tawook! The first time I made this I made entirely too much though. I found out the hard way that it freezes quite well in smaller containers and you can serve this with many savory dishes. But if you're pairing this with the Shish Tawook, make sure you throw in some Lebanese spicy lemon potatoes, too! (Hint: that's the next recipe in the book.)

Ingredients

- 1 cup long-grain brown rice
- 1 tablespoon olive oil
- ½ yellow onion finely chopped
- 2 garlic cloves minced
- 2 tbsp tomato paste
- ½ teaspoon cumin
- ¼ teaspoon cinnamon
- 1 Roma tomato seeded and finely chopped
- ½ teaspoon salt
- 1 ½ cups low-sodium vegetable broth
- ¼ cup fresh cilantro leaves for garnish (optional)

Directions

1. Place the rice in a mesh sieve and rinse with cold water while agitating the rice with your hands to release as much starch as possible, until the water runs clear. Set aside.
2. Heat oil in a large pot over medium heat. Add onions and cook, stirring occasionally, until softened, 2-3 minutes. Add garlic and cook until fragrant, one minute more. Stir in rinsed rice, tomato paste, cumin, cinnamon, chopped tomatoes, and salt, and cook until well combined, about 2 more minutes.
3. Add vegetable stock and bring mixture to a boil. Reduce heat; cover and simmer for 45 minutes, or until liquid is absorbed and rice is tender.
4. Remove from heat and allow the rice to steam covered for 5 more minutes. Uncover and fluff with a fork. Sprinkle with fresh cilantro and serve.

Lebanese Spicy Lemon Potatoes

Ingredients

- 24 small red or gold Yukon potatoes, halved
- 1 tablespoons extra virgin olive oil
- 1 teaspoon salt
- ½ teaspoon pepper

Spicy Lebanese Sauce

- 2 tablespoons extra virgin olive oil
- 3 cloves garlic (minced)
- 1 teaspoon cayenne
- ¼ cup cilantro (minced)
- 2 tablespoons lemon juice

Directions

1. Preheat the oven to 450° and line a baking sheet with foil.
2. Spread on a baking sheet in a single layer and toss with olive oil, salt and pepper. Roast until crispy, about 20 minutes.
3. About 5 minutes before the potatoes are done roasting, prepare the Spicy Lebanese Sauce.
4. Begin the sauce by heating olive oil in a small skillet over medium heat.
5. Add the garlic and heat until fragrant, about 30 seconds. Stir in the cayenne, cilantro and lemon juice and cook for another 30 seconds; remove from heat and pour sauce over the roasted potatoes. Serve warm.

Once again, watch out for the next recipe! If you're serving these potatoes with the Shish Tawook, the garlic sauce is a MUST HAVE to go with them!

Lebanese Garlic Sauce

One last thing... If you're making the Shish Tawook with tomato rice, spicy lemon potatoes, and this fabulous garlic sauce, send me a photo by email! Make me jealous! I'd love to see how yours turns out. Maybe you can inspire me to make it again. It's been a while.

Ingredients

- ½ cup garlic cloves, peeled
- ½ teaspoon kosher salt
- 1 ½ cups sunflower oil (*you may not need all of this and can substitute canola oil)
- 3 tbsp lemon juice (about ½ a lemon)
- ¼ tsp cayenne pepper

Directions

1. Place the garlic cloves and salt in a large food processor and puree until smooth. It's a good idea to scrape down the sides two or three times to ensure that all of the garlic is finely processed.
2. Turn the machine back on and add cayenne pepper. Slowly drizzle in the oil through the lid starting with ¼ cup. After the first ¼ cup has been added, pour in ½ teaspoon of the lemon juice.
3. Continue alternating between ¼ cup of the oil and ½ teaspoon of the lemon juice until you've added all of the oil and lemon juice. Alternating between the two is the key to proper emulsification which creates the light and fluffy garlic sauce. One tip is to let the machine run between oil additions to let the emulsion thicken. **NOTE: This process requires you to drizzle in the oil — not dump in the oil right away.** When you see it begin to thicken up THEN you start with the lemon juice. You know it's done when the sauce is white and thick with a similar consistency of mayonnaise. It usually takes about 10-15 minutes.

Slow Cooker Stovetop Stuffing

Ingredients

- stuffing (2x 6 oz packages Stove Top)
- 3 cups low sodium chicken broth
- 1 can cream of mushroom soup

Directions

1. Combine ingredients inside a crockpot and cook on high for 2-4 hours.
2. Fluff with fork and serve!

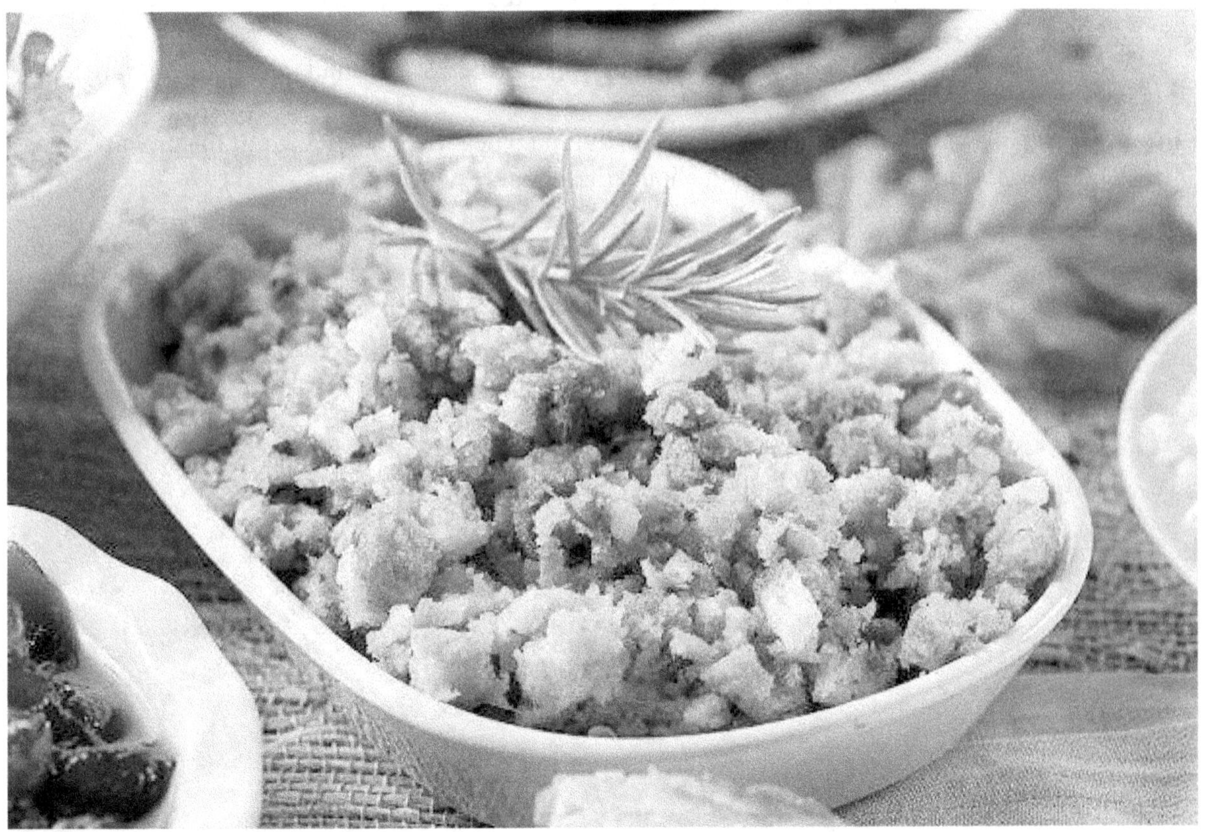

Cauliflower Spanish Rice

Ingredients

- 1 12 oz bag of riced cauliflower
- 1/2 tbsp olive oil or avocado oil
- 1/4 cup diced onion
- 2 cloves garlic minced
- 1/2 tsp cumin
- 1/4 tsp salt + more to taste
- 1 can diced tomatoes

Directions

1. Heat up a large skillet to medium heat. Add onion and saute for 3 minutes, then add garlic and saute another 1-2 minutes.
2. Add in riced cauliflower and saute for another 4-5 minutes. Stir around the veggie mixture to coat.
3. Now add in cumin, salt, and diced tomatoes. Bump up heat to medium high. If the mixture is slightly wet, continue to cook until the liquid dissolves.
4. Serve hot!

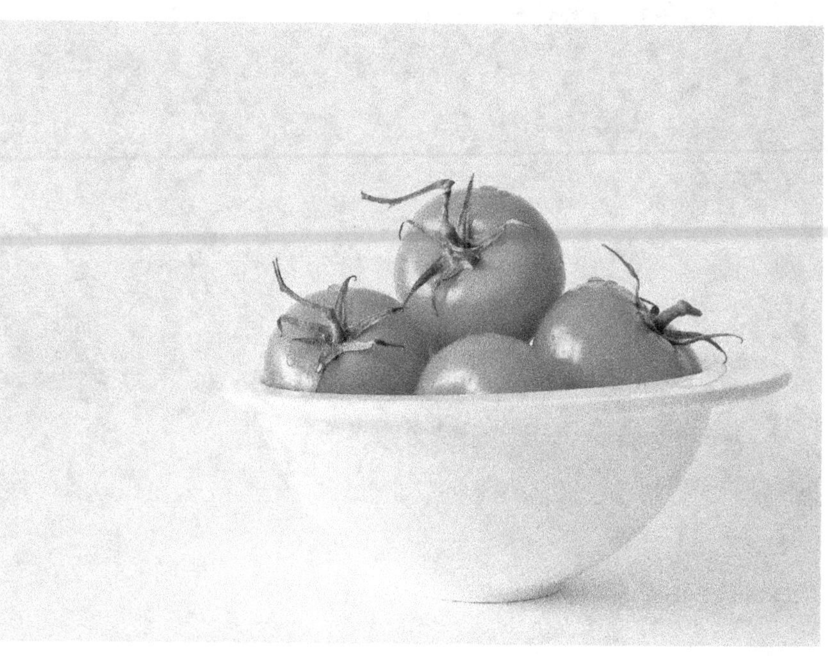

Rosemary Garlic Mashed Potatoes

These go so incredibly well with the Chicken Pierre! The flavors pair so nicely it's hard to imagine serving one without the other. If you saw the story about our cat sitter's love of the meal (shared with the Chicken Pierre recipe), this dish might have something to do with it.

These mashed potatoes can have many variations, too. If you're trying to avoid dairy, you can use 1 cup of milk alternative and exclude the sour cream. If you're not a fan of rosemary, you could try a combination of basil and thyme. To have some added flavor, you could stir in freshly cooked bacon pieces and ½ cup of delicious, shredded cheddar cheese.

Ingredients

- 4 lbs potatoes - russet or yukon gold
- ⅓ cup salted butter, melted
- 3 cloves garlic, minced
- 1 Tbsp dried rosemary
- ½ cup sour cream
- ½ cup milk, milk alternative, or cream
- Salt and pepper to taste

Directions

1. Peel and quarter potatoes. Place the potatoes in *cold* salted water. Add the garlic and turn the heat on under the potatoes to high.
2. Bring the potatoes in water to a boil, reduce heat to medium high and cook uncovered for 15 to 20 minutes until fork tender. Drain well.
3. Combine the rosemary and milk into a saucepan. Heat the milk on the stovetop until warm. Add butter to the potatoes and begin mashing. Pour in the milk and rosemary a little at a time while using a potato masher to reach the desired consistency. Season with salt and pepper, and serve hot.

Roasted Vegetable Medley

Here's another easily customisable recipe. If you don't like any of these vegetables, leave them out. If you can think of something that would be more suitable to the flavors of your household or whatever main dish you're servinging them with, add them in! In my household growing up we didn't eat much yellow squash because my father hated it. Taking it on faith that it was the most vile thing to ever grow from the ground, I didn't discover the beauty and flavor of yellow squash until some was given to me by a local grower when I was in my 30's. At that point I needed to figure out what to do with it and fast! Now it's one of my most favorite things to serve with any kind of roast bird or rabbit. The sweetness of the squash pairs beautifully with almost anything I throw at it.

Ingredients

- 1 Bell pepper
- ½ lb mushrooms
- 1 carrot
- 1 zucchini
- 1 yellow squash
- 1 onion or shallot
- 3 cloves garlic, minced
- ½ peeled butternut squash
- About 10 to 50 cherry tomatoes
- 2 Tbsp olive oil
- Fresh thyme, rosemary, and basil - minced
- Salt and freshly ground black pepper
- 1 Tbsp fresh lemon juice (optional)

Directions

1. Preheat the oven to 400° F. Line a *dark* baking sheet with foil.
2. Slice the long vegetables into strips about ¼ inch wide and 2 inches long. Leave the mushrooms whole. Halve the shallots and cherry tomatoes. Keep smaller mushrooms whole but cut any large ones in half.
3. Keep the tomatoes to the side but toss the remainder of the prepared vegetables in a bowl with the olive oil, sprinkle with the minced herbs, garlic, salt, and pepper.
4. Spread the vegetables evenly across the bottom of the roasting pan in a single layer if possible. Roast in the 400° oven for 20 minutes. Remove the pan from the oven. Add in the halved tomatoes, and return to the oven to roast for an additional 10 to 15 minutes.
5. Drizzle with lemon and serve warm!

Hawaiian Roast Veggies

Try to pair this with something else that has that traditional Hawaiian flavor to it. You could always go with a good Spam musubi, but I tend to stick with my coconut chicken. There's something great about pairing these two with the mango pineapple salsa while you're at it. The whole thing kicks off a beautiful flavor combination that just can't be beat.

Speaking of the flavors of Hawaii, have you ever heard of Waipio Valley? In 2003 I stayed in a treehouse there. An honest, real life tree house! It was equipped with an outdoor shower, a natural waterfall coming down the cliff, an ancient beheading stone I accidentally used as a bench (because I didn't know any better), and had quite the adventure. It's a hard place to get to, but if you get the chance I'd always suggest trying to visit. Just don't drive down that cliff... it's a hike, but the hike is much safer.

Ingredients

- 1 red onion
- 2 bell peppers
- 1 can pineapple chunks, juice reserved
- 1 cup carrots
- 1 cup green beans
- ½ broccoli florets
- ½ tsp fresh grated ginger
- 2 cloves garlic, minced
- 1 Tbsp soy sauce
- 1 Tbsp olive oil

Directions

1. Preheat the oven to 425° F. While the oven is preheating, cut the red onion into petals. Then cut up the bell peppers into chunks and slice the carrots on the diagonal.
2. In a bowl, combine 2 Tbsp of the reserved pineapple juice with the grated ginger, minced garlic, soy sauce, and olive oil. Whisk to combine and toss in the onion, bell pepper and carrots. Toss *only these* vegetables until they're all covered in the sauce.
3. Place the coated onion, bell pepper and carrots on a parchment lined baking sheet. Add on the *uncoated* green beans, broccoli florets and pineapple chunks.
4. Roast the vegetables in the preheated oven for about 25 minutes or until they start to get brown. Remove from the oven, allow to cool slightly, and serve hot.

Oven Roasted Asparagus

This is one of my favorite side dishes to pair with the broiled salmon and lentils. There's something so beautiful about crips, tender asparagus that pairs well with a flaky, soft fish. The added crunch of lightly salted asparagus can help to curb other cravings for salty things later in the day or evening, too! Did you know that's why so many people crave chips? In general we as humans are not getting enough fluid intake, and our brains associate crunchy things with salt intake, and our bodies are looking to retain whatever moisture we have. Try to drink more water, for sure! But also try eating more veggies that have high amounts of water in them. It makes a difference!

Ingredients

- 1 bunch of thin asparagus spears, trimmed
- 3 tbsp olive oil
- 1 ½ tbsp grated parmesan cheese
- 1 clove garlic, minced
- 1 tsp sea salt
- ½ tsp ground black pepper
- 1 tbsp lemon juice

Directions

1. Heat the oven to 425° F
2. Place the asparagus into a mixing bowl and drizzle with olive oil. Toss to coat the spears, then sprinkle with parmesan cheese, garlic, salt and pepper.
3. Arrange the spears onto a booking sheet in a single layer.
4. Bake in a preheated oven until just tender, about 12 to 15 minutes depending on the thickness. Sprinkle it with lemon juice just before serving.

Quick Sticky Rice

When you're looking for a quick and easy side dish to go with the lemon broccoli chicken or the dishes included with an island theme (coconut chicken, instant pot pineapple chicken, ect) this is going to be one of the easiest things you can throw at it. This is also absolutely *amazing* with the oven roasted salmon. Essentially just have fun with this one! You can also exclude a few tablespoons of water and substitute pineapple juice for a touch of sweetness. Another variation would be to add 2 tablespoons of sugar, and serve with sliced mango for a nice dessert that isn't overpoweringly sweet.

Ingredients

1 cup medium grain rice
1 cup water
½ tsp salt

Directions

1. In a colander, wash the rice several times until the water runs clear. Let the rice soak for a few minutes in the colander as it rests in a bowl.
2. Put rice in a pan with a tight fitting lid and add 1 cup of water. Cover and bring to a boil. Simmer over a low heat for 15 minutes.
3. Remove the pan from the heat and quickly stretch a clean tea towel over the pot. Cover this tightly with a lid and let this sit off heat for another 15 minutes. Serve warm!

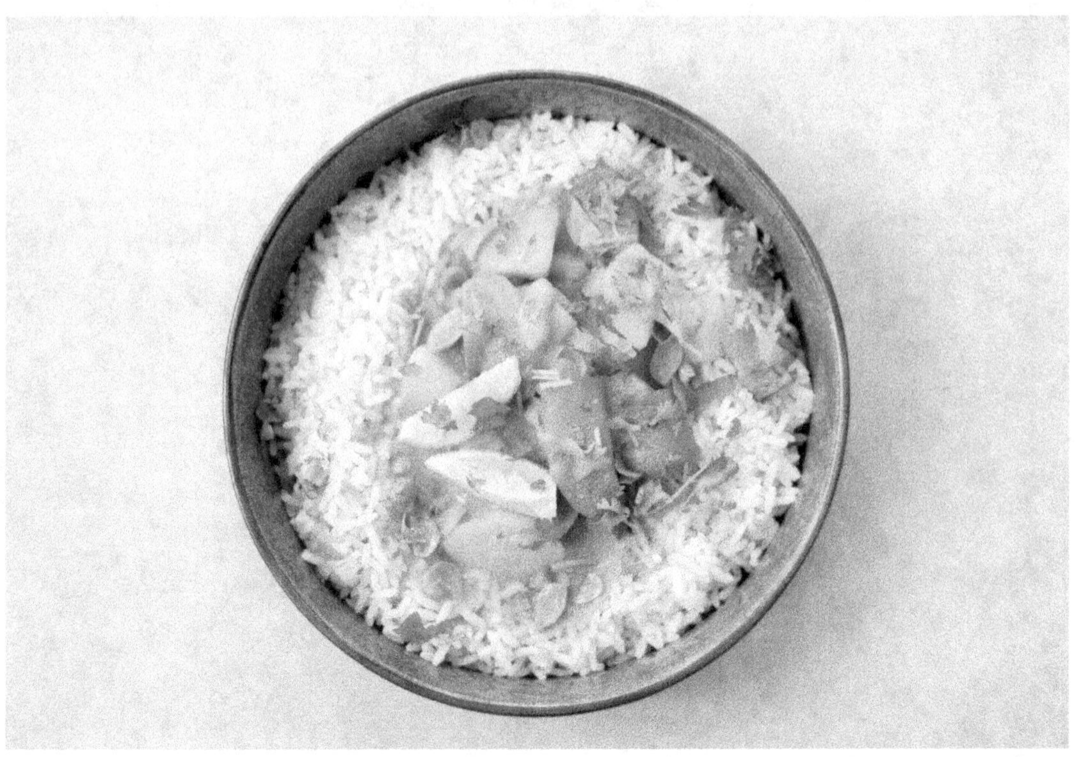

Roast Fingerling Potatoes

Ingredients

- 2 pints of fingerling potatoes
- 2 sprigs of fresh rosemary
- 2 to 3 sprigs fresh sage
- 3 sprigs of fresh thyme
- 6 cloves garlic, left unpeeled
- 1 cup Small mushrooms (optional)
- 3 Tbsp extra virgin olive oil, plus more for sheet pan
- Salt and pepper to taste

Directions

1. Preheat oven to 500°F and place a baking sheet inside to heat
2. Add potatoes, rosemary, sage, thyme, mushrooms, and garlic to a medium bowl. Drizzle with olive oil and season with salt and pepper.
3. Remove the sheet pan from the oven, lightly coat with the olive oil, and pour potatoes onto the pan. Place potatoes in the oven and reduce heat to 425° F. Roast for 20 minutes, or until the potatoes are crispy on the outside and tender on the inside.

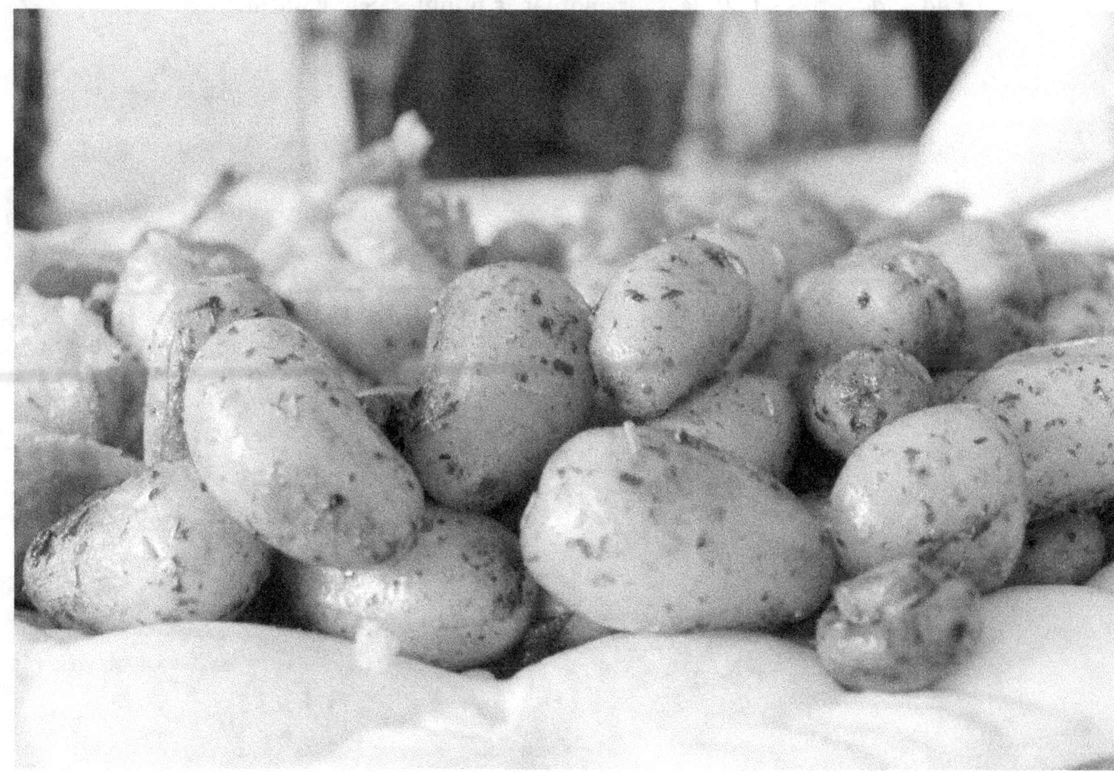

Fresh Spinach

This recipe is a GREAT base to so many other dishes. This goes incredibly well with the Mediterranean stuffed swordfish steaks, or you can create an amazing fresh spinach salad by adding some additional ingredients to the end. For the salad, don't wilt the spinach quite as much and try to only let it sit for 1 minute covered before serving.

Ingredients

- 2 tbsp olive oil
- 16 oz of fresh spinach
- 3 cloves garlic, minced
- ¼ whole lemon, freshly squeezed juice
- 2 tbsp lemon zest or peel
- Salt and fresh ground black pepper to taste

Directions

1. Heat the olive oil in the skillet on medium heat. Add the garlic when the oil is hot, and saute the garlic for about 1 minute to release the flavor, constantly stirring to keep the garlic from burning.
2. Add the spinach, a handful at a time. Add another handful as the spinach just begins to wilt. To get the best spinach results, you want to cook the spinach only enough to just wilt it. Cook, uncovered, on medium high heat for only one minute, constantly stirring, uncovered.
3. Remove from heat and cover. Let it sit for 2-3 minutes. Uncover and mix. Squeeze just a touch of the fresh lemon juice right out the lemon (using about ¼ of a small lemon), and stir to combine. *Do not use bottled lemon juice, it's too acidic!*
4. Taste the spinach and add a pinch of salt if needed, and the fresh cracked pepper. Top with lemon zest and serve!

For the gourmet warm spinach salad, add some candied walnuts, dried cranberries, diced apple pieces, and a vinaigrette, or see the separate spinach salad recipe included on the next page.

Warm Spinach Salad

Ingredients

- 8 slices bacon, cut into ½-inch pieces
- ¼ cup finely chopped shallots, from 1 to 2 shallots
- 2½ tablespoons cider vinegar
- 1½ tablespoons honey
- 1½ teaspoons Dijon mustard
- Heaping ¼ teaspoon salt
- Several grinds fresh black pepper
- 6 oz (about 8 cups) baby spinach
- 8 oz white button or baby bella mushrooms, thinly sliced (about 2 cups)
- 3 hard or soft boiled eggs, thinly sliced or cut into wedges

Directions

1. Place the bacon in a medium nonstick skillet and fry over medium heat, stirring occasionally, until crisp, 8 to 10 minutes.
2. While the bacon cooks, start the dressing: in a large bowl, whisk together the vinegar, honey, mustard, salt, and pepper. Set aside.
3. Using a slotted spoon, transfer the cooked bacon to a paper towel–lined plate.
4. Pour the bacon fat into a heatproof bowl, then return 4 tablespoons of the bacon fat to the skillet. (You can discard the remaining bacon fat or save it if you'd like it for cooking.) Add the shallots to the skillet and cook over low heat, stirring frequently, until softened, 1 to 2 minutes. Do not brown.
5. Add the bacon fat and shallots from the skillet to the vinegar mixture and whisk to combine. Add the spinach and mushrooms and toss to coat evenly. Taste and adjust the seasoning with salt and pepper, if necessary. Divide the salad between 4 plates or bowls; evenly divide the egg and cooked bacon among them. Serve immediately.

Baconated green beans

Ingredients

- 2 1/2 pounds green beans, trimmed
- Kosher salt
- 1/2 pound bacon, roughly chopped
- 1 small yellow onion, finely chopped
- 3 cloves garlic, minced
- 1 teaspoon red pepper flakes
- 1/2 cup chopped toasted pecans
- Juice of 1/2 lemon
- Freshly ground pepper

Directions

1. Toss the green beans into a large pot of boiling salted water and cook until bright green in color and crisp-tender, about 5 minutes.
2. Drain the beans and shock in a large bowl of ice water to stop the cooking. Drain the beans again and pat dry.
3. Cook the bacon in a large, heavy saute pan until crisp, about 5 minutes. Remove the bacon to a paper towel-lined plate to drain. Spoon off the excess bacon grease, leaving 2 tablespoons in the pan.
4. Add the onion to the pan and saute until soft and very tender, 4 to 5 minutes. Sprinkle in the garlic and red pepper flakes and saute until just fragrant, about 1 more minute.
5. Add the green beans back in and toss in the pecans. Cook until heated through, 5 to 6 minutes more.
6. Return the bacon to the pan, pour in the lemon juice and toss. Season with salt and pepper.

Prosciutto wrapped asparagus

Honestly this might be another of those amazing 'dinner party destroying' things. They can be served as an appetizer or as a side dish. When I do Chicken Pierre with the rosemary garlic mashed potatoes, this is often the vegetable I serve on the side. The crispness and saltiness of the prosciutto pairs incredibly beautifully with the vinegar of the chicken and buttery potatoes.

Ingredients

- Olive oil cooking spray
- 32 spears fresh asparagus, trimmed
- 16 slices prosciutto
- 8 oz cream cheese, softened to room temp

Directions

1. Preheat the oven to 450° F.
2. Line a baking sheet with aluminum foil and coat with a spray of olive oil.
3. Lay a single piece of prosciutto in the palm of your hand and spread with about 1/2 ounce of cream cheese. Place the ends of two to three asparagus spears on the end of the prosciutto and wrap the slice of prosciutto around the asparagus spears, starting at the bottom, and spiraling up to the tip.
4. Place the wrapped spears on the prepared baking sheet.
5. Bake in the preheated oven for 10 minutes. Remove, and roll the spears over. Return to the oven until asparagus is tender and prosciutto is crisp, another 5 minutes. Serve immediately.

Bleu Cheese Fries

Ingredients

- 1 (28 ounce) package frozen French fries
- 3 slices bacon, sliced into 1/4-inch pieces
- 1 tablespoon butter
- ¼ cup minced scallions or sweet onion
- 1 tablespoon minced garlic
- ½ cup blue cheese crumbles
- 2 tablespoons milk

Directions

1. Preheat the oven and cook the fries to the specification of the manufacturer.
2. Place bacon in a large skillet and cook over medium-high heat; cook and stir until evenly browned, about 10 minutes. Drain bacon slices on paper towels, reserving some of the bacon grease in the skillet. Slice into 1/4-inch strips.
3. Stir butter into the bacon grease and set skillet over medium heat; add scallions and garlic. Cook and stir until scallions are soft and browning, about 5 minutes. Add blue cheese; cook and stir with a spatula until cheese is melted, 2 to 3 minutes. Stir in half-and-half until the sauce is smooth, 2 to 3 minutes. Remove from heat and let sit for 2 minutes.
4. Arrange fries on a plate and drizzle sauce over fries. Sprinkle bacon strips on top.

Honey Lacework Cornbread

When I first went to Scotland (before the nightmare began) the family of the man who trafficked me had a surprising request. They'd all seen the movie "The Green Mile" and wanted to know more than anything what cornbread tastes like. They assumed it was a savory treat, so I knew the only way to really surprise them was to make this sweet version of the savory bread. I made a large patch of it, and within minutes the entire thing was gone. Since then I've shared my recipe dozens of times but this is the first time it's ever gone into a cookbook.

Ingredients

- 1 cup all-purpose flour
- 1 cup yellow cornmeal
- ¼ cup white sugar
- 1 tablespoon baking powder
- 1 cup heavy cream
- 2 large eggs, lightly beaten
- ¼ cup vegetable oil
- ¼ cup honey + 2 tbsp honey.

Directions

1. Preheat the oven to 400° F. Lightly grease a 9x9-inch baking pan.
2. Stir together flour, cornmeal, sugar, and baking powder in a large bowl; form a well in the center. Add cream, eggs, oil, and honey; stir until well combined. Pour batter into the prepared baking pan.
3. Drizzle the 2 tbsp honey over the batter in a zigzag pattern. Then, using a knife, create lines in the honey drizzle on the opposite zigzag pattern.
4. Bake in the preheated oven until a toothpick inserted into the center comes out clean, 20 to 25 minutes.

Jalapeno Cornbread

Ingredients

- 2 jalapeño peppers
- 1 c. fine cornmeal
- ½ c. all-purpose flour
- 1 tbsp. granulated sugar
- 1 tbsp. baking powder
- 1 tbsp. chili powder
- 1 ½ tsp. kosher salt
- ½ tsp. baking soda
- 1 c. buttermilk
- ½ c. milk
- 1 large egg
- ¼ c. vegetable shortening, melted
- 2 tbsp. salted butter

Directions

1. Preheat the oven to 425°F.
2. Stem, seed and dice one of the jalapeños. Stem the other jalapeño and slice into thin rounds.
3. Whisk the cornmeal, flour, sugar, baking powder, chili powder, salt, and baking soda in a large bowl. Whisk the buttermilk, whole milk, and egg in another large bowl. Add the buttermilk mixture to the cornmeal mixture and stir to combine. Add the melted shortening and stir to combine.
4. Melt the butter in a 9- or 10-inch cast-iron skillet over medium-high heat. Add the diced jalapeños and cook until just softened, about 2 minutes. Use a slotted spoon to transfer the jalapeños to the batter, leaving the drippings in the skillet; stir the batter to distribute the peppers. Pour the batter into the hot skillet (the batter should sizzle) and carefully spread to even out the top. Arrange the jalapeño slices on top of the batter.
5. Transfer the skillet to the oven and bake until the cornbread is golden brown and a toothpick inserted into the center comes out clean, 20 to 25 minutes. Let cool before slicing.

Baked potatoes

It might seem strange to include a basic recipe for how to bake a potato, but this is incredibly important. You'll see a million recipes that say to cook at high temps for an hour, but with this recipe, it takes longer but the skin is crispy and the inside is perfect.

Ingredients

- 4 baking potatoes
- 1 1/2 tbsp. olive oil
- Optional toppings: cheddar cheese, cooked bacon, sour cream, butter, chives, chili, etc.

Directions

1. Preheat the oven to 300°. Scrub the potatoes and dry them, then prick them across the top with a fork.
2. Rub the olive oil on the potatoes and then place the potatoes directly on the oven rack.
3. Bake until they are cooked thoroughly and soft in the center, about 2 hours.

Baked sweet potatoes

Ingredients

- 4 sweet potatoes
- 2 tablespoons olive oil
- Salt and pepper
- Toppings of your choice

Directions

1. Preheat the oven to 425°F. Thoroughly wash and dry sweet potatoes, then prick them across the top with a fork. Rub the skin with olive oil and sprinkle them with salt and pepper.
2. Bake the sweet potatoes directly on the oven rack for one hour. A fork or knife should be easily inserted into the center of the potato when it's finished baking.
3. Remove from the oven and allow the potatoes to cool for five minutes. Season with butter, brown sugar, pecans, marshmallows or any other topping of your choice.

Roast Broccolini

Ingredients

- 3 bunches broccolini
- 2 tbsp High quality olive oil
- ½ tsp garlic powder
- 1 tsp salt
- ½ tsp freshly ground black pepper

Directions

1. Preheat the oven to 375°F.
2. Trim 2 inches off the ends of the broccolini stems and cut any thick stalks in half lengthwise. Place the broccolini in a single layer on two sheet pans. (If you put them on one sheet pan, the broccolini will steam rather than roast.)
3. Drizzle each sheet pan with the olive oil, sprinkle with ½ tsp garlic powder, 1 teaspoon salt and 1/2 teaspoon pepper, and toss well. Roast for 15 minutes, until the broccolini is crisp-tender. Sprinkle lightly with salt and serve hot.

Perfect Corn on the Cob

Ingredients

- 4 quarts water
- 4 ears of corn, shucked
- 3 Tbsp sugar

Directions

1. Add the sugar to the water and bring the water to a boil. You should always have 1 quart of water per ear into your largest pot; the more room the better.
2. Once the water is at a full boil, add the shucked ears of corn.
3. After you add the corn, cover the pot and immediately turn off the heat. Let it sit undisturbed for 10 minutes.

4. The corn is ready at that point but don't feel rushed to serve it! You can wait up to an additional 10 minutes before serving without fear of it being overcooked.

Red beans and rice

Ingredients

- 2 Tbsp. vegetable oil
- 1 large onion, coarsely chopped
- 1 medium green bell pepper, coarsely chopped
- 2 stalks celery, coarsely chopped
- 1lb. dried kidney beans, soaked overnight, drained
- 3 garlic cloves, finely chopped
- 2fresh bay leaves
- 8cups (or more) low-sodium chicken broth or 4 cups low-sodium chicken broth plus 4 cups water
- ¼cup finely chopped parsley, plus more for serving
- 1 Tbsp. Cajun seasoning
- 3½tsp. Diamond Crystal or 2¼ tsp. Morton kosher salt, divided, plus more
- 1 tsp. ground sage
- 2 tsp. freshly ground pepper
- 6oz. andouille sausage, cut into ½" pieces
- 2 cups long-grain rice

Directions

1. Heat 2 Tbsp. vegetable oil in a Dutch oven or other heavy, large pot over medium. Cook 1 large onion, coarsely chopped, 1 medium green bell pepper, coarsely chopped, and 2 stalks celery, coarsely chopped, stirring occasionally, until onion is translucent, about 5 minutes. Add 1 lb. dried kidney beans, soaked overnight, drained, 3 garlic cloves, finely chopped, and 2 fresh bay leaves. Cook, stirring often, 2 minutes.
2. Pour in 8 cups low-sodium chicken broth or 4 cups low-sodium chicken broth plus 4 cups water and bring to a boil. Stir in ¼ cup finely chopped parsley, 1 Tbsp. Cajun seasoning, 1½ tsp. Diamond Crystal or 1 tsp. Morton kosher salt, 1 tsp. ground sage, and 2 tsp. freshly ground pepper. Reduce heat to medium-low and simmer, adding more broth or water (up to ½ cup) as needed to keep beans submerged, until beans are tender but still intact, 1½–2 hours. Add 6 oz. andouille sausage, cut into ½" pieces, and simmer for 30 minutes. Taste and add more salt if needed; remove and discard bay leaves.
3. Bring 4 cups of water to a boil in a medium saucepan. Add 2 cups of long-grain rice and remaining 2 tsp. Diamond Crystal or 1¼ tsp. Morton kosher salt and return to a boil. Reduce heat to low, cover, and cook rice until grains are tender and liquid is absorbed, 30–35 minutes.
4. Divide rice among bowls and ladle beans over. Top with parsley.

Best of All Brussels

When I met my husband he wasn't a big brussel sprouts fan but I loved them. I'd never had them until I was in my 20's but once I discovered them I was a fan instantly. Having avoided them for my entire childhood and never having straight boiled brussel sprouts probably helped with that in a big way. Now he enjoys them whenever I make them. He's even requested me them a few times!

Ingredients

- 1 ½ pounds Brussels sprouts trimmed and halved
- 1 tablespoon, plus 1 teaspoon extra-virgin olive oil
- ½ teaspoon kosher salt
- ¼ teaspoon black pepper
- ¼ tsp garlic powder
- Balsamic Reduction (optional) for drizzling

Instructions

1. Place a rack in the upper third of your oven and preheat the oven to 350°F.
2. Toss the Brussels sprouts in a large bowl. Drizzle with the olive oil and sprinkle with salt, pepper, and any other desired spice additions. Gently mix until the Brussels sprouts are evenly coated.
3. Spread the brussel sprouts into a single layer on a sprayed baking sheet. For even better crisping, flip the Brussels sprouts so that they are all cut sides *down.*
4. Bake for 45 minutes until the Brussels sprouts are lightly charred and crisp on the outside and tender in the center. The outer leaves will be very dark too.
5. Season with additional salt and/or pepper to taste. Drizzle with the balsamic reduction and enjoy.

Snacks & Appetizers

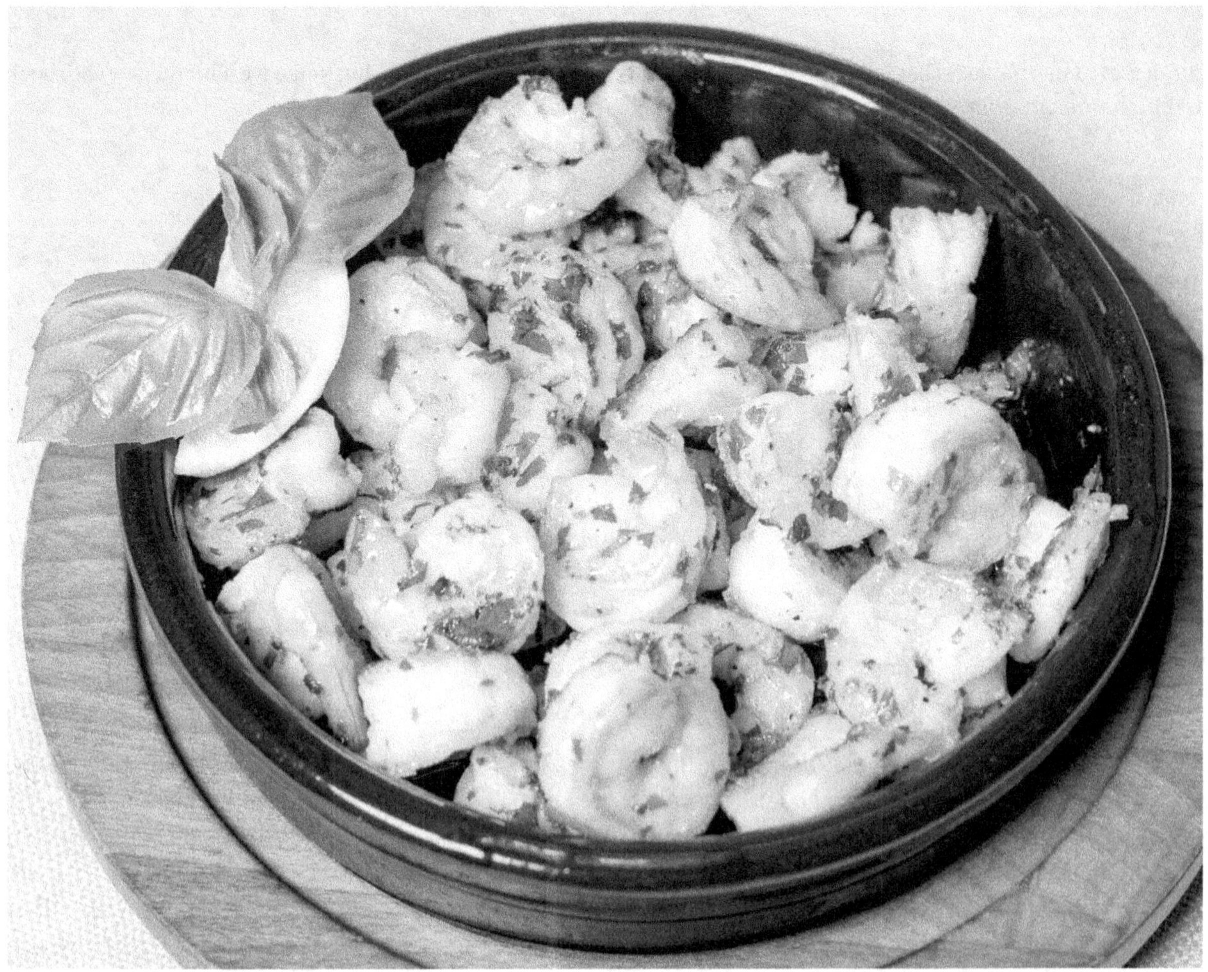

I used to have a boss who asked his dog all the time if she wanted "schnacks" when he was offering her a treat. To this day, I can't pronounce the word any other way unless I concentrate on it. But these aren't the kind of snacks you'd want to give to your dog. Maybe those neighbors you actually like, or your treasured family that comes to visit at the holidays, but definitely *not* the dog. Just watch out - that mutt might just try to steal the amazing shrimp or bacon cheeseburger sliders right off the table.

Potato Skins

The secret to these skins is baking them multiple times! It's a bit time consuming, but you have a brand new cookbook to thumb through while you're waiting for things to catch up to you!

Ingredients

- 6 medium (3 lbs) Russet potatoes
- Extra Virgin Olive Oil
- Kosher Salt
- Freshly Ground Pepper
- 6 slices bacon
- 4 oz grated cheddar cheese
- ½ cup sour cream
- 2 green onions, thinly sliced

Directions

1. Scrub the potatoes clean, then bake the potatoes in the oven at 350° F for about 2 hours until the potatoes are cooked through and give when pressed.
2. Cook the bacon! Do this while the potatoes are baking. One of the secrets to bacon is to cook it at medium heat in a skillet, but to add the bacon before the skillet heats up. It doesn't pop oil quite as bad, and your bacon has a tendency to curl less! Drain the cooked bacon on paper towels, allow it to cool, and then crumble it (or cut it, if you have super thick, chewy bacon) into small-ish pieces.
3. Remove the potatoes from the oven and let them cool enough to handle them easily. Cut in half horizontally (long ways). Use a spoon to carefully scoop out the potato from the inside, leaving about ¼ inch of potato on the skin. Save the potato for another use later on, like the Rosemary mashed potatoes I love to serve with Chicken Pierre!
4. Increase the heat of the oven to 450°. Brush or rub olive oil all over the skins, outside and in. Sprinkle each with salt. Place the skins on a baking rack in a roasting pan or broiler pan (not a cookie sheet because the high temp will warp a cookie sheet). Cook for 10 minutes on one side, then flip the skins over and cook for another 10 minutes. Remove from the oven and let them cool enough to handle.
5. Add the cheese and bacon, and bake AGAIN. Arrange the skins skin-side down on the roasting pan or rack. Sprinkle the insides with freshly ground black pepper, cheddar cheese, and bacon. Return to the oven and BROIL for an additional 2 minutes, or until the cheese is bubbly. Remove from the oven.

6. Place the skins on a serving plate (using tongs to avoid burning off your fingerprints, unless you're going for that look). Add a dollop of sour cream, sprinkle with green onions, and serve immediately.

Spaghetti Squash Pizza Bites

Ingredients

- 1 medium spaghetti squash, halved
- 1 tbsp. olive oil
- kosher salt
- Freshly ground black pepper
- 1/3 c. grated Parmesan
- 1 tsp. garlic powder
- nonstick cooking spray
- 2 c. pizza sauce
- 1 1/2 c. shredded mozzarella
- 1/2 c. mini pepperoni
- 1 tbsp. parsley, chopped

Directions

1. Preheat the oven to 400° and line a medium baking sheet with parchment paper.
2. Drizzle cut side of spaghetti squash with olive oil and season with salt and pepper. Place cut side down on a baking sheet and bake until tender, 45 minutes to an hour, depending on the size of your squash. Reduce heat to 375°F when finished baking.
3. Let cool for 10 minutes before using a fork to shred the squash into spaghetti pieces. Place into a bowl and combine with parmesan and garlic powder. Season with salt and pepper.
4. Transfer 1/4 c squash to a greased muffin pan, pressing down on bottoms and side to create cups. Place in the oven to bake, 15 minutes.
5. Spoon pizza sauce into each cup, top with mozzarella and mini pepperonis. Bake again, 8-10 more minutes, or until the cheese is melted. Top with parsley and serve.

Party Shrimp

Serve these beauties for guests who come over and they'll start requesting them in the future. They're so easy to do, I'm sure you won't even mind!

Ingredients

1 tablespoon olive oil
1-1/2 teaspoons brown sugar
1-1/2 teaspoons lemon juice
1 garlic clove, thinly sliced
1/2 teaspoon paprika
1/2 teaspoon Italian seasoning
1/2 teaspoon dried basil
1/4 teaspoon pepper
1 pound uncooked shrimp (26-30 per pound), peeled and deveined

Directions

1. In a bowl or shallow dish, combine the first 8 ingredients. Add shrimp; toss to coat. Refrigerate for 2 hours.
2. Drain shrimp, discarding marinade. Place shrimp on an ungreased baking sheet. Broil 4 in. from heat until shrimp turn pink, 3-4 minutes on each side. Serve hot!

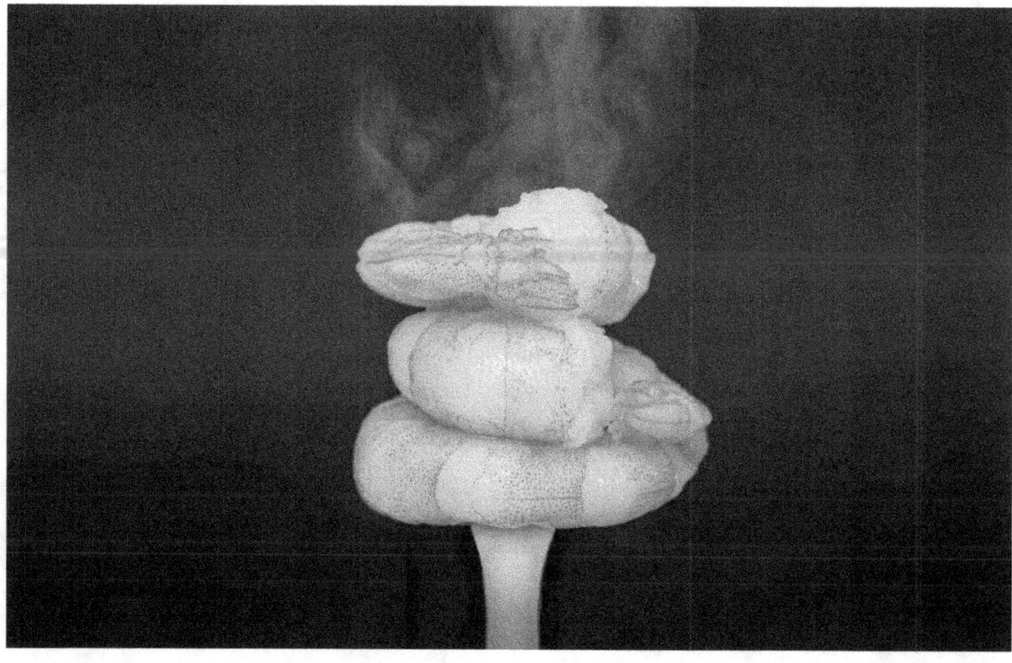

Cheeseburger Sliders

Ingredients

- 2 packages (17 ounces each) Hawaiian sweet rolls
- 22 slices American or cheddar cheese, divided
- 2 pounds ground beef
- 1 cup chopped onion
- 1 can (14-1/2 ounces) diced tomatoes with garlic and onion, drained
- 1 tablespoon Dijon mustard
- 1 tablespoon Worcestershire sauce
- 3/4 teaspoon salt
- 3/4 teaspoon pepper
- 24 bacon strips, cooked and broken into 1-inch pieces

GLAZE:
- 1 cup butter, cubed
- 1/4 cup packed brown sugar
- 4 teaspoons Worcestershire sauce
- 2 tablespoons Dijon mustard
- 2 tablespoons sesame seeds

Directions

1. Preheat the oven to 350°. Without separating rolls, cut each package of rolls horizontally in half; arrange bottom halves in 2 greased 13x9-in. baking pans. In each pan, place 5 slices of cheese on bottom halves of rolls. Bake until the cheese is melted, 3-5 minutes.
2. In a large skillet, cook beef and onion over medium heat until beef is no longer pink and onion is tender, breaking beef into crumbles, 6-8 minutes; drain. Stir in tomatoes, mustard, Worcestershire sauce, salt and pepper. Cook and stir until combined, 1-2 minutes.
3. Spoon beef mixture evenly over rolls; top with bacon and remaining cheese. Replace tops. For glaze, in a microwave-safe bowl, combine butter, brown sugar, Worcestershire sauce and mustard. Microwave, covered, on high until butter is melted, stirring occasionally. Pour over rolls; sprinkle with sesame seeds. Bake, uncovered, until golden brown and heated through, 20-25 minutes.

Caprese Skewers with Balsamic Drizzle

Ingredients

- 2 cups balsamic vinegar
- 10 oz cherry tomatoes
- 8 oz small round mozzarella cheese (known as Ciliegine or Cherry size mozzarella)
- 8 oz fresh basil leaves
- Salt and pepper
- Toothpicks

Directions

1. For the balsamic drizzle: add the balsamic vinegar to a small saucepan over high heat, then bring to a boil. Turn the heat down to medium then simmer until vinegar is the consistency of thin syrup. This takes about 20 minutes. You'll know it's done when you can see the bottom of the pan for a second or two after scraping a spatula across. Pour the balsamic reduction into a small bowl and set aside to cool. (You could also use a store bought balsamic reduction if you're short on time.)
2. Thread a cheese ball onto a toothpick, followed by a basil leaf folded in half or quartered if large. Finish this with a cherry tomato then place onto a serving platter. Repeat with remaining ingredients. Just before serving, sprinkle the skewers with salt and pepper, then drizzle with your homemade and cooled balsamic reduction. Serve these right away!

Baked Mushrooms

I once ruined a dinner party with these beauties. The long and short of it is that a young couple invited my then boyfriend and myself to their home one night for dinner. They didn't tell anyone until we'd arrived that they had decided to become vegetarian, and we certainly were not. If memory serves, we stopped at a fast food joint on the way home for burgers afterward. About a week later, we invited the two of them over for dinner at our place to reciprocate. When they walked in I'd arranged these mushrooms as an appetizer beside the baked brie (see below) with apple and pear slices, then served the apple walnut salad with raspberry vinaigrette, followed by a choice of traditional or vegetarian hand rolled lasagne (because I wanted to be a good host and have options). Much to my surprise, they chose the traditional! Just when they thought it was over I'd prepared some poached pears in an orange muscat wine with cobbler cake and vanilla bean ice cream. I guess they felt that my menu that evening made it too difficult for them to remain vegetarian, and we never saw them again. I can assure you, that was never my intention.

Ingredients

- Cooking spray for the pan
- 1 ½ lbs baby mushrooms
- 2 Tbsp butter
- 2 cloves garlic, minced
- ¼ cup breadcrumbs
- Kosher salt
- Freshly ground black pepper
- ¼ cup freshly grated parmesan cheese, plus more for garnish
- 4 oz cream cheese, softened to room temperature
- 2 Tbsp freshly chopped parsley
- 2 Tbsp freshly chopped thyme

Directions

1. Preheat oven to 400° F
2. Grease a baking sheet with cooking spray. For easier cleanup, line with foil and spray the foil.
3. Remove stems from mushrooms and roughly chop the stems. Place the unchopped mushroom caps on the baking sheet, cup side up.
4. In a medium skillet over medium heat, melt butter. Add the chopped mushroom stems and cook until most of the moisture is out, about 5 minutes. Add garlic and cook until fragrant, about 1 minute. Add breadcrumbs and let toast slightly, about 3 minutes. Remove from heat and let cool slightly.
5. In a large bowl mix together mushroom stem mixture, parmesan, cream cheese, parsley, and thyme. Season with salt and pepper. With a small spoon, spoon the mixture into the mushroom caps and sprinkle with a bit more parmesan. Bake at 400° F until mushrooms are soft and the tops are golden, about 20 minutes.

Baked Brie

You can wrap the wheel of brie in pastry and keep it refrigerated for up to a day before baking and serving. The prep for this appetizer is so minimal that this "make-ahead" tip might sound silly, but when I'm planning a whole party, it's always nice to be able to check small steps off my list and know that all I have to do before the party is put the brie to the oven to bake.

Ingredients

- 1 sheet puff pastry, thawed but still cold
- All-purpose flour, for rolling
- 1 (8 to 12-ounce) round brie cheese (5- to 7-inches in diameter)
- 1 large egg, beaten
- Jalapeno Jelly
- Crushed walnuts
- Cooked bacon

Directions

1. Heat the oven to 400°F. Line a baking sheet with parchment and set aside, or bake your brie in a pie plate.
2. Dust a work surface with a small amount of flour. Unwrap the puff pastry and place it on the flour. Coat a rolling pin with a little flour and roll out the puff pastry into a rough 11-inch square. No need to get out a ruler; it's fine to estimate.
3. Place the jalapeno jelly and then the walnuts in the center of the pastry, roughly the same shape as the brie. Place the round of brie in the middle of the pastry and place the bacon on top of it. Fold the corners over the brie, forming a neat package. Use your hand to gently press the edges against the brie and neaten up the sides. Turn the brie over, leaving the jalapeno jelly and walnuts to top the brie, and the bacon to rest on the bottom seam beneath the brie.
4. Place the wrapped brie to the baking sheet or pie plate. If the pastry has warmed and is no longer cool to the touch at this point, place it back into the fridge for 10 minutes, or until you're ready to bake and serve.
5. Brush the pastry all over with the beaten egg. Be sure to get the sides and around all of the folds. Try not to let the egg puddle under the brie.
6. Bake until the pastry is deep golden-brown, 35 to 40 minutes.
7. Set aside to cool for 5 to 10 minutes. This gives the hot cheese time to firm up a little. Cut into the brie early and most of it will gush right out — which is still delicious, but much less visually appealing.
8. Use the parchment paper to transfer the brie to a serving plate. If you baked it in a pie plate, serve straight from the plate, but double check that the plate has cooled enough to handle.
9. Arrange thin apple and pear slices around the brie with a plate of crackers or sliced warm baguette next to it and serve warm.

Mango Pineapple Salsa

As mentioned with the Hawaiian Roast Veggies, try to pair this with the coconut chicken or another tropical influenced dish. The combo will blow your mind and make you wonder why you'd never cooked like this before.

Ingredients

- 1 cup chopped peeled mango
- 1 cup pineapple chunks
- 1 tsp grated ginger
- Fresh mint
- ½ cup diced sweet red pepper
- 1 Roma tomato, seeded and chopped
- 3 Tbsp minced fresh cilantro (optional)
- 2 green onions, sliced
- 2 Tbsp lime juice
- 1 Tbsp lemon juice
- Salt to taste
- Dash of cumin
- 1 Jalapeno, finely chopped.

Directions

1. Finely dice all of the ingredients to approximately the same size.
2. Stir it together and serve!

It really is that simple. This is great with that coconut chicken, but it's also amazing with something super simple like a bag of tortilla chips on a hot day.

Not Your Mama's Deviled Eggs

These are always a hit when I bring them around. Whenever I post them on social media I'm flooded with questions about why they're referred to as "Adult deviled eggs" or "Not your Mama's Deviled Eggs" but they have enough complex flavors in these little beauties that they kind of speak for themselves.

Ingredients

- 12 large eggs
- 1/4 cup mayonnaise
- 1/4 cup mustard
- 1/2 teaspoon Parsley Flakes
- 2 strips cooked bacon, crumbled
- Pickled jalapenos, dried slightly on a paper towel.
- 1/4 teaspoon Seasoned Salt
- Smoked Paprika

Directions

1. Place the eggs in a single layer in a large saucepan and add enough cold water to cover by 1 inch. Cover and quickly bring eggs to a boil over high heat. Immediately remove the pan from heat and let it stand for 15 minutes for large eggs (18 minutes for extra-large eggs and 12 minutes for medium eggs). The residual heat in the water cooks the eggs. Cool with an ice bath and peel.
2. Slice the eggs carefully in half lengthwise. Remove yolks and place the yolks in a bowl.
3. Mash the yolks with a fork or potato masher.
4. Stir in mayonnaise, mustard, parsley and seasoned salt until smooth and creamy. Fold in the bacon crumbles.
5. Spoon or pipe the delicious yolk mixture into the egg white halves. Sprinkle with paprika and top with a single pickled jalapeno,
6. Refrigerate 1 hour or until ready to serve.

TIPS TO BOIL EGGS

- You can remove your eggs from the fridge at least 30 minutes before you plan to cook them. This will help them cook evenly and prevent the shell from cracking.
- Older eggs are best for hard-boiling. Eggs that are close to their best-by date will peel much easier than fresh eggs.
- Avoid a green ring around your yolks by diligently timing how long the eggs cook.
- Don't skip the ice bath. Not only does the ice bath prevent your eggs from overcooking, but it also helps loosen the shell and make them easier to peel!

Desserts

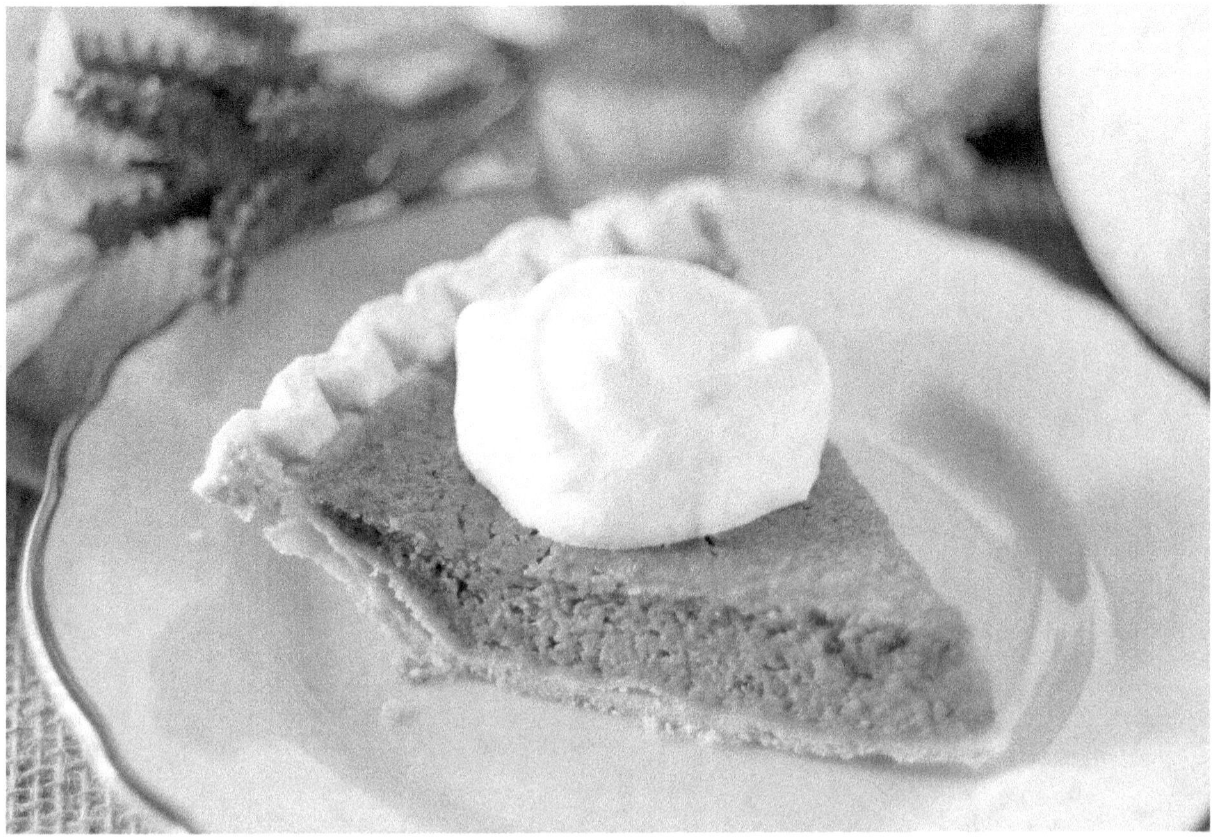

If you don't have a sweet tooth, we can't be friends. I'm only half way kidding. The first time I ever sat down with the woman who is now my best friend it was over a slice of pie and a meeting of the minds, trying to put together a charity event in 2018. It was a weeknight, I needed to work in the morning, and yet we stayed there for seven hours. I was exhausted in the morning, but it was the best pie I'd ever had. It became a ritual of ours for a while, going out for pie. I miss those days. Maybe that's why I included my version of the exact pie I had that night in this recipe book. So many comfort foods we have are built on the memories we associate with them. Pie will always remind me of Collette for the rest of my life.

Stay Soft Chocolate Chip Cookies

I've never been a fan of hard, powdering, crumbling cookies. Since childhood I've always loved soft cookies.

Ingredients

- 8 tablespoons of salted butter
- 1/2 cup white sugar (I like to use raw cane sugar with a coarser texture)
- 1/4 cup packed light brown sugar
- 1 teaspoon vanilla
- 1 egg
- 1 1/2 cups all purpose flour (more as needed – see video)
- 1/2 teaspoon baking soda
- 1/4 teaspoon salt (but I always add a little extra)
- 3/4 cup chocolate chips (I use a combination of chocolate chips and chocolate chunks)

Directions

1. Preheat the oven to 350°. Microwave the butter for about 40 seconds to just barely melt it. It shouldn't be hot – but it should be almost entirely in liquid form.
2. Using a stand mixer or electric beaters, beat the butter with the sugars until creamy. Add the vanilla and the egg; beat on low speed until just incorporated – 10-15 seconds or so (if you beat the egg for too long, the cookies will be stiff).
3. Add the flour, baking soda, and salt. Mix until crumbles form. Use your hands to press the crumbles together into a dough. It should form one large ball that is easy to handle (right at the stage between "wet" dough and "dry" dough). Add the chocolate chips and incorporate with your hands.
4. Roll the dough into 12 large balls (or 9 for HUGELY awesome cookies) and place on a cookie sheet. Bake for 9-11 minutes until the cookies look puffy and dry and just barely golden. Warning, friends: DO NOT OVERBAKE. This advice is probably written on every cookie recipe everywhere, but this is essential for keeping the cookies soft. Take them out even if they look like they're not done yet. They'll be pale and puffy.
5. Let them cool on the pan for a good 30 minutes or so (I mean, okay, eat four or five but then let the rest of them cool). They will sink down and turn into these dense, buttery, soft cookies that are the best in all the land. These should stay soft for many days if kept in an airtight container. I also like to freeze them.

Stay Soft Sugar Cookies with Frosting

Be warned: If you like the sugar cookies that retain their shape when baking, these are not them! You can cut them into cute little snowmen or Santa shapes if you want, but you won't be able to tell Rudolph from a lightbulb when you're done. "Stay soft" cookies don't keep those sharp, crisp edges because of the ingredients required to keep them soft. However, if you're truly an artist with a piping bag, what does it matter? You can still make them look like something special.

Ingredients

- 2 ¾ cup all purpose flour
- 1 tsp baking soda
- ½ tsp baking powder
- ½ tsp salt
- 1 cup unsalted butter, room temp
- 1 cup + 2 tbsp granulated sugar
- 2 tbsp brown sugar
- 1 egg
- 2 tsp vanilla extract
- ¼ cup sugar (for rolling)

Directions

1. Preheat the oven to 350°F. Line baking sheets with parchment paper or silicone baking mats. Set aside.

2. Combine the flour, baking soda, baking powder and salt in a medium sized bowl and set aside.

3. Cream the butter and sugars together in a large mixer bowl on medium speed until light in color and fluffy. You should be able to see the change in color happen and know it's ready.

4. Add the egg and mix until well combined.

5. Add the vanilla extract and mix until well combined.

6. Add the dry ingredients and mix until the dough is well combined. It will be thick and shouldn't be sticky. Do not over mix. Once it's well combined, use a rubber spatula to help it come together to form a more cohesive ball.

7. Create 1 1/2 tablespoon sized balls of cookie dough. Gently roll into a ball, then roll each ball in the additional sugar to coat. Set the balls on the baking sheet.

8. Bake cookies for 7-8 minutes. The cookies will spread and the centers will look soft, but should look done. Remove just before the edges begin to turn golden. Don't over bake. The cookies will be a little puffy when you take them out of the oven but will fall a bit as they cool.

9. Remove from the oven and allow to cool on baking sheets for 4-5 minutes before transferring to a wire rack to cool completely.

Sugar Cookie Frosting

Ingredients

- 8 oz (226g) cream cheese, room temperature
- 6 tbsp (86g) salted butter, room temperature
- 4 cups (460g) powdered sugar
- 1 tsp vanilla extract
- CREAM CHEESE FROSTING FOR CAKES
- 16 oz (452g) cream cheese, room temperature
- 3/4 cup (172g) butter, room temperature
- 10 cups (1150g) powdered sugar
- 2 tsp vanilla extract

Directions

1. Add the cream cheese and butter to a large mixer bowl and beat until well combined and smooth.

2. Add about half of the powdered sugar and mix until well combined and smooth.

3. Add the vanilla extract and mix until well combined.

4. Add the remaining powdered sugar and mix until well combined and smooth. Add more or less powdered sugar, as desired, for consistency purposes.

Banana Bread Cookies

Ingredients

- 1 cup butter flavored shortening
- 1 cup white sugar
- 2 eggs
- 1 teaspoon vanilla extract
- 1 banana, peeled and mashed
- 2 cups all-purpose flour1 teaspoon baking soda
- ½ teaspoon salt
- 3 tablespoons butter
- ⅓ cup powdered' sugar
- 1 tablespoon milk
- 1 teaspoon vanilla extract

Directions

1. Preheat the oven to 350°F. Lightly grease baking sheets.
2. In a medium bowl, cream together shortening and white sugar until smooth. Beat in eggs, vanilla extract, and banana.
3. In a separate bowl, combine flour, baking soda, and salt; blend thoroughly into the shortening mixture to make a sticky batter.
4. Drop by rounded tablespoons onto the prepared baking sheets, bake for 10 to 15 minutes in the preheated oven, or until lightly browned. Keep the remaining dough refrigerated between batches.
5. In a medium bowl, blend butter, powdered sugar, milk and vanilla extract. Adjust the amount of milk as necessary to attain a drizzling consistency. Drizzle over warm cookies and serve!

Oatmeal Raisin Cookies

Ingredients

- 1 cup all-purpose flour (spooned & leveled)
- 1/2 teaspoon ground cinnamon
- 1/2 teaspoon baking soda
- 1/4 teaspoon salt
- 1/2 cup unsalted butter, softened to room temperature
- 1/2 cup brown sugar
- 1/4 cup granulated sugar
- 1 large egg
- 1 teaspoon vanilla extract
- 1 and 1/2 cups old-fashioned rolled oats
- 1 cup raisins

Directions

1. In a large bowl, whisk together the flour, cinnamon, baking soda, and salt. Set aside.
2. In the bowl of a stand mixer fitted with the paddle attachment, or in a large mixing bowl using an electric mixer, cream together the butter, brown sugar, and granulated sugar for 1-2 minutes until well combined. Add the egg and vanilla extract and mix until fully combined.
3. Slowly mix in the flour mixture and continue mixing until just combined, then mix in the oats and raisins until fully combined, making sure to scrape down the sides of the bowl as needed.
4. Cover the cookie dough tightly with plastic wrap and refrigerate for 30 minutes.
5. Meanwhile, preheat the oven to 350°F. Line two large baking sheets with parchment paper or silicone baking mats and set aside.
6. Once the dough is chilled, remove it from the refrigerator. Using a 1.5-2 tablespoon cookie scoop, scoop the cookie dough and drop onto the prepared baking sheets. Roll the cookie dough into balls and very gently press down with your hand to flatten each ball of cookie dough slightly (make sure not to flatten them completely, just slightly). Make sure to leave a little room between each ball of cookie dough as they will spread a little while they bake.
7. Bake in separate batches at 350°F for 10-12 minutes or until the edges of the cookies are lightly golden brown and the top is set. Remove from the oven and cool on the baking sheet for 5 minutes, then transfer the cookies to a wire rack to finish cooling.

Pumpkin Pie

Ingredients

- 1 (15 ounce) can pumpkin
- 1 (14 ounce) can Sweetened Condensed Milk
- 2 large eggs
- 1 teaspoon ground cinnamon
- 1/2 teaspoon ground ginger
- 1/2 teaspoon ground nutmeg
- 1/2 teaspoon salt
- 1 (9 inch) unbaked pie crust

Directions

1. Preheat the oven to 425 ° F. Whisk pumpkin, sweetened condensed milk, eggs, spices and salt in a medium bowl until smooth. Pour into the crust. Bake for 15 minutes.
2. Reduce oven temperature to 350 ° F and continue baking 35 to 40 minutes or until a knife inserted 1 inch from the crust comes out clean. Cool. Garnish as desired. Store leftovers covered in the refrigerator.

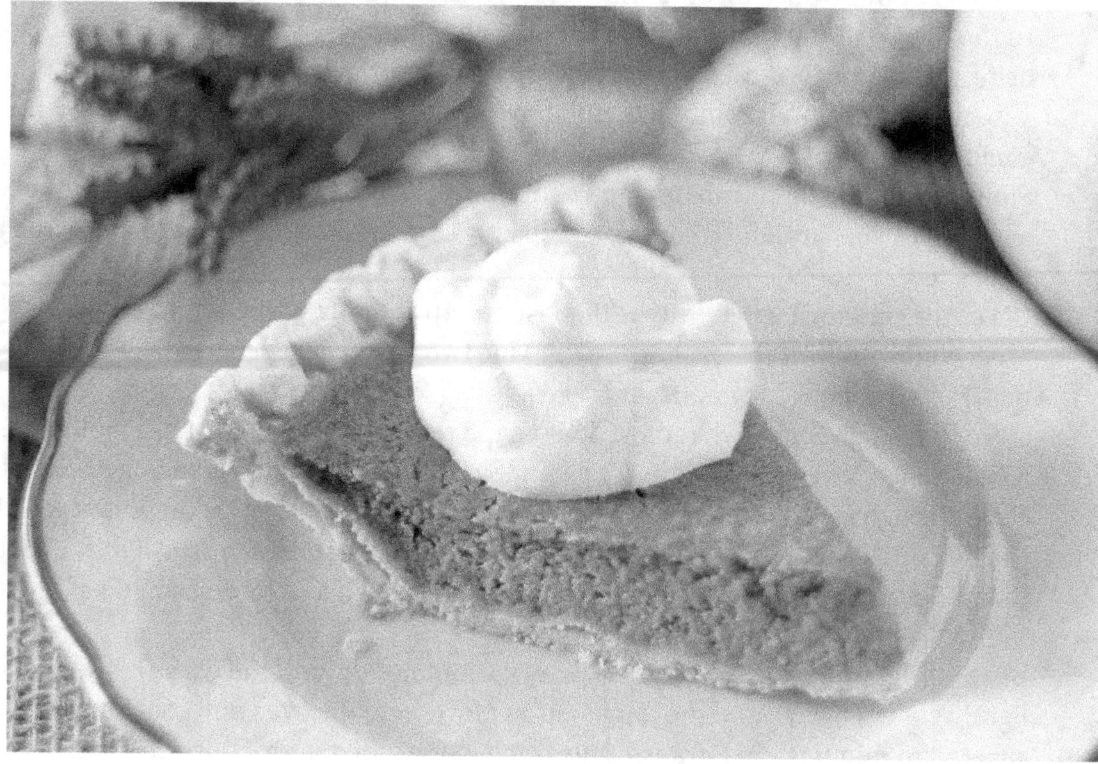

Peach Cobbler

We had a peach tree in the backyard when we moved to Utah. I was only twelve at the time but quickly learned the value of fresh fruit. There were many late summer afternoons when I could be found climbing the thin branches of that favorite tree to pluck a juicy peach for an afternoon snack. My dog Cookie would climb the tree with me by jumping from one limb to another and sit with me as I bit into the fuzzy fruit and watched the peach juice drip from my elbow. To this day I can't purchase peaches in the grocery store because the flavor just isn't there and I'm always left extremely disappointed. This old fashioned Peach Cobbler recipe is not only extremely easy to make from scratch, but it's made with fresh *or* canned peaches in case there are no truly fresh, ripe, soft, juicy peaches available.

Ingredients

- 4 cups of peaches that have been peeled, cored and sliced (or two large cans)
- 3/4 cup granulated sugar
- 1/4 teaspoon salt

For the batter:
- 6 Tablespoons butter
- 1 cup all-purpose flour
- 1 cup granulated sugar
- 2 teaspoons baking powder
- 1/4 teaspoon salt
- 3/4 cup milk
- ground cinnamon

Directions

1. Add the sliced peaches, sugar and salt to a saucepan and stir to combine. *(If using canned peaches, skip steps 1 & 2 and follow the directions starting at step 3)
2. Cook on medium heat for just a few minutes, until the sugar is dissolved and helps to bring out juices from the peaches. Remove from heat and set aside.
3. Preheat the oven to 350°F. Slice butter into pieces and add to a 9x13 inch baking dish. Place the pan in the oven while it preheats, to allow the butter to melt. Once melted, remove the pan from the oven.
4. In a large bowl mix together the flour, sugar, baking powder, and salt. Stir in the milk, just until combined. Pour the mixture into the pan, over the melted butter and smooth it into an even layer.

5. Spoon the peaches and juice (or canned peaches, if using) over the batter. Sprinkle cinnamon generously over the top. Bake at 350°F for about 38-40 minutes. Serve warm, with a scoop of ice cream.

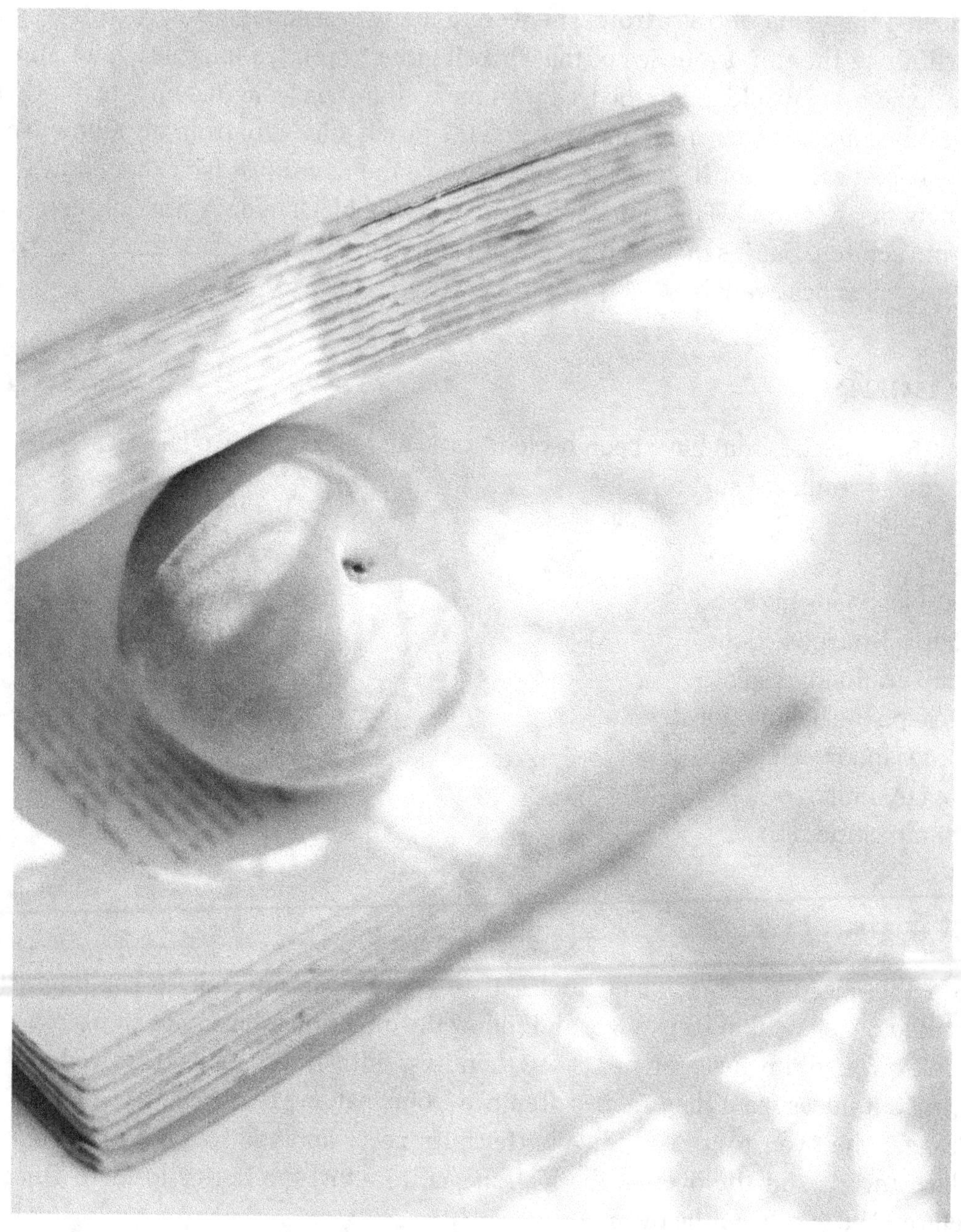

Blackberry Cobbler

You can change this recipe up by substituting blueberries, raspberries, strawberries, peaches, or a combination of mixed berries. My husband's favorite fruit is blackberry, so that's what I traditionally make for his birthday. We aren't big cake people.

Ingredients

- 1 cup Sugar
- 1 cup Self Rising Flour
- ¼ cup Butter
- 2 cups Blackberries
- ¼ cup additional sugar, plus 2 Tbsp.
- Vanilla Ice Cream

Directions

1. Combine the 1 cup sugar and 1 cup self-rising flour. Add 1 cup whole milk and 1/2 stick melted butter.
2. Add to a (9 x 9) casserole dish and top with 2 cups of blackberries. A 9 x 9 inch pan works well for this recipe. If using a 9 x 13 pan, consider doubling the recipe for thicker results.
3. Sprinkle 1/4 cup sugar on top and bake at 350° F for 50 minutes.
4. Add 2 Tablespoons sugar and bake for 10 more minutes.
5. Serve with vanilla ice cream.

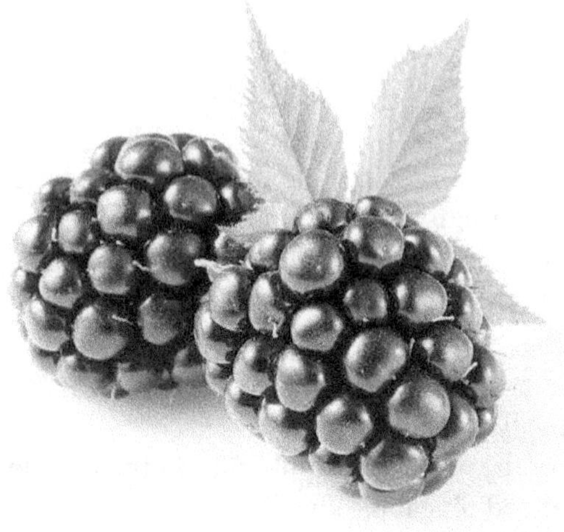

Best Yet Pineapple Upside Down Cake

Years ago I dated a man whose mother made a Pineapple Upside Down Cake for him every year for his birthday. After she passed, he was determined to continue getting his favorite cake for his birthday, so that was his major criteria in deciding he wanted to date me. He knew I liked to cook and would take up the challenge. Shortly after his birthday he broke up with me (he really only liked me for my cooking) and I wished him good riddance when I learned why. Just about a year later I got a message from him asking if I'd make this cake for him again because it was the best he'd ever had, and even offered to pay for the ingredients. I'm assuming his dating exploits had failed to produce another passable Pineapple Upside Down cake.

Ingredients

- 1/2 cup unsalted butter
- 3/4 cup light brown sugar, packed
- one 20-ounce can pineapple slices
- about 12 maraschino cherries
- 1 cup all-purpose flour
- 3/4 cup granulated sugar
- 2 teaspoons baking powder
- pinch salt, optional and to taste
- 1 large egg
- 1/2 cup buttermilk
- 1/3 cup sour cream, lite is okay (plain Greek yogurt may be substituted)
- 3 tablespoons canola or vegetable oil
- 2 teaspoons vanilla extract

INSTRUCTIONS

1. Preheat the oven to 350°F.
2. In a small, microwave-safe bowl, melt the butter, about 1 minute on high power.
3. Pour the butter into a 9-inch springform cake pan. Use your finger to run a bit of butter around the side of the pan so it's well-greased. Evenly sprinkle the brown sugar over the butter.
4. Add 1 whole pineapple slice to the center of the pan. Halve the remaining slices vertically. Stagger them in a fan-like fashion going around the cake. I used 12 slices.
5. Place the remaining slices as evenly as possible around the sides of the cake pan with the curved side pointing down toward the bottom of the pan.
6. Place 1 cherry in the center of the whole pineapple slice in the middle of the pan. Place 1 cherry in the center cutout of all the fanned pineapple slices; set pan aside.
7. In a large bowl, whisk together flour, granulated sugar, baking powder, optional salt; set aside.
8. In a separate small bowl, whisk together the next 5 wet ingredients (through vanilla).
9. Add the wet mixture to the dry, mixing lightly with a spoon or folding with a spatula until just combined. Small lumps will be present, don't overmix or try to stir them smooth.

10. Gently turn the batter out into the prepared pan, being careful to not disturb the pineapple slices on the sides or bottom. Fill the pan only to about 3/4-full. If you have a little extra batter, discard it rather than overfilling your pan.
11. Place the pan on a cookie sheet (to catch anything that does overflow) and bake for about 40 minutes, or until the center is set and not jiggly, and a toothpick inserted in the center comes out clean or with a few moist crumbs, but no batter. Only go down about 1-inch with the toothpick, not all the way to the bottom where you'll hit gooey pineapple juice.
12. Place the pan on a wire rack and allow the cake to cool for at least 30 minutes before inverting, slicing, and serving. I allowed the cake to cool overnight, covered with a sheet of foil, before inverting. Cake will keep airtight at room temperature for up to 5 days.

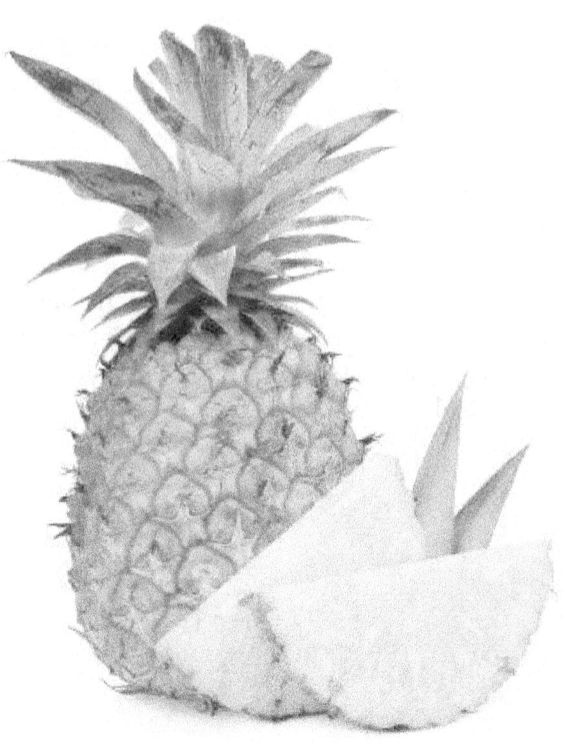

CINNAMON ROLL RICE CRISPY TREATS

These things never fail to be a big hit! People who say they don't even like Crispy Treats love these things. I've made entire batches as Christmas gifts and never heard a sour note about it.

INGREDIENTS

- 1 c. (2 sticks) butter, plus more for pan
- 24 oz of marshmallows (2x 12 oz bags)
- 2 tsp. cinnamon, plus more for dusting
- 1/4 tsp. salt
- 10 c. Rice Krispies

Icing

- 3 oz. cream cheese, softened to room temperature
- 3/4 c. powdered sugar
- 1/2 tsp. pure vanilla extract
- 2 tsp. heavy cream, optional

DIRECTIONS

1. Grease a 9"-x-13" baking pan with butter. In a large pot over medium heat, melt butter. Add marshmallows and stir until completely melted. Stir in cinnamon and salt, then remove from heat and stir in Rice Krispies.
2. Pour into the pan and gently smooth top. (If you use cooking spray on your hands this is easier!)
3. Let cool for 10 minutes, then cut into 12 squares. Use your hands to round the edges and shape Rice Krispies into rounds. Let cool completely.
4. Meanwhile, make glaze: In a medium bowl, combine cream cheese and beat until smooth. Add powdered sugar and vanilla and beat again until smooth. If icing is too thick, add heavy cream teaspoon by teaspoon until desired consistency is reached. Transfer to a piping bag or plastic bag.
5. Cut a small hole in a corner of the plastic bag or use a piping bag and pipe swirls of frosting onto each Rice Krispies treat. Dust with cinnamon and serve.

Double Layer Pumpkin Cheesecake

Ingredients

- 2 (8 ounce) packages cream cheese, softened
- 1/2 cup white sugar
- 1/2 teaspoon vanilla extract
- 2 eggs
- 1 (9 inch) prepared graham cracker crust
- 1/2 cup pumpkin puree
- 1/2 teaspoon ground cinnamon
- 1 pinch ground cloves
- 1 pinch ground nutmeg
- 1/2 cup frozen whipped topping, thawed

Directions

1. Preheat the oven to 325° F
2. In a large bowl, combine cream cheese, sugar and vanilla. Beat until smooth. Blend in eggs one at a time. Remove 1 cup of batter and spread into the bottom of the crust; set aside.
3. Add pumpkin, cinnamon, cloves and nutmeg to the remaining batter and stir gently until well blended. Carefully spread over the batter in the crust.
4. Bake in a preheated oven for 35 to 40 minutes, or until the center is almost set. Allow to cool, then refrigerate for 3 hours or overnight. Cover with whipped topping before serving.

Brownie Batter Dip

Ingredients

- 1 package (8 ounces) cream cheese, softened
- ¼ cup butter, softened
- 2 cups powdered' sugar
- ⅓ cup baking cocoa
- ¼ cup 2% milk
- 2 tablespoons brown sugar
- 1 teaspoon vanilla extract
- M&M's minis, optional
- Animal crackers, pretzels *and/or* sliced apples

Directions

In a large bowl, beat cream cheese and butter until smooth. Beat in powdered' sugar, cocoa, milk, brown sugar and vanilla until smooth. If desired, sprinkle with M&M's minis. Serve with dippers of your choice. Super simple and ALWAYS a hit!

Peach Pie Smoothie

Ingredients

- 1 cup unsweetened frozen peaches
- 1 tbsp honey (plus more, to taste)
- ¼ tsp vanilla extract
- ⅛ tsp ground cinnamon
- Pinch ground nutmeg
- Pinch ground ginger
- ½ cup milk or unsweetened milk alternative
- ½ cup nonfat plain yogurt

Directions

Add all the ingredients into a blender and blend until smooth. Done!

Do you know what it means to be a book author? It means the same thing as running a small business. Do you know what a small business needs to survive? People. Customers. Word of mouth. Product reviews. All authors depend on readers and reviewers to survive!

If you've enjoyed this book please consider taking the time to leave a written review through your favorite book retailer online.

Please also feel free to reach out to me through Facebook and let me know what your favorite recipe is, or if you altered it to fit your family's taste buds better. I love hearing about creative people who make something their very own!

https://www.Facebook.com/amandablackwoodsurvivor

LOW-COMPLEXITY CLASSIFIER FOR ACCURATE DIAGNOSIS OF BONE MARROW CANCER CELLS

First Edition September 2024

Written by KAVITHA R

LOW-COMPLEXITY CLASSIFIER FOR ACCURATE DIAGNOSIS OF BONE MARROW CANCER CELLS

KAVITHA R

LIST OF TABLES

LIST OF SYMBOLS AND ABBREVIATIONS

A	-	Accuracy
A(i)	-	Accuracy at i^{th} new iteration
ALL	-	Acute Lymphoblastic Leukemia
AML	-	Acute Meyloid Leukemia
AMF	-	Adaptive Median Filter
ASR	-	Age-Standardized incidence
ACS	-	American Cancer Society
AI	-	Artificial Intelligence
ANN	-	Artificial Neural Networks
O	-	Bias factors
BM	-	Bone Marrow
BMC	-	Bone Marrow Cancer
CNS	-	Central Nervous System
CCD	-	Charge-Coupled Device
CLL	-	Chronic Lymphocytic Leukemia
CML	-	Chronic Myeloid Leukemia
CBC	-	Complete Blood Count
CT	-	Computed Tomography
CAD	-	Computer-Aided Diagnosis
$\oplus$	-	Concatenation operation
CSO	-	Cat Swarm Optimization algorithm
CL	-	Convolutional layers
CNN	-	Convolutional Neural Networks
CMYK	-	Cyan, Magenta, Yellow, and Key (Black).
DICOM	-	Digital Imaging and Communications in Medicine
DL	-	Deep Learning

DNN	-	Deep Neural Network
DWT	-	Discrete Wavelet Transform
ELM	-	Extreme Learning Machines
FN	-	False Negative Values
FP	-	False Positive and
FFNN	-	Feed-Forward Neural Network
FF	-	Fitness Function
FF(i)	-	Fitness of the cat at the time i
FAB	-	French-American-British
FCL	-	Fully Connected Layers
GLCM	-	Gray Level Co-occurrence Matrix
HSV	-	Hue, Saturation, Value
I_0	-	Initial value of intensity at the source and the attractiveness
x	-	Input
$_I$	-	i^{th} position of the firefly
KNN	-	K-Nearest Neighbours
α	-	Learning rate
LBP	-	Local Binary Pattern
ML	-	Machine Learning
MRI	-	Magnetic Resonance Imaging
FFmax	-	Maximum fitness function
MGG	-	May-Grünwald-Giemsa
MAE	-	Mean Absolute Error
FFmin	-	Minimum fitness function value,.
H*	-	Moore−Penrose generalized inverse
MLL	-	Munich Leukemia Laboratory
NB	-	Naive Bayes
NN	-	Neural Networks

L	-	Next filter
μ	-	No of Epochs
NHL	-	Non-Lymphoma Hodgkin's
FF(b)	-	Number of cats
T.N	-	Number of Pixels
H(x)	-	Output hidden layer
OL	-	Output Layers
	-	Output weight vector
PB	-	Peripheral Blood
PBS	-	Peripheral Blood Smears
PL	-	Pooling Layers
PNN	-	Probabilistic Neural Network
RBFNN	-	Radial Basis Function Neural Network
RBC	-	Red Blood Cells
RGB	-	Red, Green, Blue
S(k)	-	Saliency maps
k	-	Size of each filter layers
SGD	-	Stochastic Gradient Descent
SVM	-	Support Vector Machine
p	-	Total pixels.
TN	-	True Negative Values
TP		True Positive Values
$_{i+1}$	-	Value of attraction
WBC	-	White Blood Cells
WHO	-	World Health Organization
Y	-	y-dimensional pre trained vectors

CHAPTER 1

INTRODUCTION

1.1 PRELIMINARY BACKGROUND

The most common type of blood cancer among all age groups, particularly among youngsters, is leukemia. It is an abnormal phenomenon caused by uncontrolled blood cell growth and proliferation, which can damage immune system function, bone marrow, and red blood cells.

In India, where more than 60,000 new cases of cancer were reported in 2018, leukemia represents more than 3.5% of all new cancer cases. Before spreading to vital biological tissues, malignant white blood cells, or lymphoblast, go through the blood to other organs such as the spleen, brain, liver, and kidneys. (Hegde *et al.* 2019; Namayandeh *et al.* 2020)).

Hematologists at cell transplant facilities can diagnose and differentiate between different types of leukemia based on microscopic images. If the slide is properly stained, some types of leukemia can be more easily identified and distinguished from one another, but further instruments are needed to determine the underlying leukemia. The stained slides for the most prevalent kinds of leukemia are shown in Figure 1.1 (Wolach *et al.* 2017).

Leukemia early diagnosis has always been difficult for hematologists, clinicians, and researchers. The swelling of the lymph nodes, pallor, fever, and weight loss are leukemia signs, although they can also be seen in other conditions. Since the signs of early leukemia are typically mild, making a diagnosis can be difficult. The examination of Peripheral Blood Smears (PBS) under a microscope is the approach used most frequently to diagnose leukemia. The gold standard for diagnosing leukemia, however, merely requires the collection and analysis of bone marrow samples (Xing *et al.* 2017).

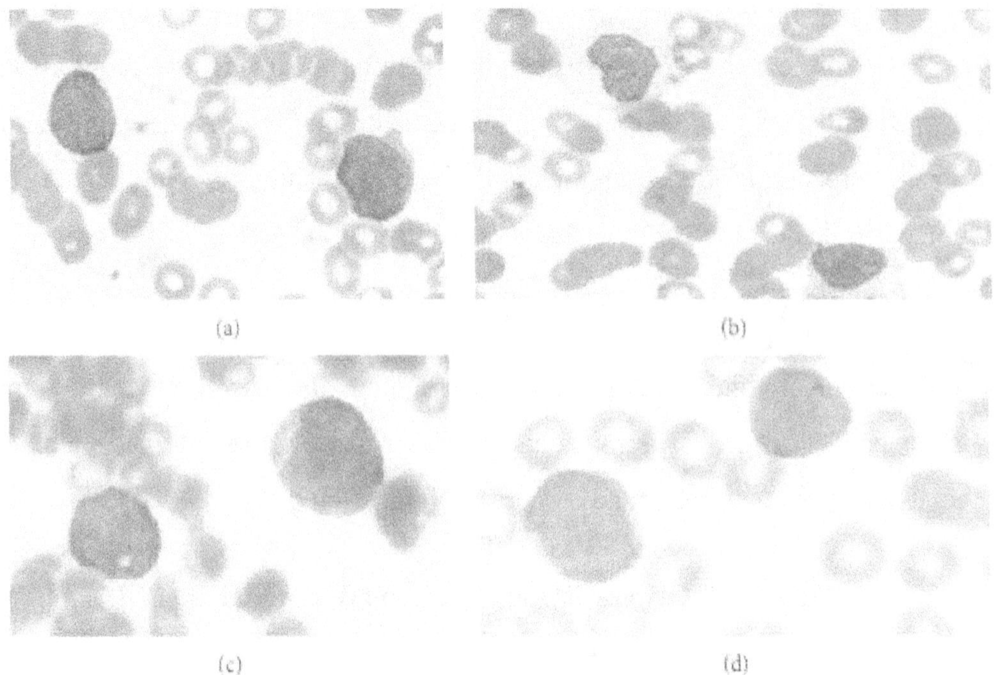

Figure 1.1   **(a) AML (M1), (b) AML (M2), (c) B-ALL (pre-A), and (d) B-ALL (pro-B)**

Over the past 20 years, a number of researchers have used machine learning (ML) and computer-aided diagnostic methods for laboratory image analysis in an effort to overcome the limitations of a late leukaemia diagnosis and pinpoint its subgroups.

Blood smear images are evaluated for the goal of identifying, differentiating, and counting the cells in various kinds of leukaemia.

(Wen *et al.* 2018). The well-known artificial intelligence subject known as machine learning (ML) involves mathematical correlations and algorithms that have been widely used to the field of clinical research.

With ML, machines can be programmed without explicit training and learn from it. When analyzing medical data, these algorithms have produced astounding findings, and they have proven incredibly successful in identifying disorders. (Obermeyer *et al.* 2016; Ehrenstein *et al.* 2017).

According to the research, Machine Learning (ML) approaches significantly help challenging medical decision-making processes in medical image processing by extracting and then analyzing the features of these images (Ghaderzadeh *et al.* 2013; Zhao *et al.* 2017).

The proliferation of medical diagnosis instruments and the massive production of high-quality data necessitated the development of more advanced data processing systems. Such a vast amount of data cannot be analyzed or its patterns found using traditional methods.

1.2 DETECTION OF BONE MARROW CANCER (BMC) USING INTELLIGENT METHODS

Artificial intelligence (AI), which has the express objective of computationally simulating human intelligence, consists of a variety of tools and techniques. By applying a number of algorithms from the subfields of Machine Learning (ML) or Deep Learning (DL), AI may improve the computerization of the tasks carried out by human specialists. This has the potential to have a substantial and immediate influence on the healthcare sector.

Recently, the application of AI in medicine has gone beyond clinical research to encompass translational medicine and therapeutic therapies for a variety of conditions, including cancers (Yu *et al.* 2018; Jiang *et al.* 2017; Reddy *et al.* 2018; Chen *et al.* 2019).

In general, ML seeks to provide accurate assessments by identifying patterns in data using numerical algorithms, with the benefit that these techniques may automate the process of developing hypotheses. The traditional statistical approaches are changed and merged with ML algorithms in some cases (Lynch *et al.* 2018).

The so-called Artificial Neural Networks (ANN) used in Deep Learning (DL) are a subset of machine learning that takes their structure cues from the human brain. In essence, it organizes algorithms into layers to produce Convolutional Neural Networks (CNN), which are capable of learning and making wise judgments on their own.

DL really more closely resembles the functioning of a genuine "brain" than ML does, giving it an almost "human-like" AI technology. The algorithm won't need any form of human input, unlike ML, and will be able to assess the accuracy of a particular prediction using its own CNN. Although DL approaches require a larger amount of computational resources overall, analysis of their results has shown that they frequently perform better than other, more traditional ML techniques (Gupta *et al.* 2018).

The difficulty of anticipating therapeutic effects in many types of tumors has been addressed by the development and application of DL structures for the identification of tumors (Chen *et al.* 2016; Koh *et al.* 2017; Baptista *et al.* 2020). Because ML algorithms and DL techniques have the potential to manage cancer patients using a combination of proteomic, genomic, histology, or pictures, their usage in the last few years to identify tumors has steadily expanded(Libbrecht *et al.* 2015; Jones *et al.* 2017; Wainberg *et al.* 2019; Zou *et al.* 2018).

However, the objective of ML or DL is to improve oncologists' ability to make decisions in their practice as opposed to replacing human capacity (Walsh *et al.* 2019). These treatments have been shown to offer helpful assistance not only in the treatment of solid tumors but also in the care of patients with hematological disorders.

1.3 IMAGE PROCESSING AND MACHINE LEARNING FOR DETECTING BMC

Image recognition software has become quite popular over the past several years. They now play a crucial role in a variety of industries, including science, engineering, and medicine. The ability to see is man's most developed sense.

The capacity to gather information about the issue being studied, however, something that is difficult for a human to do without the aid of computerized systems thanks to the concepts of image processing and Machine Learning (ML). To put it another way, there are occasions when this information is difficult for the eye to discriminate (Fabijańska *et al.* 2009).

One way that image processing and machine learning techniques have benefited medicine is by enabling the investigation and study of a wide range of phenomena using digitalized medical images.

Medical images in digital format enable further investigation that can lead to a more precise diagnosis, enabling the best possible patient care. Digital medical images of peripheral blood (PB) smears taken under a microscope are the major works in this experiment. Examining blood components and their changes are one of the common diagnostic techniques used in clinical regular practice.

In this study, digital image processing and ML techniques are used for medical picture analysis and recognition, namely haematology.

The objective of this research is to develop a method for identifying acute leukemia and classifying it according to cell morphology into acute lymphoblastic leukemia (ALL) and acute myeloid leukemia (AML). For this study, the PB smear pictures rather than the Bone Marrow (BM) sample have been used for a variety of reasons, including:

1) First Leukemia diagnosis procedure is carried out. On the basis of the results of the first diagnosis, additional laboratory tests will be performed.

2) Peripheral Blood (PB) is commonly used for periodic therapy evaluations since drawing blood from a vein is substantially easier, less expensive, and less unpleasant than drawing blood from the bone marrow (BM).

White Blood Cells (WBCs) are affected by leukemia, a blood cancer, which is a most deadly illnesses that kill individuals, especially in affluent nations (Kothari*et al.* 1996). The three main types of blood cells are platelets, which are the specialized cells in-charge of blood clotting, white blood cells (WBCs/Leukocytes), which fight infections, and red blood cells (RBCs/Erythrocytes), which carry oxygen.

They are all produced in the bone marrow, which also gives rise to several WBC subtypes in the lymph nodes. They are subsequently released into the bloodstream once they have reached their full development. WBCs turn malignant in leukemia for reasons that are yet not fully understood (Lavelle *et al.* 2004).

Leukemia can develop in one of the numerous types of WBCs. They may occur in lymphoblast, which are lymphoid cells that are still forming and produce ALL, a disease that manifests suddenly. Alternatively, when the neoplasm (abnormally rapid cell division) affects mature cells, Chronic Lymphocytic Leukemia (CLL), which is frequently more latent, is the designation used.

Chapter two will cover various medical and cellular jargon as well as a full description of blood parts. The characteristics of leukemia, techniques of diagnosis, and treatments will also be fully explained. Leukemia is available especially among youngsters, according to information provided by the American Cancer Society (ACS) (American Cancer Society, 2013).

According to the American Childhood Cancer Organization (2012), the distribution of the most common childhood cancers among children in the United States between the ages of one and 14 is depicted in the graph below in Figure 1.2.

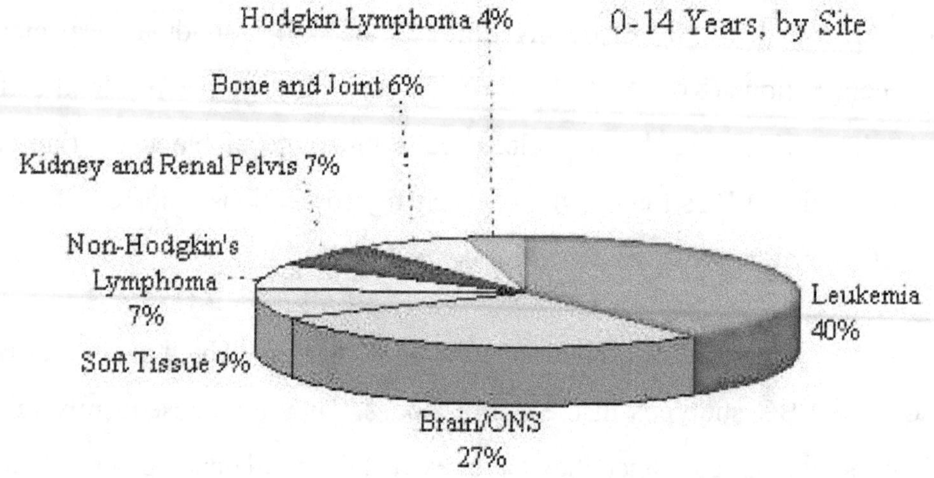

Figure 1.2 Most prevalent childhood cancer in the US

The distribution of the most prevalent childhood malignancies among children in the United States between the ages of one and 14 is shown in the graph above in Figure 1.2, according to the American Childhood Cancer Organization (2012).

Men had an annual crude rate of 100.2 percent per 100,000 persons, while women had a crude rate of 132.1 percent. Table 1.1 displays the cancer incidence per 100,000 by gender (Lim *et al.* 2008).

Table 1.1   Cancer incidence per 100,000 people and age-standardized incidence (ASR), by gender (Lim 2008)

Gender	No.	%	CR	ASR
Male	29596	43.7	100.2	136.9
Female	38196	56.3	132.1	156.4
Both Genders	67792	100	116.0	145.6

The most prevalent cancers were divided into gender categories in the 2008 National Cancer Registry report (Lim *et al.* 2008). Males are more likely to develop the following cancers than females: leukaemia, lymphoma, prostate cancer, stomach, liver, bladder, large intestine, lung, nasopharyngeal cancer, and other skin cancers as shown in Figure 1.3.

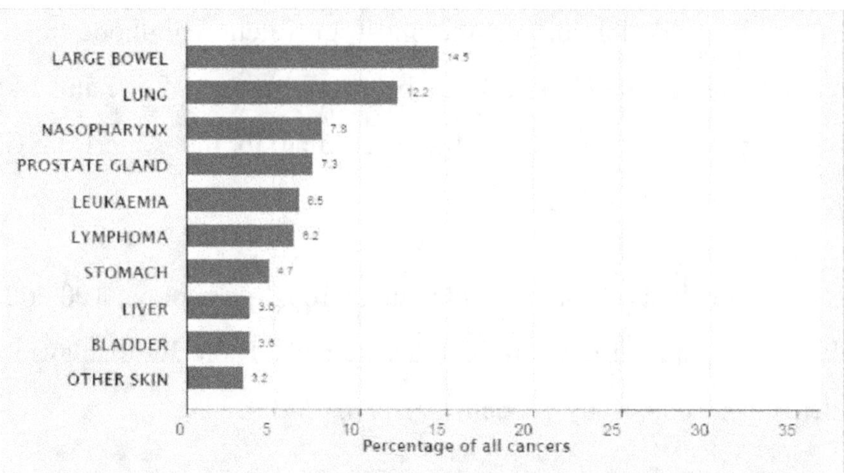

Figure 1.3 Most Common Cancers among Male

Leukemia, lung, lymphoma, corpus uteri, thyroid gland, breast, cervix, large bowel, ovary, lymphoma, and stomach are the most prevalent malignancies in females, in order of frequency as shown in Figure 1.4.

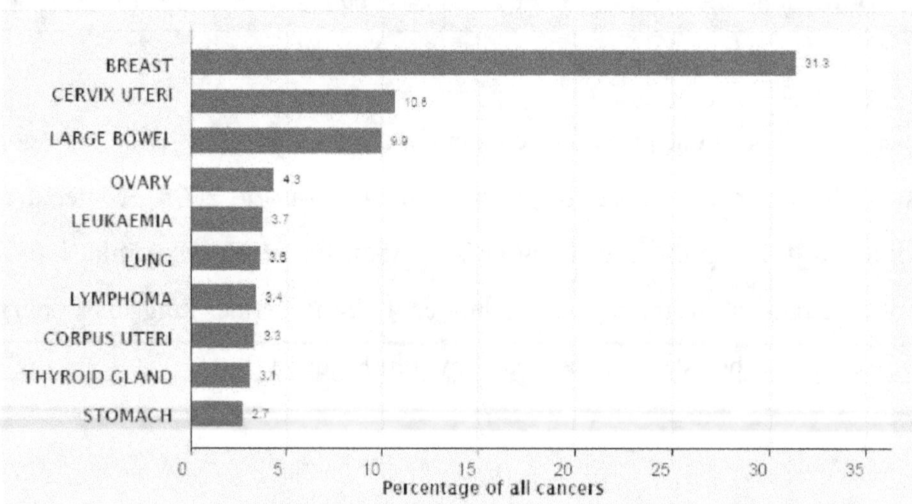

Figure 1.4 Most Common Cancers in Women's Bodies

Leukemia was discovered to be highly prevalent among male cancers, which was unexpected given that leukemia was reported to be the second most prevalent cancer type overall and among men in the Kelantan Cancer Registry Report 1999–2003.

The incidence of leukemia per 100,000 people is shown in Table 1.2 by race and gender (Lim *et al.* 2008).

Table 1.2 Age-Standardized incidence (ASR) and leukemia cancer incidence per 100,000 people, by ethnicity and gender (Lim 2008).

Ethnic group	Male				Female			
	No.	%	CR	ASR	No.	%	CR	ASR
Malay	220	67.9	3.6	4	111	55.5	1.8	2
Chinese	86	26.5	3.2	3.3	72	36	2.8	2.6
Indian	18	5.6	2	2.2	17	8.5	1.9	1.9

Due to advancements in diagnosis and therapy over the past 40 years, leukemia survival rates have significantly risen. The total 5-year survival rate for all forms of leukemia was roughly 14% in 1960. It has however recently risen to 70%. (Johnson *et al.* 2018). Consequently, determining the correct kind of leukemia is essential for early detection and treatment. (Lim *et al.* 2008).

1.4 PROBLEM BACKGROUND AND PROBLEM STATEMENTS

A malignancy of the BM and WBCs called leukemia. Despite the fact that leukemia is regarded as a deadly kind of cancer, recent developments in diagnostic equipment and therapeutic alternatives have led to a cure rate of approximately 70% (Johnson *et al.* 2018). Leukemia generally comes in two different forms: acute and chronic. Clinically and physiologically, acute leukemia differs from chronic leukemia.

Acute leukemia is characterized by the aggressive and rapid development of immature cells, particularly blast cells. On the other hand, chronic leukemia develops gradually over several years. Before considering treatment, chronic leukemia is occasionally observed over time to guarantee the therapy's maximum efficacy. However, acute leukemia needs to be treated right away because, if it is not, it can cause death within a few weeks (Silverstein *et al.* 2006).

According to Döhner *et al.* (2010) and Gökbuget *et al.* (2009), acute leukemia is a collection of diverse disorders that can afflict people of various ages. The French-American-British (FAB) and World Health Organization (WHO) categories are the most often used procedures for acute leukemia diagnosis (Tkachuk *et al.* 2007). Using the blast cell's precursor as a basis, both classification protocols basically divide acute leukemia into ALL and AML.

Because acute leukemia is so aggressive, it has to be treated right away. Additionally, ALL is treated differently from AML. It is important to determine whether the cell of origin is lymphoid or myeloid as soon as possible in order to deliver the appropriate treatment in a timely manner (Riley *et al.* 1999). We view acute leukemia as the present area of interest for our study.

Utilizing a range of laboratory techniques, including microscopic morphological analysis of PB slides and BM aspiration, acute leukemia is clinically diagnosed and distinguished. Additionally, cytogenetic and immunephenotypic testing are performed on the BM.

The initial diagnostic step is often a microscopic morphological examination of the PB smear.This is because the PB smear test is frequently conducted before the patient undergoes any painful or invasive therapies, such BM biopsy, and is seen to be the most economical method for initial screening of acute leukaemia (Angulo *et al.* 2006).

The morphological analysis of PB smears for the diagnosis of leukemia has a number of advantages, including the capacity to identify a likely diagnosis or range of diagnoses, the capacity to choose which more pertinent additional tests are necessary, and the capacity to avoid laborious and unnecessary procedures that are difficult to interpret, like immunophenotyping.

A PB smear test is therefore crucial since it enables quick diagnosis and targeted therapy (Bain 2005). Labor-intensive laboratory procedures are one drawback of this approach. It also requires the employment of highly skilled professionals since it is prone to human error or inter-observer variance (difference in diagnosis among various observers) (Scotti 2005; Briggs *et al.* 2009; Mohapatra *et al.* 2013).

The numerous forms of normal leukocytes flowing in the blood stream can only be identified by the equipment, which include haematology analyzers, which lack the ability to categorize aberrant cells despite the recent, significant advancements in haematology instruments. Recent developments include the CellaVision DM96 automated microscope (Briggs *et al.* 2009).

With the use of this device, stained blood slides can be scanned, prospective WBCs can be located, and then high-magnification digital photos may be captured. A computerized neural network that is trained on a cell database then classifies the WBC pictures. In cases when the DM96 fails to accurately identify the WBCs, the user must either manually reclassify the WBCs in the appropriate category or check the cell categorization.

Recent research that looked at the usage of DM96 revealed that DM96 was capable of detecting blast cells. However, based on research done by Billard *et al.* (2010), only 74% of ALL and 73% of AML could be classified by the DM96, indicating that a sizable portion of cells were misclassified by the DM96.

Even though, the number of blast cells was underestimated while the number of lymphocytes was overstated. These studies showed that for the initial leukemia diagnosis, laboratory staff should employ conventional microscopy. Due to this, it is still challenging to use these analyzers to reliably distinguish immature and aberrant cells, such as blast cells and atypical lymphocytes (Billard *et al.* 2010; Briggs *et al.* 2009).

Because it permits scanning of a greater number of PB slides than manual inspection (Escalante *et al.* 2012), time is saved by using image processing and machine learning approaches in computer-aided microscopic morphological evaluation. It also increases accuracy by removing human mistake, such as errors brought on by repetition, weariness, lack of expertise, and so on.

The phases of computer-aided PB screening for the purpose of acute leukaemia diagnosis and classification include blast cell location and segmentation, feature extraction and selection, and eventually blast cell classification. The diagnosis and classification of acute leukemia are discussed in this study. Every stage that was previously mentioned is so present.

When creating a computer-aided system for identifying haematological malignancies, isolating the target cells (blast cells) from the stained blood picture backdrop is a key technological challenge.

PB segmentation is crucial since the accuracy of the subsequent steps, feature extraction and classification, completely hinges on the accurate segmentation of the interest cells (Liao *et al.* 2002; Joshi *et al.* 2013).

The segmentation stage is therefore regarded as the most difficult and complex task due to the following reasons:

1. The PB slide presentation illustrates the cells' intricate structure (Liao *et al.* 2002). The variety in cell size, shape, and aspect accounts for this challenges.

2. Localization of each particular cell and sub-image extracting for feature extraction, sub-images with a single nucleus per picture are crucial (Mohapatra 2011). In many instances, the blurry borders between the cell of interest and the backdrop impair accurate cell localization and extraction (Nee *et al.* 2012).

3. It is practically impossible to attain the same imaging quality because the acquisition stage's imaging quality varies on the varied illumination levels, light, the staining procedure, and the ability of the laboratory staff who manufacture the PB smear (Markiewicz *et al.* 2005).

4. Cell proximity and superimposition obtaining appropriate segmentation results are typically difficult, especially when separating cells that are touching or overlapping.

Once all of the blast cells have been correctly segmented, it is crucial to extract the right diagnostic characteristics that may be expressed as a numerical value and define the blasts (Duda *et al.* 2012). Blast cells are classified as lymphoid or myeloid depending on these traits. There are various methods for creating characteristics that will help classify acute leukemia. Form, texture, or color are the three categories into which the traits typically fall (Sinha *et al.* 2003).

These three groupings may be used to extract hundreds of characteristics. Not all of them, nevertheless, are helpful for the categorization procedure. The categorization procedure may not be aided by comparable feature values shared by various blood cells, such as when two cells have the same area size. Determining the ideal combination of discriminative traits is therefore crucial in order to get the most effective recognition outcomes (Osowski *et al.* 2009).

It has been determined from the thorough literature study that is undertaken (presented in chapter 2) that there are relatively few scientific publications that are specifically indicating the issue of acute Leukemia diagnosis and classification. There is still a lot of need for additional work and researches in this area despite the efforts of a number of scholars (Scotti 2006; Markiewicz *et al.* 2005; Supardi *et al.* 2012; Nasir *et al.* 2013).

Despite the fact that every image analysis system consists of three fundamental stages: segmentation, feature extraction, and classification, this study focused on just one, namely segmentation (Sadeghian *et al.* 2009; Madhloom *et al.* 2012).

Several other researchers, like the works by (Piuri *et al.* 2004; Theera-Umpon *et al.* 2007), Rezatofighi & Soltanian-Zadeh 2011) and others, concentrated on various blood counts of WBCs but not Leukemia, whereas others, like the study by (Piuri & Scotti 2004), exclusively focused on ALL (Scotti 2005). Chapter 2 will discuss the most recent studies in this sector, along with their benefits and drawbacks.

1.5   BMC CLASSIFICATION DATASETS

The spongy material found inside some of our bigger bones is sampled and examined via a bone marrow biopsy. The ability of the bone marrow to produce healthy blood cells can be evaluated using this biopsy. Medical practitioners use these techniques to identify and keep track of malignancies, blood and marrow disorders, and unexplained fevers.

More than 170,000 de-identified, expertly annotated cells from bone marrow smears of 945 individuals stained with the May-Grünwald-Giemsa/Pappenheim stain are included in the Kaggle dataset. The sample was included in significant laboratory that had a focus on leukemia diagnoses, as evidenced by the cohort's diagnosis distribution, which included a variety of haematological disorders.

The photos were captured using a bright field microscope with a 40x magnification and oil immersion. The Fraunhofer IIS-developed scanners and post-processing software both were used to process all of the samples in the Munich Leukemia Laboratory (MLL).

1.6   PROBLEM STATEMENT AND OBJECTIVES OF THE RESEARCH

The goal of this study is to create a diagnostic approach for acute Leukemia blast cells by utilizing image processing, ML and DL on PB smear pictures. In order to determine the best strategy for the acute Leukemia diagnostic procedure, we first examine the pertinent image processing and ML and DL approaches in this thesis.

The goal of this study is to use image processing and Machine Learning (ML) and Deep Learning approaches to improve the diagnostic precision of acute Leukemia for the best categorization of ALL and AML.

The Problem Statement for the proposed research work is as follows.

- To develop a bio-inspired and Deep Learning-based classification system that can diagnose bone marrow cancer cells with high accuracy and speed.

The following are the objectives of the research work:.

- Conventional Neural Network (CNN) hyper- parameters are determined

- CAT Swarm algorithm optimizes the CNN hyper- parameters

- To improve the accuracy and speed of identifying various forms of bone marrow malignancies, a more reliable and straightforward Deep Learning classifier is being developed. Performance of the classifier is validated

1.7 RESEARCH CONTRIBUTION

In the real world, a haematologist or laboratory expert examines the microscopic features of the PB smear to find blast cells and ascertain their type. Even a skilled operator could find it challenging to manually differentiate between the many types of blast cells based on morphology (Kawthalkar 2012). Additionally, the error rate for manually detecting blast cells varies from 30% to 40% depending on the operator's level of skill (Reta *et al.* 2010).

As was already mentioned, the goal of this research is to increase the accuracy of acute leukemia diagnosis for the best categorization of ALL and AML by using image processing and ML & DL techniques. In order to get the desired results, the study is carried out in four main steps: 1) image acquisition, 2) image segmentation, 3) feature extraction and selection, and finally 4) classification. The four main modules of a Computer-Aided Diagnosis (CAD) system are made up of these four components.

This research expanded on the findings of past studies and offers the following crucial contributions:

- Nucleus and cytoplasm of a single blast cell are separated from other blood cells, such as RBCs, platelets, and plasma, and other blood components.

- A thorough examination of colour channels to determine the best colour space and colour channels for segmentation, producing the best possible segmentation quality. For this, two separate databases of PB images are chosen.

- Comparing the blast cell segmentation method used in PB images to a ground truth of manually segmented PB images, an objective evaluation is made. The nucleus/cytoplasm separation and blast cell extraction results of the suggested segmentation approach are both impressively high at 94% and 96%, respectively.

- A comparison with two cutting-edge blast cell segmentation techniques demonstrates the suggested method's superiority.

- Three different types of features are created with guidance based on shape, texture, and color data obtained.

- The suggested method successfully categorizes acute leukemia blast cells with 99.5% accuracy utilizing classification engines, namely the Cat Optimized CNN. The results are remarkably comparable to and better than the vast majority of cutting-edge methods detailed in the literature.

In terms of productivity and quality control, the presented study findings also significantly enhance the medical laboratory's everyday operations. Additionally, when seeing each blast cell independently on the screen, it enables the haematologist or laboratory professional to automatically allocate the blast cells.

The difficulty of manually screening PB slides is greatly diminished. The ability to store photographs allows for comparison and evaluation in the future. This approach may assist in the education and training of new laboratory professionals and, as an added bonus, be an effective teaching tool.

The suggested method not only streamlines laboratory operations but also offers the expert significant help in identifying and categorizing blast cells. Most patients first go to their primary care physician for medical care, since initial symptoms of acute Leukemia are ambiguous and might match those of other beginning conditions, such as viral infection.

As a result, having a tool to aid in the early screening of children suspected of having acute leukemia would be beneficial to doctors and laboratories outside of large hospitals. The recommended technique is used to address the research problem and provide answers to the research questions by logically adopting many phases. Furthermore, it describes how the research's data will be gathered.

Acute Leukemia is often diagnosed and categorized through a number of phases. Picture capture, image segmentation, feature extraction, feature selection, and classification are a few of them. A diagrammatic example of the proposed study is provided in Figure 1.5. In order to diagnose acute Leukemia, the research's initial stage must be picture capture.

The following parts offer a succinct discussion of the contributing chapters and the outcomes. A brief summary of the planned research project and its findings is shown in Figure 1.5.

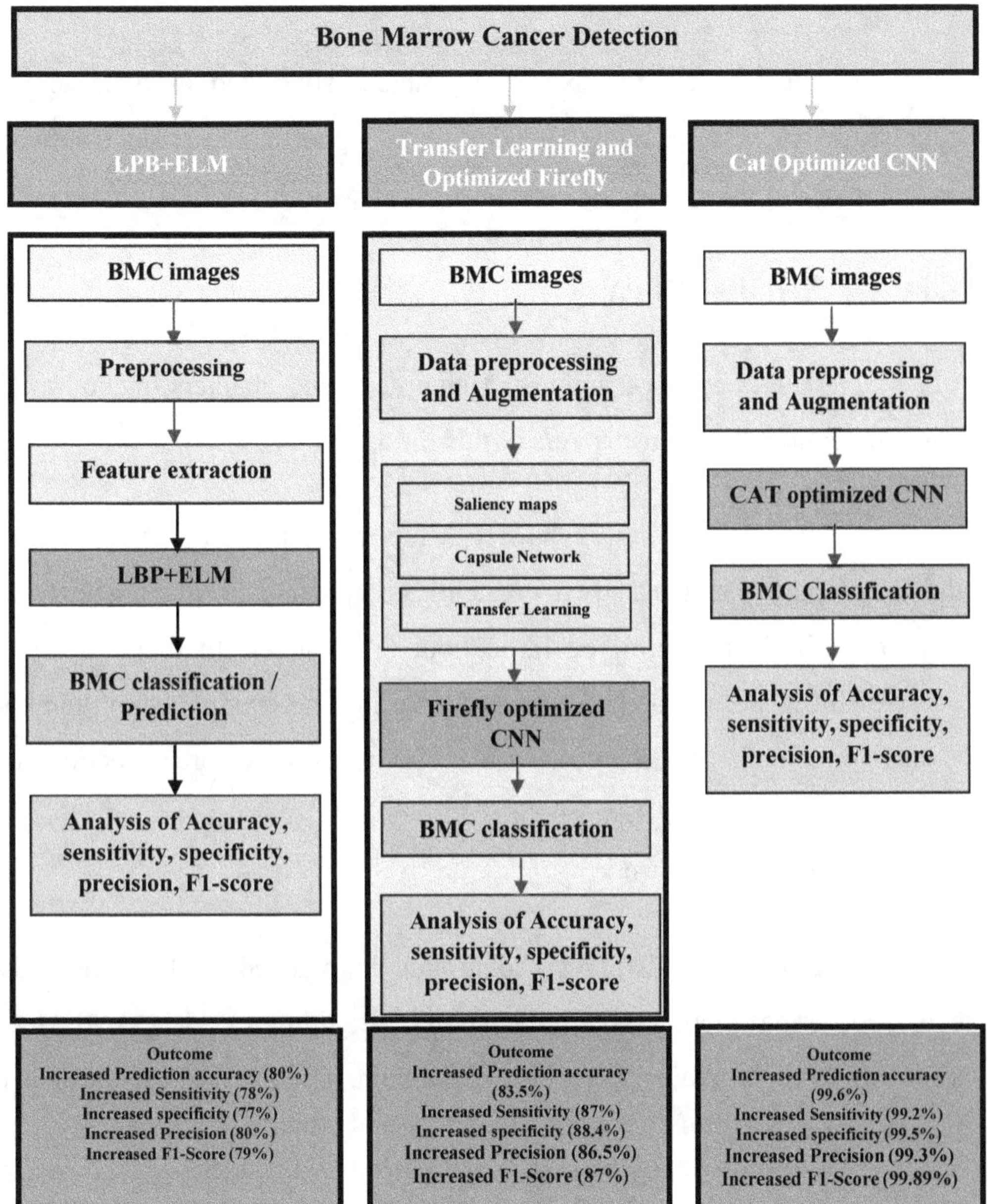

Figure 1.5 Schematic of research work carried out

A Local Binary Pattern (LBP)-based ELM framework is suggested for categorizing BMC in the early stages of the research. However, this architecture does not handle large-scale networks. The second phase is thus suggested in order to use firefly neural networks based on transfer learning for the BMC prediction; however it is unable to do so due to the complexity it adds.

A cat-optimized CNN is ultimately suggested as a solution to address the issues raised above. In addition to supporting large-scale networks and simplifying the system, this framework categorizes BMC effectively.

1.8   THESIS OVERVIEW

This opening chapter and the next six chapters make up the logically organized seven chapters of this thesis.

Literature Review, **Chapter 2** the major methods and algorithms that are employed in this study to create the computer-aided diagnostic system are emphasized and described throughout the chapter. In this chapter, an overview of recent research on computer-based Leukemia detection methods is also presented. Segmentation, feature extraction, feature selection, and classification are just a few of the key elements of such systems that are covered in this research work.

Additionally, it gives background knowledge on Leukemia blast cells and normal blood cells in "Leukemia." It addresses ALL, AML, CLL, and CML, the four major subtypes of Leukemia. The focus of the thesis is on both ALL and AML.

This chapter also describes the common diagnostic techniques for Leukemia currently in use. Additionally, it provides a thorough explanation of the FAB and WHO categorization systems for Leukemia. A brief explanation of the prognosis and available treatments for Leukemia is given toward the conclusion of this chapter.

Chapter 3 With the LBP and ELM approach, deep learning-based methods are covered. First, a proposed approach's design is shown. After that, the conditions for picture acquisition are described. Following the feature extraction and feature selection procedures, the prerequisites for image processing and image segmentation are also covered.

The criteria for classifying and identifying acute leukemia blast cells are further discussed in this chapter. The effectiveness of the measurements used to assess and test the suggested approach is then explained.

Chapter 4 Proposed firefly optimized transfer learning neural network architecture and algorithm is presented. The various stages of the development process are discussed, and each stage's results are provided in depth.

Chapter 5 Cat inspired CNN for Bone Marrow Cancer Cell detection is presented.

Chapter 6 Presents the Results and discussion of the proposed framework

Chapter 7 This section presents conclusion and future work. Along with the important findings and importance of the research, the accomplishments of the study in relation to the outcomes of the experiments are highlighted. The influence and relevance of the suggested strategy on the haematology community in particular and on society in general are also covered in this chapter.

CHAPTER 2

BACKGROUND AND LITERATURE SURVEY

The benefits and drawbacks of the current categorization scheme for bone marrow cancer are discussed in this chapter. Figure 2.1, which is shown as follows, depicts an overview of this chapter.

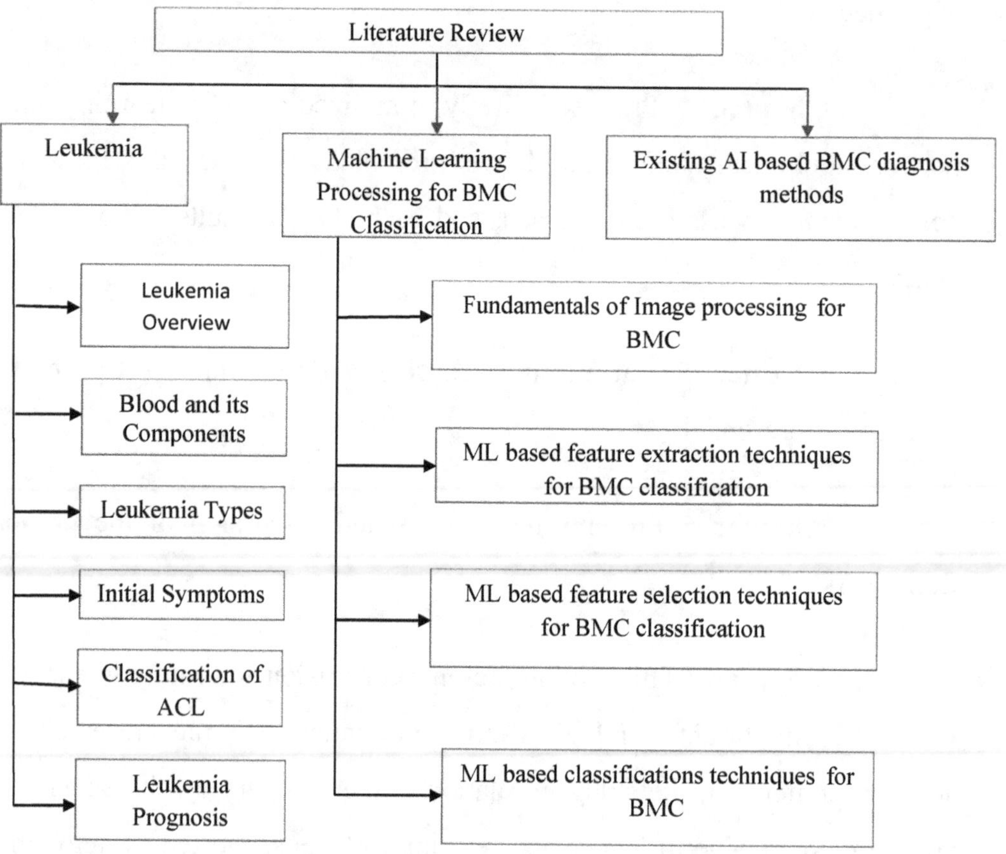

Figure 2.1 Literature Review Summary

2.1   LEUKEMIA- A SUMMARY

A variety of blood-related malignancies with varying etiologies, pathophysiology, prognoses, and therapeutic responses make up leukemia (Bain 2010). Leukemia is among the top 15 most prevalent kinds of cancer in adults. The descriptions of blood cell lineage, different forms of leukemia, current diagnostic techniques, available treatments, and prognostic variables are all covered in the parts that follow to help readers better understand leukemia.

2.2   COMPONENTS OF BLOOD

The heart and blood vessels (veins and arteries), as seen in Figure 2.2, pump the crimson, life-sustaining fluid known as blood throughout the body. The blood circulates throughout the body, supplying nutrition and oxygen to the tissues (Bain 2010). Four primary components of blood are shown in Table 2.1.

Lymphoid and myeloid hematopoietic stem cells are the source of all blood cells, which develop from the BM (Ciesla 2007). Figure 2.3 shows the maturation process of several blood cells.

Table 2.1 Four major blood components (Paul 2006).

Components of Blood	Explanation
RBCs **Erythrocytes**	RBCs is to transport oxygen from the lungs to the body's tissue and organs and to return carbon dioxide to the lungs.
WBCs **Leukocytes**	The immune system, which WBCs are a components of, protects the body against both illnesses and foreign objects
Platelets **Thrombocytes**	At the location of an injury, platelets are in charge of assisting with blood clotting and subsequent wound healing
Plasma	Numerous vital components, including gases, waste products, nutrition, and antibodies, are carried by blood plasma

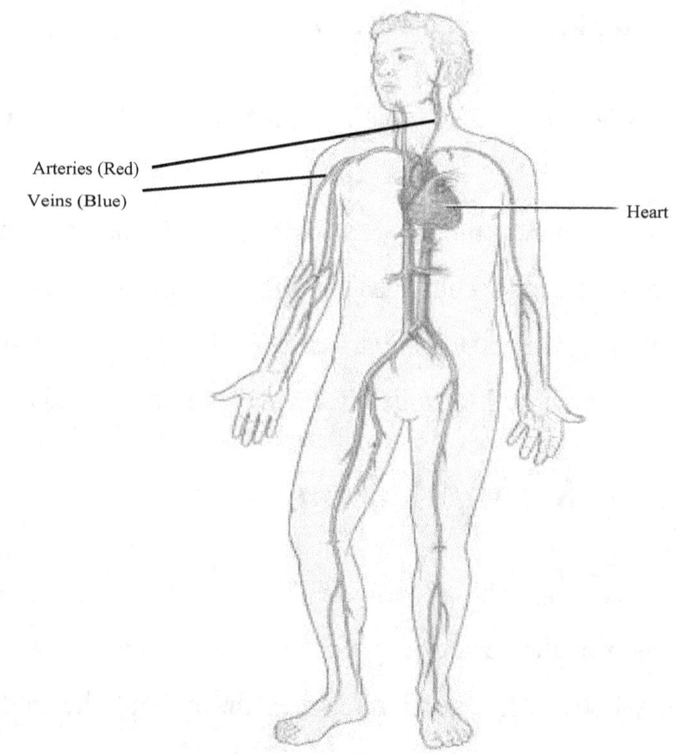

Figure 2.2 Human Body Blood Flow System (Ciesla, 2007)

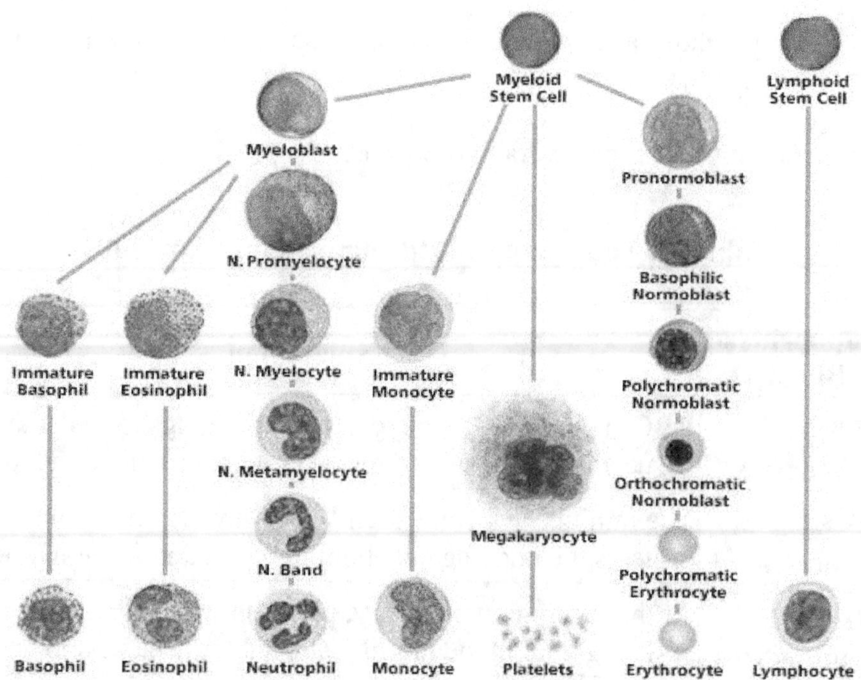

Figure 2.3 Development of Blood cell and flow diagram (Lofsness 2008)

2.2.1   Basics of Leukocytes

WBCs typically have a bigger size than platelets and RBCs. According to Esteridge *et al.* (2000), WBCs are the least abundant blood cell component, with only 5000–10,000 present in each microliter of blood, compared to 150,000 platelets.

Neutrophils, monocytes, lymphocytes, basophils and eosinophils are the five kinds of WBCs found in human blood, as indicated in Table 2.2. The percentages of each kind of WBC in healthy human blood are as follows: neutrophils 5070%, eosinophils 1-4%, basophils 0-1%, monocytes 2-8%, and lymphocytes 20.40%. Calculating the ratio of several types of WBC is the procedure of differential.

Table 2.2 Types of WBCs

WBCs Type	Description
Monocyte	Compared to other PB leucocytes, they are often bigger. Defense against bacteria, fungi, virus, and a foreign substance is the primary role of monocytes.
Eosinophil	In terms of size, nuclear morphology, chromatin pattern, and nuclear/cytoplasm ratio, eosinophils are comparable to neutrophils. The fundamental distinction between them is the existence of eosinophil cytoplasmic homogeneous, coarse, and red granules. They offer defense against parasites and aid in removing fibrin that is produced during inflammation
Basophil	One can only find basophil cells in healthy blood plasma. Heparin and histamine are found in the numerous black granulocytes that cover the nucleus of these cells.
Lymphocyte	These immune-competent cells support phagocytes in the body's defense against infection and other external invaders. The immune system's capacity to produce antigenic specificity and phenomena of immunological memory are two distinctive traits.
Neutrophil	A whitish cytoplasm surrounds the nucleus, which contain two to five lobes. The granules are separated in to primary and secondary, with the former appearing at the promyelocyte stage and the latter predominating in the adult neutrophil. Neutrophils in blood have a 10h.

2.3   LUEKEMIA TYPES

The numerous blood cell maturation processes and the steps they go through before becoming adult cells and entering the circulation are depicted in Figure 2.4.

Leukemia is often divided into two categories asacute leukemia and chronic leukemia (Bain 2010). Refer to Figure 2.3 for additional classification of leukemia based on predominant PB and BM cell types, which are classified as either myeloid or lymphoid depending on cell lineage (Ciesla 2007).

Types of leukemia are acute lymphoblastic leukemia (ALL), acute myeloid leukemia (AML), chronic lymphocytic leukemia (CLL), and chronic myeloid leukemia (CML).The four leukemia kinds are displayed in Table 2.3.

Table 2.3 Types of Leukemia

Progression	Stem Cell	Type	Description
Acute	Lymphoid	ALL	For children, leukemia is most prevalent. Adults over 65 years are also affected.
	Myeloid	AML	It grows in both children and adults.
Chronic	Lymphoid	CLL	It mostly affects adults only.
	Myeloid	CML	Adults over 55 are affected most frequently. Younger people may occasionally have it, although children are rarely affected

2.4   LEUKEMIA'S EARLY SIGNS

Many signs and symptoms could be there for leukemia. The symptoms are non-specific and typically include fever, weight loss, and appetite loss.

The typical symptoms of acute and chronic leukemia, which can harm the spleen, muscles, skin, lungs, bones, and joints, are shown in Figure 2.4. When the full constellation is missing, the non-specific signs and symptoms of leukemia are easily confused with other benign illnesses, like viral infections.

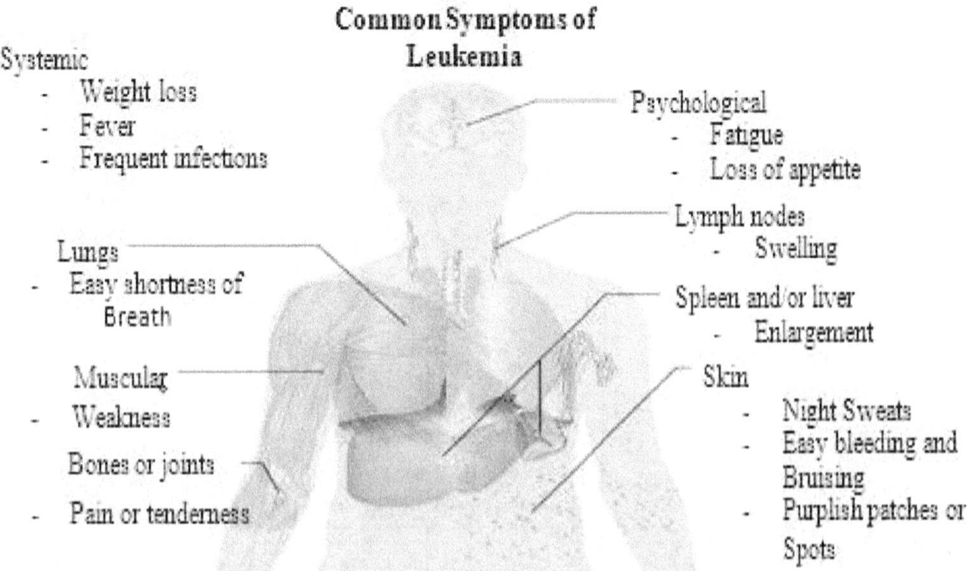

Figure 2.4 Leukemia Common Symptoms (Häggström 2009)

2.5   ACUTE LEUKEMIA LABORATORY DIAGNOSIS

Multiple laboratory tests are needed to diagnose acute leukemia. A routine physical examination will be performed on the subject to check for any abnormalities, such as swollen lymph nodes and bleeding areas. The PB will be subjected to a microscopic morphological investigation if the clinician detects acute leukemia (Please Refer to Section 2.5.2).

Based on the results of the microscopic morphological examination, BM examination along with other laboratory tests, such as BM aspirate morphological examination, immunophenotyping, and cytogenetics analysis (please refer to Sections 2.5.3, 2.5.4, and 2.5.5, respectively), would be necessary. (2012) (American Cancer Society).

Figure 2.5 illustrates the critical steps a haematologist must take to diagnose a patient with acute leukemia. Each step in Figure 2.5 is explained in Table 2.4.

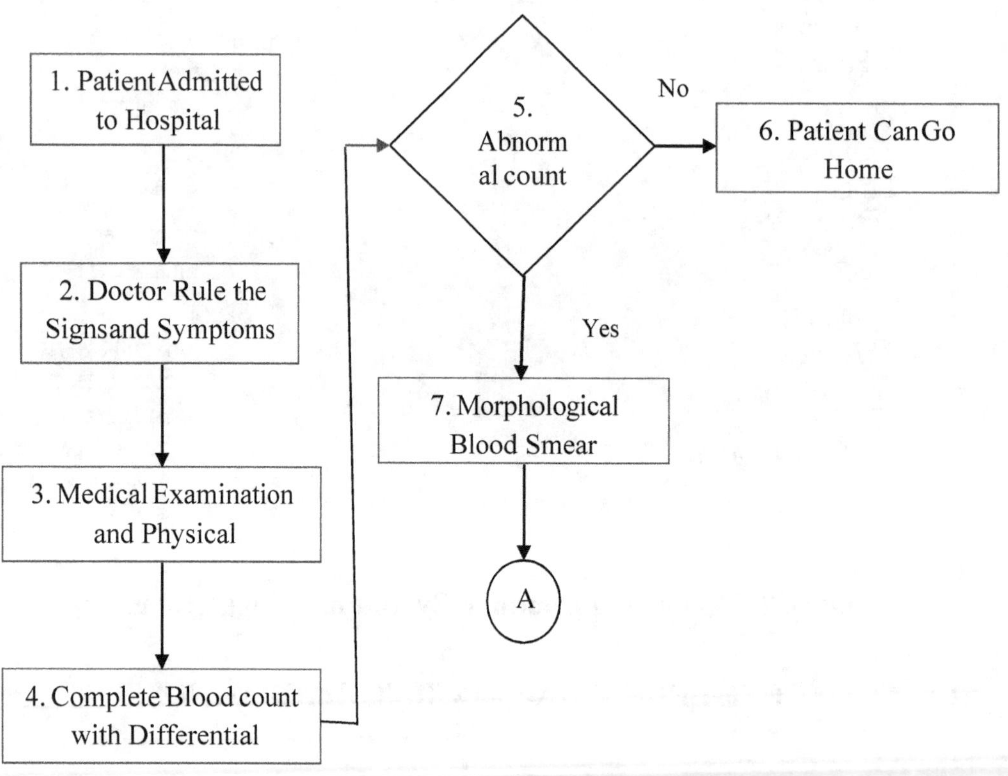

Figure 2.5 (a) Diagnosis Steps to Confirm Acute Leukemia (Part A)

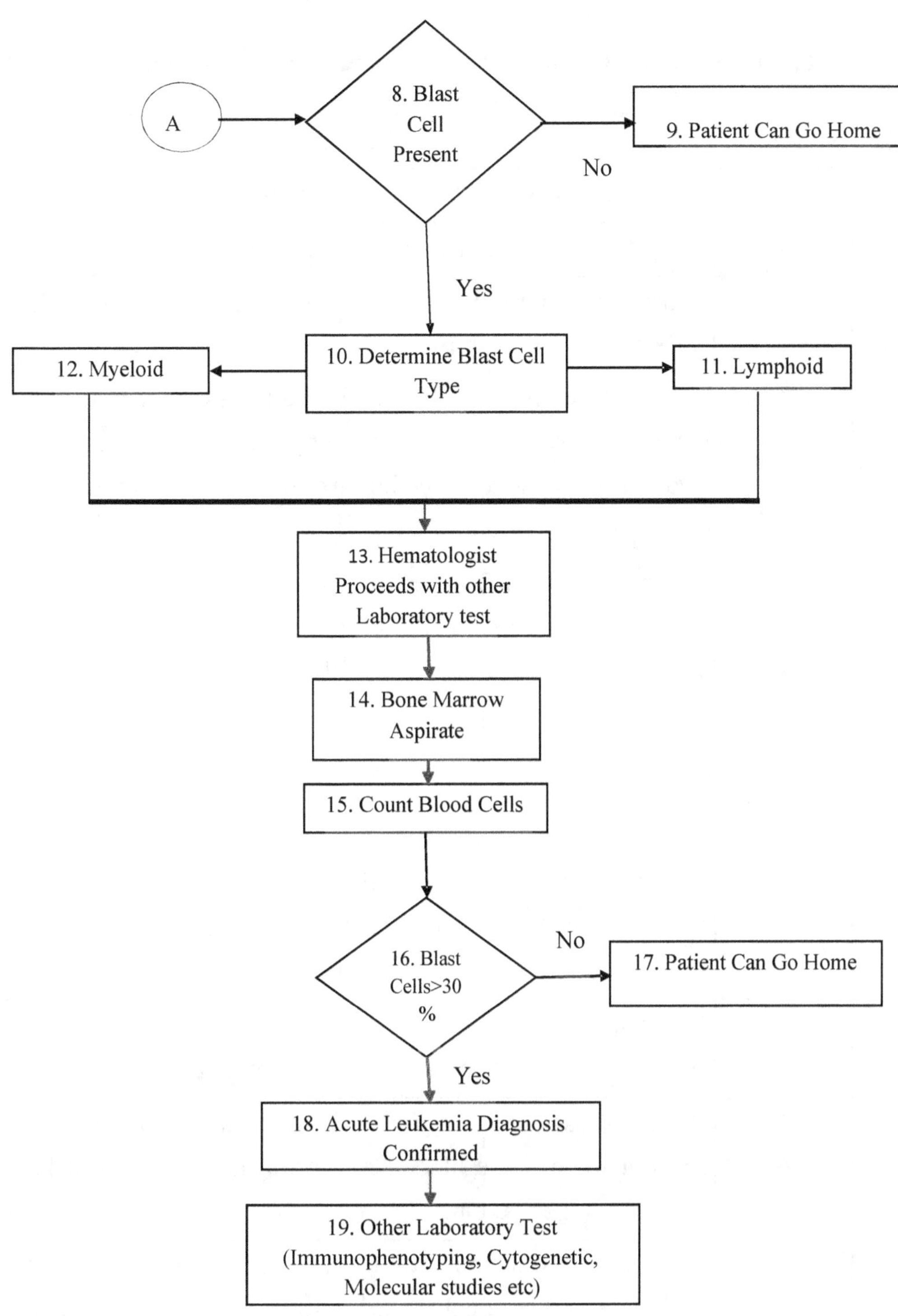

Figure 2.5 (b) Diagnosis Steps to Confirm Acute Leukemia (Part B)

Table 2.4 Details of each step in the acute leukemia diagnosis process

Step	Description
1	A person undergoing hospital treatment
2	The patient's symptoms will be questioned by the doctor
3	In order to determine the symptoms, the doctor will look up the patient's medical history. At this stage, the physician will do a physical examination of the patient in order to search for any further symptoms, such as swollen lymph nodes, bleeding wounds, skin rashes, etc.
4	To determine if there is an aberrant blood count, a Complete Blood Count with Differential is necessary. We'll check the white blood cell, red blood cell, and platelet counts. The proportion of WBCs in healthy persons is as follows: • Neutrophils 50-70% • Eosinophils 1-4% • Basophils 0-1%, • Monocytes 2-8% • Lymphocytes 20.40%. Typically, the haematology analyzer will perform the blood count and a venous blood sample will be obtained.
5	The Hematology Analyzer does the blood count, and it also examines the counts of the five different kinds of WBCs
6	Other illnesses must be looked into and the patient can probably be discharged if the blood test shows no indication of leukemia and a normal cell count
7	A PB smear is made and the slide is given to a haematologist or laboratory professional for microscope morphological inspection of the PB smear in the event that clinical concerns exist and/or a haematology analyzer detects certain abnormalities in blood count.

Table 2.4 (Continued)

Step	Description
8	To determine if there are any blast cells in the smear, a microscope morphological analysis is carried out.
9	In the absence of any indication of blasts in the PBF from the blood count, other illnesses need to be looked into before the patient is likely allowed to return home.
10	If PB smear contains blast cells, it is important to identify the lineage of the blast cells.
11	Lymphoid: Planning and management for **ALL** treatment
12	Myeloid: Planning and management for **AML** treatment
13	The doctor does further laboratory tests to validate the initial diagnosis based on the findings of the morphological analysis of the PB smear.
14	Bone Marrow biopsy is taken from the patient
15	Determine the proportion of blast cells in the bone marrow.
16	According to the WHO classification, blasts should make up roughly 30% of cells to indicate the existence of leukemia. 5% or less is regarded as usual.
17	The presence of additional illnesses must be looked into if the proportion of blast cells is within the normal range advised by the WHO, after which the patient can likely return home.
18	Once the kind of acute leukemia is identified in order to provide the appropriate therapy, the diagnosis of acute leukemia is established if the proportion of blast cells is greater than 30%.
19	Additional laboratory testing (cytogenetic, immunophenotyping, Studies on molecules, etc.)

2.5.1 Complete Blood Count (CBC)

The CBC is one of the lab tests most frequently used in standard medical practice. This test measures WBCs, RBCs, platelets, haemoglobin, differential WBC count, etc. CBCs are frequently performed in laboratories using automated machines known as haematology analyzers. Figure 2.6 depicts the Sysmex automated haematology analyzer (Diamond Diagnostics, 2013).

In automated haematology analyzers, the "flow cytometry" principle is employed, which makes use of a specific pressure and aperture configuration to force blood samples through a small aperture. The cells and other elements of the blood sample are released one at a time through the hole. Cells passing through the aperture produce a variety of signal types, which are subsequently collected and transformed to digital form for transformation, counting, histogram accumulation, and other analyses.

To count a very small number of white cells, however, automated counts can fall short. (Bain 2010).

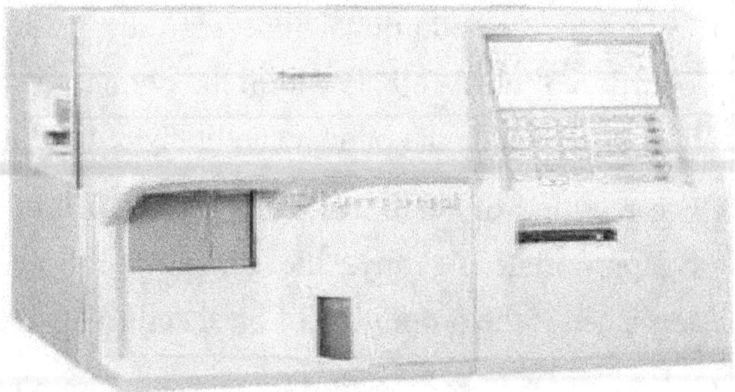

Figure 2.6 Hematology Analyzer Sysmex KX21N

Automated cell counts have a number of significant limitations, including the fact that the information they generate about cell morphology is quite restricted (the shape, structure, form, and size of cells). They are also unable to accurately categorize blast cells. Results are automatically highlighted when irregularities are found in the blood sample, though. In this instance, a microscopic morphological evaluation of the diseased cells is necessary (please refer to Section 2.5.2).

2.5.2   Analyzing a Peripheral Blood Smear's Morphology

In order to differentiate between ALL and AML, the diagnosis of acute leukemia still significantly relies on microscopic morphological examination of stained PB and BM aspirates smears.

The PB smear may be sufficient to establish a diagnosis in some cases, but reviewing the smear is an important adjunct to additional clinical findings. (Bain 2010).

Figure 2.7 outlines the steps for taking a patient's blood sample and making a PB smear. Blood samples are often taken from the vein in order to diagnose acute leukemia. On a glass microscope slide, a drop of colored blood is applied. (Riley *et al.* 2012).

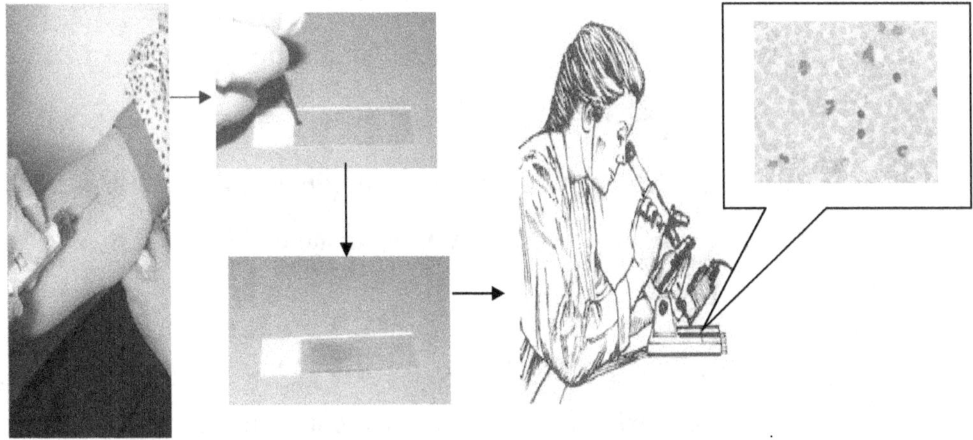

Figure 2.7 Description of PB smear preparation and examination

The following limitations may make it difficult to manually examine the PB smear's morphology:

- Uncleanly made or discolored blood streaks.

- Time commitment. The PB smear test cannot be considered a quick procedure, even when carried out by a skilled professional, because the operator must carefully examine the morphology of the blast cells (size, shape, nucleus chromatin structure) in order to make the correct diagnosis and ensure that the proper therapy will be given. Human mistake is possible during the process.

There might be a backlog and delays if there is a requirement for microscopic morphological analysis of PB smears but not enough qualified staff to perform it.

Following is a summary of the contribution made by the microscopic morphological analysis of PB smear:

- It provides details about the patient's status, with each WBC type's count potentially indicating a different disease. For instance, a patient has leukemia if their blast cell count is greater than 30%.

- To determine the patient's prognosis, the doctor might need to do a cytogenetic test, for instance, if the PB smear reveals blast

- It serves as a manual for treatment. On the eighth day of treatment for leukemia patients, the PB smear must be inspected in order to count the quantity of circulating blast cells.

- Patients who are classified as "poor-risk" and will receive more intensive chemotherapy, whereas patients who are classified as "good-risk" and will receive less intensive treatment (Madhloom *et al.* 2012b).

- It serves a warning sign for the negative consequences of chemotherapy and radiation treatment. The doctor should thus closely follow this problem with a PB smear morphological investigation.

2.5.3 Examination of the Morphology of Bone Marrow Aspirates

In a few major bones, there is a specific type of fatty tissue called BM that contains stem cells (please see Figure 2.8). Undeveloped stem cells and excess iron are present in this unique tissue. When it comes time to replace aberrant, weak, or injured cells, stem cells do not differentiate.

A sample of BM cells that belong to AML may be shown in Figure 2.8. Figure 2.9 illustrates the procedure for collecting a BM sample visually.

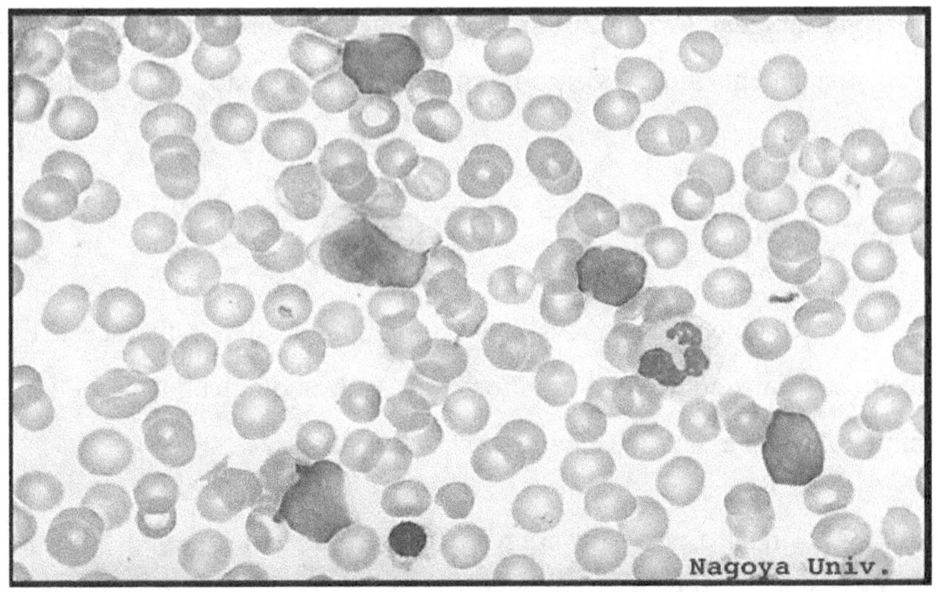

Figure 2.8 Sample of Bone Marrow (Ichihashi *et al.* 2013)

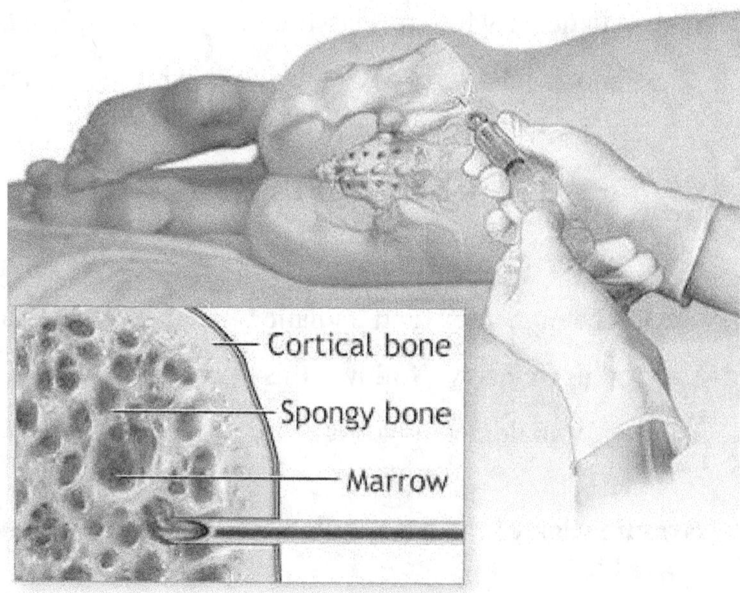

Figure 2.9 Bone Marrow Blood (Dugdale 2010).

2.5.4   Immunophenotyping

Cells are recognized by a procedure called immunophenotyping that takes into account the different antigens or markers that they have on their surface. It is possible to identify leukemia cell differentiation by using the right antigens (Wang 2014).To guarantee proper classification, all acute leukemia patients must undergo immunophenotyping, according to the current gold standard of care.

2.5.5   Cytogenetics

Cytogenetics analysis is an additional laboratory test used to diagnose leukemia in addition to morphological inspection and immunological assays (Reaman 2011).

Under a powerful microscope, chromosomes (small bits of DNA) are often examined for alterations during a cytogenetic examination. 23 pairs of chromosomes, each of a specified size and stain, may be found in a normal human cell. Chromosome alterations may be seen in some kinds of leukemia.

By recognizing the translocations, certain ALL and AML subtypes can be recognized, and the prognosis (outlook) can be determined (American Cancer Society 2012). The next section provides more information on how acute leukemia is classified.

2.6   ACUTE LEUKEMIA CATAGORIZATION

The classification are based on cytomorphology, cytochemistry, immunophenotyping, immunogenetics, and molecular cytogenetic. However, according to Reaman *et al.* (2011), the first categorization of acute leukemia is done primarily on morphology.

The best available treatment options are still enough distinct from one another, in addition to the natural history, for an inaccurate classification to have a negative impact on prognosis (Bain 2010). Laboratory haematology now uses two categorization approaches to divide acute leukemia into lymphoid and myeloid subtypes. The qualities of each categorization category are described in the sections that follow.

2.6.1   Classification system by French-American-British (FAB)

The FAB Cooperative Group has created standardized criteria to define acute leukemia's features and further subtype it. The morphological and cytochemical traits of both PB and BM smears are the only factors taken into consideration for the FAB categorization.

ALL is categorized into three subtypes (L1-L2-L3) according on the FAB classification, whereas AML is divided into eight subtypes (M0-M1-M2-M3-M4-M5-M6-M7). Tables 2.5 and 2.6, respectively, provide a summary of the morphological traits of cells belonging to the two types (ALL, AML) (Cairo & Perkins 2012).

Table 2.5   FAB   categorization   system-based   morphological characteristics of ALL subtypes

Acute Lymphoblastic Leukemia (ALL)					
Morphology	**Classification**	**Description**	**Nucleus**	**Chromatin**	**Cytoplasm**
	L1	Minimal to little cell-to-cell variation and small blasts with little cytoplasm	Round, homogeneous	Little reticulation and champing of the per nucleoli	Scant blue
	L2	Spherical nuclei with many nucleoli; larger cells with more cell-to-cell variance	Irregular, inhomogeneous	Fine	Moderate pale
	L3	Strongly basophilic cytoplasm, large cells, frequently having vacuoles, and many nucleoli	Round to oval homogenous	Coarse with clear Para-chromatin	Moderate blue Prominently vacuolated

Table 2.6   AML subtypes' morphological characteristics based on the FAB classification system

Acute Myeloid Leukemia (AML)					
Morphology	Classification	Description	Nucleus	Chromatin	Cytoplasm
	M0	Acute myeloblastic leukemia with little differentiation	Round to oval	Fine to coarse	Scant ace granulated
	M1	With just Spacadic granules, acute myelocytic leukemia cells are extremely undifferentiated	Round to oval	Fine	Scant Variably granulated
	M2	Acute myelocytic leukemia: more specialized cell that frequently have acute rods and granules	Round to oval	Fine	Moderate aerophilic granules with or without auet rods
	M3	Acute promyelocytic leukemia hyper granular promyelocytes	Round to indented lobed	Fine	Prominent aerophilic granules and/or multiple Auer rods
	M4	Acute promyelocytic leukemia: Myclocytes and monocytes co-dominase	Round to indented folded	Fine	Grey to blue is shade perhaps granular

Table 2.6 (Continued)

Acute Myeloid Leukemia (AML)					
Morphology	**Classification**	**Description**	**Nucleus**	**Chromatin**	**Cytoplasm**
	M5	Acute monocytic leukemia: monoblasts having cytoplasm that is mostly agranular	Round to indented folded	Variable lacy or ropy	Scant to moderate gray-blue, dust like lavender granules
	M6	Red blood cell precursors are the predominant kind of cell in erythroleckemia, while myeloid blasts can also be present	Single to bizarre	Open megaloblastoid	Abundant Red to blue

2.6.2 Classification framework by The World Health Organization (WHO)

The World Health Organization (WHO), the Society for Hematopathology, and the European Association of Hematopathology have all published a new classification system for acute leukemia. The principles that underlie this consensus categorization are derived from numerous published clinical and scientific investigations as well as from the cumulative experience of more than 100 pathologists, physicians, and scientists from around the world (Harris *et al.* 1999).

Table 2.7 Classification system of *ALL* by WHO

Precursor B-cell ALL/LBL
Cytogenetic subgroups t(9;22)(q34,q11),BCR/ABL t(v;11q23);MLL rearranged t(1;19)(q23;p13);PBX1/E2A t(12;21)(p13;q22);TEL/AML1
Hypodiploid
Hyperdiploid, >50 Precursor T-cell ALL/LBL
Mature B-cell leukemia/lymphoma

Table 2.8 Classification System of *AML by* WHO

Acute Myeloid Leukemia (AML) and Related Precursor Neoplasm
AML with recurrent genetic abnormalities
AML with t(8:21)(q22;22q); RUNX!-RUNX1T1
AML with inv(16)(p13.1q22)or t(16;16)(p13.1;q22);CBFB-MYH11
Acute promyelocytic leukemia with t(15;17)(q22;q12);PML-RARA
AML with t(9;11)(p22;q23);MLLT3-MLL
AML with inv(3)(q21q26.2) or t(3;3)(q21;q26.2);RPN1-EVI1
AML with mutated NPM1
AML with mutated CEBPA
AML with myelodysplasia-related changes
Therapy-related myeloid neoplasms
Myeloid sarcoma
Myeloid proliferations related to Down syndrome
Transient abnormal myelopoiesis
Myeloid leukemia associated with Down syndrome
Blastic plasmacytoid denderitic cell neoplasm

The FAB categorization system principally bases its assessment of the blast cells on their morphological characteristics, as was earlier stated in section 2.6.1. But the WHO classification system demands additional evaluation of the blast cells using molecular analysis and flow cytometry (Angelescu *et al.* 2012). Table 2.7 and Table 2.8 briefly describe the new categorization of *ALL* and *AML* similarly as suggested by WHO.

2.7   OPTIONAL THERAPIES FOR LEUKAEMIA

Several significant factors affect the acute leukemia therapy choices. When creating a treatment plan, it's need to consider the cytogenetic abnormalities of the blasts as well as clinical traits, such as the patient's age and involvement of the central nervous system (CNS). Chemotherapy is the core of treatment, and some regimens also include cranial irradiation for kids with CNS disorders.

2.8   DIAGNOSTIC FOR LEUKEMIA

Prognosis, according to Webster's New World Medical Dictionary, is the likelihood of a recovery. Another element of prognosis is the possibility of a disease's progression and end (Celik *et al.* 2006).

The survival rates at 5 years are typically used by doctors to gauge the prognosis of an illness. Patients who live five years following diagnosis are included in the survival statistics, regardless of whether they are in remission, that is, when their disease's symptoms have subsided.

These are typical variables that affect the prognosis of acute leukemia:

1.   The patient's age

2.   Gender

3.   WBCs are counted at the presentation.

4.   Cancer has spread to other body organs, like the brain.

5.   Genetic, immunological, and morphological subtypes

6.   The treatment's initial reaction

7.   Cytogenetic anomalies

The most prevalent type of cancer in youngsters is ALL. These tumors make for one-fourth of all pediatric cancers. Individuals older than 45 years old are more likely to develop it than younger adults. The recommended course of treatment for this illness is chemotherapy.

But owing to contemporary medical techniques, around 80% of the injured youngsters are fully recovered. The likelihood of a full recovery in adults has been estimated at 40%. (Greer *et al.* 2013).

AML, in contrast, has worse outcomes and is less common in children. There have been reports of a 50–60% event-free survival rate for childhood **AML** over the course of five years. Although the period of treatment is shorter for **AML** patients, they require more intense chemotherapy than **ALL** patients do.

Leukemia and blood are explored before to this chapter. The background information on leukemia and the many forms are then discussed. The two acute leukemia categorization systems were then discussed together with the detailed leukemia symptoms and the current diagnosis techniques with the benefits and drawbacks (FAB and WHO). The chapter's conclusion included the prognosis and available leukemia reatments.

2.9   IMAGE PROCESSING AND MACHINE LEARNING PROCESS

The purpose of this section is to highlight the significant techniques and procedures used in this investigation. The fundamental concepts of digital image process and machine learning techniques used in applications for the detection of acute leukemia are also discussed. Following is a summary of related research in the area, including studies that employed ML-based and image processing methods.

2.10   IMAGE PROCESSING BASICS

Understanding the concept of digital image processing is certainly required in order to properly comprehend the approaches discussed in this thesis. Focus is placed particularly on image segmentation methods.

2.10.1   Digital Representation of Microscopically Obtained Blood

A discrete two-dimensional function with spatial coordinates and is the typical definition of a digital picture. The value at any coordinates is referred to as the image element (pixels).

The bottom right corner of a digital picture is represented by the spatial coordinate 1, whereas the top left corner is represented by the spatial point 0, 0. An example microscopic PB picture is displayed in Figure 2.10 on a grid, with a focus on the upper-left and lower-right corners.

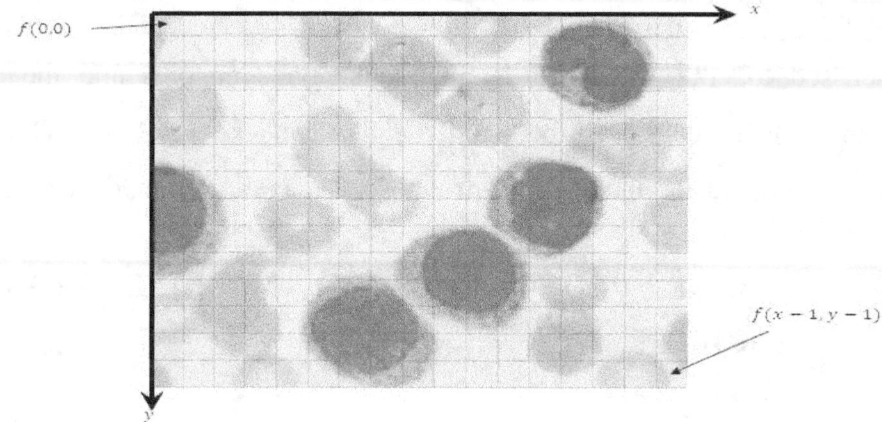

Figure2.10 Illustration of Microscopic PB digital image

In essence, there are various categories of digital photos. Binary, grayscale, and color are the three most used types. (Umbaugh 2010).

Two pixels constitute a binary image, and each of them can either be black (pixel value = 0) or white (pixel value = 1). Pixels with a value of 1 are used to represent the foreground, whereas pixels with a value of 0 are used to represent the background. The Mona Lisa picture is shown in binary format in Figure 2.11 (a).

A binary image consists of two pixels, which, depending on the image, can either be black (pixel value = 0) or white (pixel value = 1). Pixels with a value of 1 are used to represent the foreground, whereas pixels with a value of 0 are used to represent the background.

Each pixel in a colour image is given three values, which stand for the light's brightness and chrominance. Each of the pixels in this plane are thought of as 3-D vectors. Figure 2.11 depicts the Mona Lisa's colour rendition (c). The three most used colour spaces are Lab (Luminance, Chromatic Components), HSV (Hue, Saturation, Value), and RGB (Red, Green, Blue).

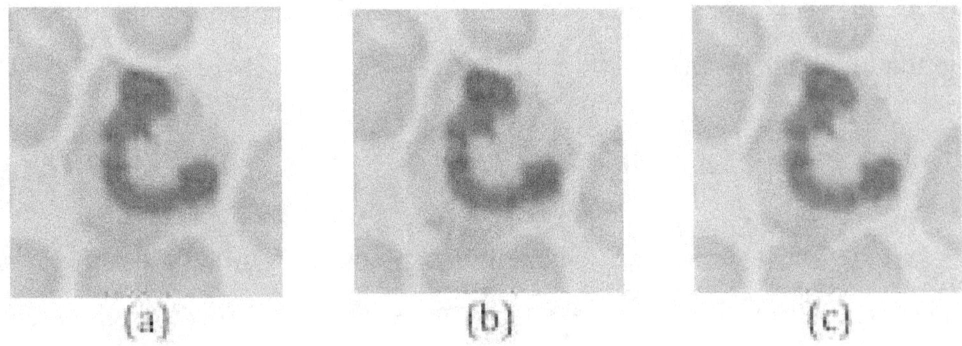

Figure 2.11 Types of Digital image (a) Color image (b) Grayscale image (c) Binary image

2.10.2 Microscopic Blood Images

The bulk of medical imaging techniques used in the first half of the 20th century, such as computed tomography (CT), magnetic resonance imaging (MRI), and X-rays, provide grayscale images. As a result, applications for medical image processing neglect color attributes.

Colour image processing might be viewed as a new field when contrasted to grayscale image processing. Because of this, processing colored medical images presents significant hurdles for researchers because many methods created for binary images are frequently inappropriate for processing colored medical images.

Colors can be represented as tuples of numbers, often with three components. This representation is explained by an abstract mathematical model known as a "color space" (Pise *et al.* 2010). Careful color space selection is essential for the implementation of picture segmentation.

While PB images are frequently captured in RGB colour space, multiple studies have revealed that other colour spaces, like HSV and Lab, may be more efficient than RGB in terms of extracting blast cells (Madhloom *et al.* 2012). The best colour schemes for identifying blast cells are discussed in the following sections.

2.10.2.1 Image Segmentation

The technique of segmenting a picture involves dividing it into discrete, relevant parts that are both homogenous and distinct based on factors like colour, texture, and other factors. It is nearly probable that mistakes in the segmentation procedure result in errors in any later analyses.

It is thought to be the most challenging phase in creating a computer-based acute leukemia diagnosis. It is essential that the blast cells are accurately recognized because if any component of the blast cell is excluded, shape, colour, and texture-based information may be lost.

Since AML and ALL blast cells have different morphologies, as shown in Tables 2.5 and 2.6, the form and structural properties of the blast cells are crucial for diagnosis (Cairo & Perkins 2012).

Blast cells may be segmented using a variety of visual attributes, including as colour, grey level intensity, shape, and texture. As a result, many techniques for extracting blast cells from PB pictures have been devised. The existing blast cells segmentation algorithms are : (1) Pixels-based threshold, employed in studies by Scotti (2005) deciding on a threshold value or values that designate the ROI as the foreground and the rest of the image as the background (Nasir *et al.* 2009; Madhloom *et al.* 2012) (2) Edge-based methods, which identify the borders between the foreground and background regions using edge operators, are (Scotii 2005) (3) Techniques that aggregate the pixels into homogenous areas using algorithms for region-merging and regionsplitting (Osowski *et al.* 2004; 2009; Markiewicz *et al.* 2005) (4) Color-clustering techniques that use unsupervised clustering algorithms to divide the colour space into homogenous sections, used by (Sabino *et al.* 2003); (5) Morphological techniques that employ a preset seed and either erosion, dilation, or a mix of both to find the ROI have been employed in works by (Scotti 2005; Khashman & Al-Zgoul 2009, Madhloom *et al.* 2012). (6) Active-contour techniques, such as snakes, establish the shape's contours by the use of curve evolution techniques. It is evident that the majority of the earlier works may be categorized using different segmentation approaches.

This fact suggests that a significant number of earlier investigations integrated the findings of several segmentation methods. Scotii (2005) developed a blast cell segmentation technique that integrates edge detection, mathematical morphology, and application to grayscale PB images to recover leukocytes and separate the nucleus from the cytoplasm.

In our initial study, we removed lymphoblast from PB images with many blast cells using a mix of mathematical morphology and a pixels-based threshold applied to HSV colour space. (Madhloom *et al.* 2012).

2.11   EXTRACTION AND ANALYSIS OF FEATURES

The identification of appropriate characteristics that can accurately distinguish distinct patterns is a fundamental problem in any pattern classification system (Osowski *et al.* 2009). Typically, feature extraction involves analyzing an image's visual data to yield characteristics including shape, texture, and colour as shown in Figure 2.12.

It is widely known that there is not a single effective set of traits that can be applied to all applications (Esposito & Malerba 2001). However, in order to improve detection accuracy, one or more traits are commonly combined (Akilandeswari *et al.* 2012).

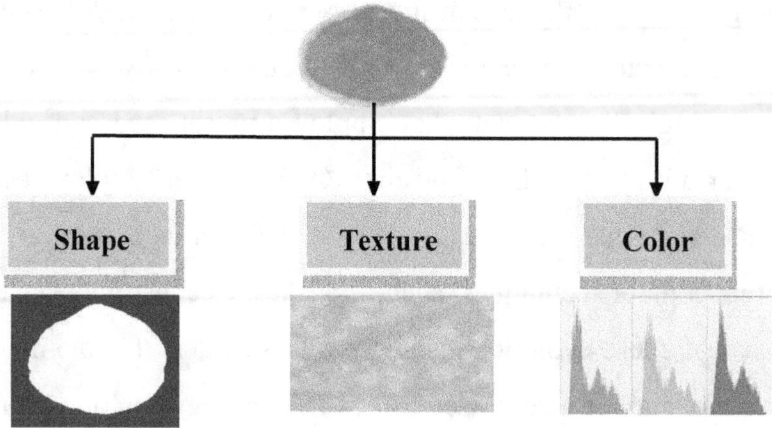

Figure 2.12 Image features representation

Acute leukemia is divided into two primary kinds for the problem of diagnosis and categorization (***ALL*** and ***AML***). Each acute leukemia type is categorized according to the FAB classification based on certain morphological traits.

Shape, texture, and colour were the three categories of attributes used in this investigation. The next sections go into great length on the theoretical information for each feature group.

2.11.1   Features Based on Shape

Shape is a noticeable visual characteristic and is one of the essential characteristics for object recognition. However, describing key form characteristics and determining how similar two shapes are to one another can be highly challenging tasks.

Furthermore, noise, imperfection, and occlusion frequently have an impact on form (Zhang & Lu 2004). The hierarchy of form types is shown in Figure2.13.

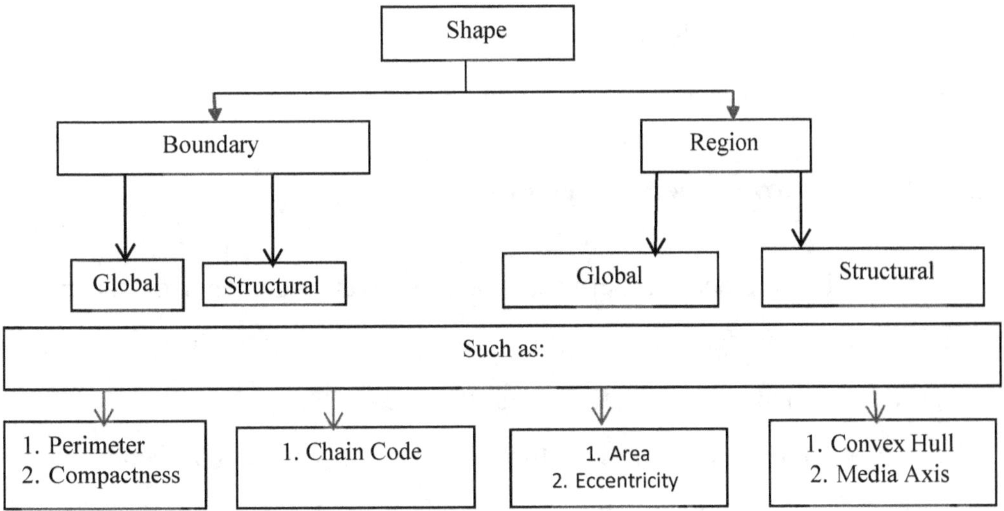

Figure 2.13 Techniques for categorizing form representation and description

Boundary-based approaches solely utilize the ROI's contour data; they entirely neglect interior features like perimeter, circularity, eccentricity, etc. As opposed to this, the region-based method considers both the inner and exterior features of the ROI, including the area size and the lengths of the major and minor axes.

Many methodologies are divided into subcategories within each class, such as global approaches and structural approaches. This subclass includes shapes that are represented as a whole, in segments, or in parts (primitives). (Zhang & Lu 2004).

Despite the fact that they are rarely necessary for classification, these traits can be utilized to distinguish between various types of cells (Rodenacker & Bengtsson 2003). The reader is advised to for more details on shape and size issues (Costa & Cesar 2000). The characteristics of the blast cells include size, shape, cytoplasm content, nucleus size and shape, and cytoplasm constituents (Ismail *et al.* 2010).

In this work, attention has been given to a subset of shape attributes from the two previously mentioned categories to determine how much they can aid in the identification of acute leukemia blast cells.

2.11.2   Features Based on Texture

The interactions between the spatial arrangements of the picture pixels in digital images serve as a representation of texture. They are seen as variations in pattern strength or grey tones (Osowski *et al.* 2004). The two fundamental types of texture are tactile textures and visual textures. An illustration of how tactile textures relate to the sense of touch is the sensation we get when we touch a smooth or rough surface.

Visual textures are small-scale variations in colour, direction, and intensity that occur locally inside an image. They are what texture looks like to a human viewer (Wilson & Moore 2010). Figure 2.14 shows several examples of various texture feature patterns.

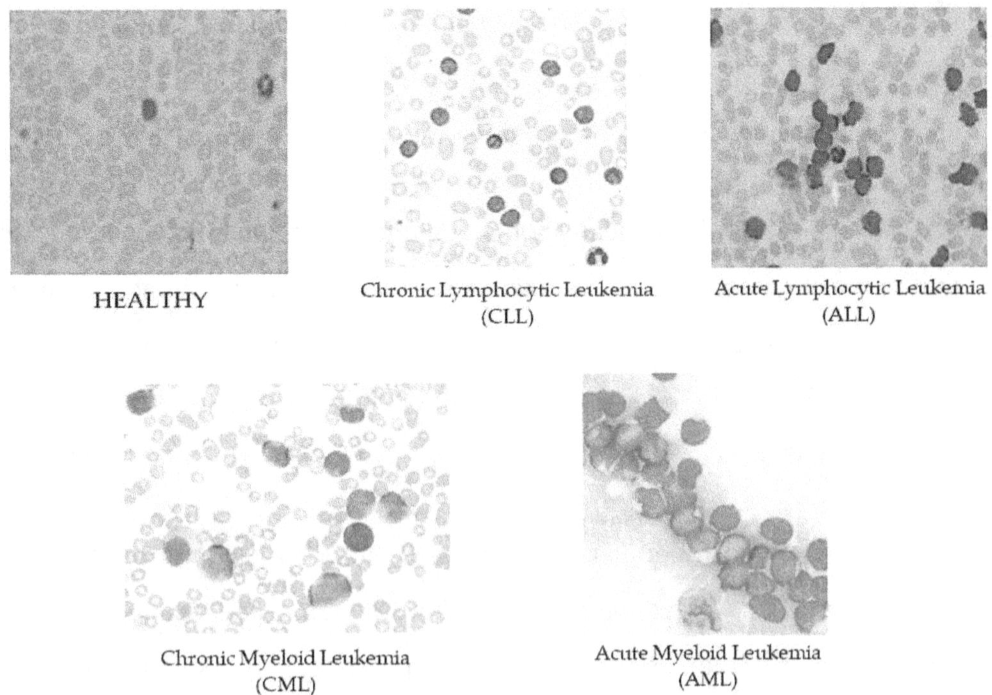

Figure 2.14 Samples of textures

The four basic types of texture feature extraction approaches are structural, model, transform, and statistical. In this study, two statistical feature extraction methods—the Gray Level Co-occurrence Matrix (GLCM) and Histogram-based statistics are used.

Depending on how many pixels make up the local feature, statistical approaches can be categorized as first-order (one pixel), second-order (a pair of pixels), or higher-order (three pixels or more). First-order statistics estimate properties (such as average and variance) of individual pixel values by ignoring the spatial interaction between image pixels, whereas second-order and higher-order statistics estimate properties of two or more pixel values occurring at specific locations relative to each other.

The co-occurrence matrix serves as the source of the most often used second-order statistical characteristics for texture analysis. It has been shown that second-order statistical techniques, or statistics provided by pairs of pixels, outperform power spectrum techniques. (transform-based) and structural methods in terms of discriminating rates (Castellano *et al.* 2004).

In general, medical photos contain a large quantity of texture data that may be crucial for clinical diagnosis. The classification of acute leukemia and other damaged tissues, such as the liver, thyroid, breasts, kidneys, prostate, heart, brain, and lungs, have all benefited by the addition of texture information (James *et al.* 2001; Sinha *et al.* 1997; Osowski *et al.* 2009).

The most popular texture-based analysis techniques in medical pictures are those based on statistics. Furthermore, statistical techniques to texture analysis outperform other approaches, such as structural or transform methods, and have attained higher discrimination indices (Castellano *et al.* 2004).

In this study, texture features are extracted using two alternative statistical-based methods: the Histogram-based methodology and the Gray Level Co-occurrence Matrix (GLCM). The next sections provide a theoretical underpinning for the chosen texture analysis techniques.

2.11.3 Approach Based on Histograms

An image's histogram is generated using the frequency at which each unique gray-level intensity value appears in the picture. The histogram, then, contains the first-order statistical data about the image. (Srinivasan & Shobha 2008; Selvarajah & Kodituwakku 2011).

A picture with 16 grey level intensity values is shown as a histogram in Figure 2.15(a–b). Gray level intensity levels are represented by the histogram element's indices (0–15). The number of pixels with a certain intensity value is indicated by each bin in the histogram. Figure 2.15 (a) displays the histogram bins, whereas Figure 2.15 (b) displays the number of pixels in each grey level intensity.

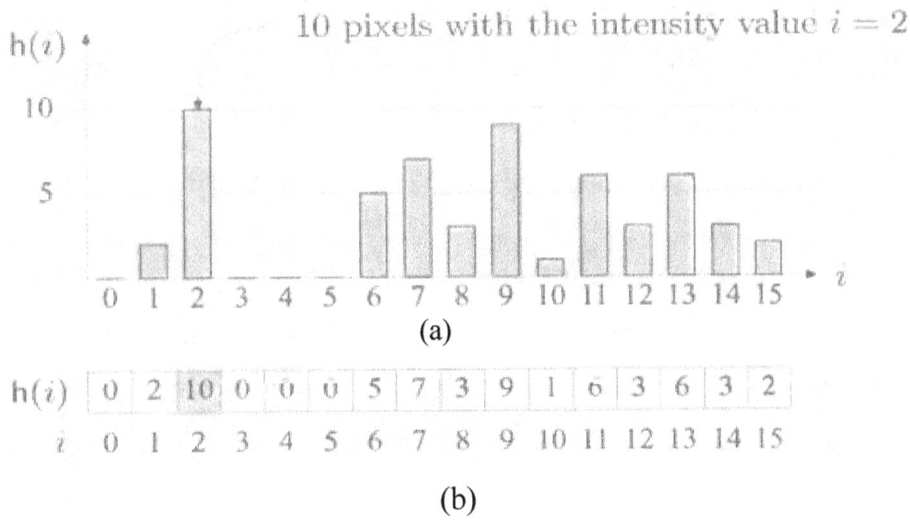

Figure 2.15 Histogram of image with 16 gray-level intensity (a) Histogram bins (b) Number of pixels in each gray level intensity (Burger & Burge 2009)

Based on the histogram statistics, it is possible to determine a variety of textural qualities, such as mean, standard deviation, average energy, entropy, skewness, and kurtosis (Suematsu *et al.* 2002). The histogram's dispersion is measured by the standard deviation, and the average intensity of the image is represented by the mean. The skewness and kurtosis, respectively, assess the dissymmetry and flatness of the grey level distribution.

Many medical applications, particularly in the diagnosis of cancers like cervical cancer, breast cancer, lung cancer and acute leukemia, have shown the value of the texture characteristics retrieved from picture histogram.

2.12 SELECTION OF FEATURES

In order to accurately describe the phenomena under research, it is typical to extract the broadest feature set during pattern categorization. This approach is typically thought to be successful. However, a lot of features could cause issues (Kuncheva 2004). Now, the idea of feature selection is put into action. Choosing a strong collection of characteristics to properly classify the target classes is the process of feature selection. The terms variable selection, attribute selection, and subset selection are also used to describe it.

However, if feature selection is not done on the dataset, these traits would still be present in the dataset and would negatively affect the performance of the classifier. Many features in pattern recognition are typically redundant or unneeded. Additionally, a high dimensionality of attributes makes it challenging to categorize data due to a phenomenon known as the "curse of dimensionality."

The following are some benefits of feature selection: (1) dimensionality reduction to decrease processing costs; (2) noise reduction to increase classification accuracy; (3) extra interpretable traits or characteristics to aid in identifying and tracking the phenomena being studied (Ding & Peng 2005).

The three basic classifications used to categorize feature selection procedures are filter methods, wrapper methods, and embedding methods. How the feature selection search is combined with the classification engine's design will determine how this categorization is achieved (Guyon & Elissee 2003).

The classifier's characteristics are ignored by filter methods since it uses statistical tests to rank the features. Low-scoring features are subsequently eliminated after the feature set is organized according to the score (Guyon & Elissee 2003).

Filter methods ignore feature dependencies; this may lead to worse classification performance when compared to other types of feature selection techniques such as wrapper or embedded methods (Saeys *et al.* 2007).

The feature selection procedure is encircled by the learning algorithm in the second feature selection strategy, known as the wrapper. Benefits of wrapper techniques include the interaction between feature subset search and model selection as well as the ability to take feature dependencies into consideration. However, compared to filter approaches, these strategies depend more on the classifier and need more computation (Guyon & Elissee 2003; Saeys *et al.* 2007).

Embedded approaches make up the third category of feature selection techniques. When using embedded approaches, the learning and feature selection phases are combined. Instead of treating the classifier as a black box to evaluate classification accuracy, it directly uses the classifier's parameters. Like wrapper methods, embedding methods also depend on the classifier (Guyon & Elissee 2003; Saeys *et al.* 2007).

2.13 CLASSIFICATION OF PATTERNS

Pattern classification is the process of categorizing input patterns (like blast cells) into one of a predetermined list of classes (like ALL, AML) according to the traits that are discovered during the feature extraction phase (e.g. shape, texture, Color) (2006) Patel and Marwala.

2.14   REVIEW ON DIAGNOSIS AND CLASSIFICATION OF COMPUTER-BASED ACUTE LEUKEMIA

The initial stage in the sequence of the leukemia diagnosis process is typically microscopic morphological examination of the peripheral blood (PB) smear, despite the availability of alternative cutting-edge diagnostic procedures like flow cytometry, immunophenotyping, and cytogenetic analysis.

The accuracy of the manual technique, on the other hand, is only predicted to be between 60% and 70%, making this diagnostic procedure still difficult and having a restricted degree of precision (Nasir *et al.* 2013).

Many researchers have used ML and image processing approaches to address this issue. Compared to a subjective manual technique, a computer-based acute leukemia diagnosis gives a quantitative and objective assessment of the blast cells.

It reduces inter-observer variability, enabling repeatable diagnosis. Additionally, by automating the analysis, it lessens the amount of time that the haematologist or laboratory professional must spend on boring and repeated activities.

As a result of improvements in microscope imaging technology and image processing techniques as well as because of the morphological variations between blast cells, which make it an ingratiating topic to work on, there has been a significant increase in interest in the development of computer-based acute leukemia diagnostic systems. In the subsections that follow, the techniques for diagnosing and classifying acute leukemia based on the morphological characteristics of blast cells are critically discussed.

2.14.1   Acquisition of peripheral blood images

Any image recognition system's initial stage is often regarded as picture acquisition. For both medical professionals and non-professionals, getting a picture with the right lighting intensity, high resolution, clarity, and accuracy is a challenging process because of the sophisticated settings for the video camera and the microscope (Madhloom *et al.* 2012).

Prior to the early 1990s, the majority of microscopic applications that required image capture were carried out using closed-circuit television (CCTV) cameras and frame grabbers (Rajendran *et al.* 2008).

Present days, Charge-Coupled Device (CCD) cameras, which are mounted atop microscopes, have taken the role of the analogue cameras. Figure 2.16 depicts a modern microscope with a mounted digital camera linked to a computer.

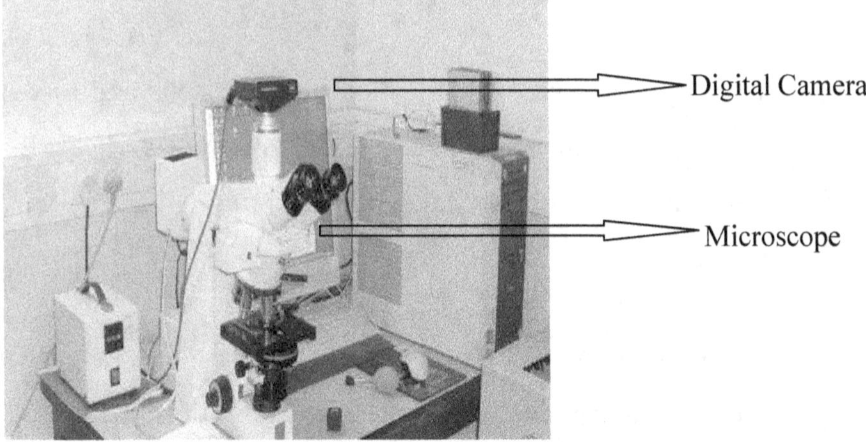

Figure 2.16 Digital camera in Microscope (Zephyris 2007)

The light microscope, in which the specimen and lenses are directly illuminated by visible light, is the most common microscopic apparatus used in clinical laboratories (Estridge & Reynolds 2011). A light microscope has at least three objective lenses. These magnifying glasses frequently make things bigger by 10, 40, and 100 times, respectively (Pommerville 2009).

A 100x objective lens must be used to take the blood smear image in order to perform a thorough visual inspection. High-quality blood smear photography requires a variety of considerations, such as a well-prepared blood smear, balanced lighting, and the ideal evaluation region of the blood smear from which to take pictures (Rodak *et al.* 2007).

The mechanics of how blood photographs were taken were left out of several earlier literary works (Osowski *et al.* 2004, Markiewicz *et al.* 2005, Osowski *et al.* 2009).This may be because the researchers did not participate in the acquisition procedure when they acquired the digital blood imaging data sets from the hospital. While this was going on, other researchers talked in depth about the setup and tools used to get blood smear images.

2.14.2   Segmentation of Blast Cells

Image segmentation is used to find the blast cells and to separate them from background components like plasma and RBCs. It is thought to be the system's most difficult stage for identifying acute leukemia (Patil *et al.* 2012).

The most modern methods for segmenting blast cells are covered in this section. The techniques described in the literature do not fully address three important blast cells segmentation issues; these issues are as follows:

1. Recognizing the blast cells in the PB image and isolating them into a single sub-image

2. The proximity and overlap of cells.

3. Adjustment to variations in colour, lighting, and staining

Finding a blast cell and cropping it into a sub-image is a helpful step that enables each blast cell to be separately evaluated and categorized as either ALL or AML. (Problem1) One frequent issue resulting from the PB smear preparation process is the heterogeneous dispersion of cells in the sample (Nee *et al.* 2012).

The segmentation method should not include any clustered cells that are close to the cell of interest because otherwise the neighboring cell(s) and the cell of interest would be considered as a single item since there is no way to guarantee the quality of the cell allocation. This could lead to the retrieval of inaccurate characteristics (Problem 2). (Liao *et al.* 2002).

Additionally, blood images obtained using diverse types of capture device must not alter the segmentation approach (Problem 3). Markiewicz *et al.* (2005), according to the literature review, the current blast cells segmentation algorithms may be generally classified into six main techniques based on their underlying methodologies. There are six ways to do it: There are six different ways: (1) pixel-based threshold approaches, (2) edge-based approaches, (3) region-based approaches, (4) color-clustering approaches, (5) mathematical morphology approaches, and (6) active-contour based approaches. But the majority of the suggested algorithms in the literature incorporated a number of methods to remove blast cells from the picture.

Leukocytes and one type of leukemic cell, CLL, should be separated using a two-step semi-automatic segmentation technique, according to (Sabino *et al.* 2003). (Chronic Lymphocytic Leukemia). A sub-image was cropped using the Green channel threshold once the nucleus was identified. The nucleus, the cytoplasm, the erythrocytes, and the plasma were then separated from the pixels using the Bayesian Supervised Learning Algorithm based on the RGB colour pixels.

The segmentation was susceptible to changes in lighting and frequently restricted to a selection of photos with comparable staining characteristics. Additionally, cropping a single cell sub-image using the nucleus bounding box might result in an incomplete cell with omitted cytoplasm.

The watershed approach was applied by (Osowski *et al.* 2004) to segment blast cells in bone marrow aspirate pictures. After being converted to grayscale, binary, and then treated using morphological closure and erosion, the watershed was applied to the original picture. This method failed to differentiate a whole blast cell from the background, especially at the cytoplasmic boundary, according to (Osowski *et al.* 2004).

This could be because the erythrocytes close to the cytoplasm of the blast cell have the same values for the grey level. Later, the strategy outlined by Osowski *et al.* (2004) was utilized in a variety of research, including the works of (Markiewicz *et al.* 2005; Osowski *et al.* 2009). The study by used a mathematical morphology operator along with Canny edge detection (i.e. dilation and erosion).

A single lymphoblast cell in a gray scale blood smear image is recognized (Scotti 2005). Edge connecting is necessary to finish the contour of areas after edge detection; however this operation is quite difficult because it is unknown which edges are crucial and which are not (Zhang *et al.* 2004). The application of morphological dilation to link the edges was made possible by the premise that the edge size might vary within a given range (Scotti 2005).

The erroneous cell identification, however, can happen if the edge value is beyond the predicted range. Later, (Scotti 2005) suggested using the Otsu Threshold to divide the cytoplasm from the nucleus. Other researchers, used their segmentation algorithms to quickly isolate a single blast cell in a sub-image that had been meticulously cropped. (Khashman & Al-Zgou 2009).

The fundamental goal of this was to physically divide the cytoplasm from the nucleus. However, the sub-image was first processed using canny edge detection, then a gradient vector flow (GVF) active contour was used to identify the nucleus, and finally the Zack threshold was used to define the cytoplasm portion. In the study by Khashman & Al-Zgou (2009), the nucleus and cytoplasm were separated using a pixel-based threshold.

A segmentation method (M2-M3-M5) is utilized to divide acute leukemia blast cells into five distinct subtypes, including ALL (L1-L2) and AML. Both the Lab color space and the 2-D world decomposition texture model were used. The Markov Random Field was utilized to represent the color and texture data and to decide the positions of cell elements.

Using a rule-based classifier with reference to color and form features, the cytoplasm and nucleus were divided. Additionally, a conical shape was developed for a cell overlapping separation procedure employing linear interpolation in the polar space. Edge linking is a particularly challenging operation since it is unclear which edges are of relevance and which are not produced by this overlapping separation technique (Zhang *et al.* 2004).

The blood smear picture was segmented into blast cells using algorithms that, like those developed by, employed a preset threshold value (Patil *et al.* 2012; Halim *et al.* 2011).

A specified threshold value cannot be utilized to successfully segment all photos since the blood smear image may have originated from several sources, which causes a drop in segmentation performance due to a manually determined threshold. Due to constant absence of the cytoplasm area, none of these methods that employed a set threshold value were successful in extracting a full blast cell.

In our early research (Madhloom *et al.* 2012), we proposed a novel method that integrated morphological reconstruction with color features for the location and isolation of lymphoblast cells. According to the findings of our research, this strategy was able to localize the whole lymphoblast cell population; nevertheless, the adjacency issue was not resolved. In addition, this method did not further divide the cytoplasm from the nucleus.

(Nee *et al.* 2012; Huey Nee *et al.* 2012) used same method for morphological reconstruction as described in (Madhloom *et al.* 2012). Three types of *AML* were the subject of a colour segmentation approach presented by (Nee *et al.* 2012). (M2-M5M6). Through the saturation band of the HSV color space, the original image was used to generate a mask and marker, and the cell was then reconstructed using morphological reconstruction.

Other researchers employed unsupervised clustering segmentation techniques such as fuzzy c-means and K-means clustering. In this context, a segmentation approach to distinguish between lymphocytes and lymphoblast, two types of blood cells.

The blood smear image is divided into four sections based on lab color space: erythrocyte, nucleus, cytoplasm, and plasma. An approximate K-mean clustering was used to divide a blood smear image into four separate parts. This approach outperformed fuzzy c-mean clustering and K-means in terms of performance.

They recommended using a two-step clustering approach. A sub-image of the whole cell is then cropped in accordance with the nucleus bounding box after the blood smear image has first been segmented using K-mean clustering based on RGB color space to locate the nucleus area.

Separate areas of the image based on colour or intensity using unsupervised clustering and segmentation techniques. When there is a clear distinction in the colour or intensity of the several zones, this strategy works well. However, it struggles when distinct parts of the picture are given with the same colour, such as when erythrocytes and cytoplasm have equal brightness levels (Won et al. 2005). Because of this, researchers have shown that the cytoplasm and erythrocytes are grouped together in the same cluster.

This condition can also appear in clumped (overlapping) cells that clustering methods are unable to separate. In the paper, a WBC identification method was suggested (Putzu & Ruberto 2013)

Leukocytes were identified, clustered leukocytes were separated, and nucleus and cytoplasm were chosen as the final two steps of the algorithm.

Applying the Zack threshold to the CMYK colour model component allowed for the detection of leukocytes. The watershed technique was then used to separate the leukocyte groups after this. On every leukocyte sub-image, the Otsu approach was used in a threshold-based procedure.

The threshold-based procedure was applied to an intensity image created by fusing the green component of the RGB color space with the component of the Lab color space.

The ALL-IDB1 database, which served as the basis for the method's evaluation, is the same dataset-B used in this study (Labati *et al.* 2011). (Please refer to Section 4.2.2). 33 PB pictures with a total of 267 cells were used as the sample set. The method was able to identify 245 of the 267 cells with an average accuracy of 92%.

Using images of peripheral blood and bone marrow, the study proposed a unique technique for segmenting both healthy WBC and acute lymphoblastic leukemia blast cells.

In order to test the algorithm, 650 WBCs were used. In spite of the algorithm's ability to distinguish 637 cells from a total of 650, it occasionally failed to do so because some false positive items, such as RBCs or dead cells, had colorations and forms that were comparable to those of lymphoblasts.

2.14.3   Feature Extraction, Selection and Classification

A procedure known as feature extraction involves taking certain distinguishing characteristics from a picture and using them to create a collection of useful descriptors. The aim of the feature extraction stage is to extract the features from a blood image that best represent a specific blood cell.

This section analyses the most significant articles in the literature from the perspectives of the three main processes—feature extraction, feature selection, and classification. All of these procedures are presented collectively since it is impossible to evaluate feature extraction and selection effectiveness without also taking classification accuracy into account.

We only incorporated earlier studies that documented these three phases together. As was previously mentioned, the goal of the study is to use peripheral blood smear pictures to categorize acute leukemia blasts into *ALL* or *AML*. This is the first time that we are aware of that acute leukemia blast cells have been classified using images from peripheral blood smears. The majority of literary works have little bearing on the research presented in this thesis.

Some studies attempted to differentiate between acute leukemia blast cells and normal WBCs. (Madhloom *et al.* 2012; Nasir *et al.* 2011). While others developed a system for categorizing one of the kinds of acute leukemia (i.e. *AML*) into their sub-types such as the work by (Osowski *et al.* 2004; Markiewicz *et al.* 2005; Scotti 2005; Osowski *et al.* 2009). The literature on acute leukemia categorization only contains a relatively small number of efforts. But in each of these attempts, BM smear photographs were focused (Nasir *et al.* 2011)

However, all of the above methods have been tested utilizing bone marrow imaging data. But, it was discovered that there are no changes between blast cells in PB and BM sample in terms of morphological characteristics, cytochemistry, or immunophenotyping. Additionally, the primary method of leukemia diagnosis still involves microscopy evaluation of stained PB smears.

Clinically, the desire to spare the patient from an invasive and unpleasant procedure as well as the intuitive notion that the PB and BM blast cells in the same patient at any given time are comparable are the driving forces behind the use of PB smears rather than BM. (Almarzooqi *et al.* 2011).

Sabino *et al.* 2004) developed a system for categorizing ***CLL*** and normal leucocytes. Every cell's nucleus and cytoplasm yielded 62 attributes in total, including colour, texture (5 GLCM), and basic form parameters like area, perimeter, etc (first-order histogram features based on RGB colour space).

Utilizing wrapper approaches, including the Sequential Forward Selection, the top 12 characteristics were chosen (SFS). The method's accuracy was reported to be 89.07% after testing 718 samples using Naive Bayes classifiers. Later, the identical approach used in the earlier work by (Ushizima *et al.* 2005) was replicated (Sabino *et al.* 2004). SVM was used to classify the data, nevertheless. SVM beat Nave Bayes with 95.14% average accuracy, according to the results.

In their study, the authors suggested a classification method based on SVM for identifying various myelogenous blast cells in BM pictures while accounting for the myelogenous blast cells' various maturation degrees (Osowski *et al.* 2004; Markiewicz *et al.* 2005; Osowski *et al.* 2009).

Numerous characteristics of each blast cell were obtained, including geometrical, textural, and color data based on the RGB color histogram. The comparison of various feature selection techniques was the main focus. (Osowski *et al.* 2004) used two filter methods (correlation analysis, mean and variance measures) and chose the top 70 characteristics from a set of 99 features in order to distinguish 12 groups of myelogenous blast cells.

(Markiewicz *et al.* 2005) used a wrapper of a linear support vector machine (SVM) for selecting characteristics from a vector of 87 dimensions in order to distinguish between 10 groups of myelogenous blast. Later, Markiewicz *et al.* (2005) tested two filter strategies (correlation analysis, mean and variance measures), as well as one wrapper of a linear Support Vector Machine, for selecting features from a vector of 164 dimensions (SVM).

The most successful method combined the linear SVM ranking with the relationship between the feature and the class. A genetic algorithm-based feature selection strategy was put out in the works by (Osowiski *et al.* 2009). In this method, chromosomes were used to represent each conceivable collection of traits.

Using genetic operations like mutation and crossover in accordance with a fitness function that was given as the classification error on the validation data set, the best solution(s) were found. The findings showed that wrapper features selected using a linear SVM outperformed features selected using this technique in terms of classification.

Scotti (2005) looked at the K-Nearest Neighbour (KNN), the Feed-Forward Neural Network (FFNN), and the Nave Bayes as three different classifiers for the categorization of ALL. The mean and standard deviation of the gray scale image were utilized as texture characteristics, and each cell contained information on 23 simple shape properties, such as area, perimeter, circularity, and others.

The sequential forward selection wrapper approach was used to choose the top three characteristics. According to the results, the FFNN provided the best classification performance. A method is described to classify acute leukemia blast cells into ALL and AML based on blast cell shape. Weka's basic shape feature, first-order statistics based on grey level, and RGB color histogram were used to evaluate 27 properties of the five different classifiers KNN, Random Forest, Simple Logistic, Sequential Minimal Optimization, and Random Committee (Hall *et al.* 2009).

The Sequential Minimal Optimization produced the classification accuracy of 92.20%, which was the highest of the classifiers.

In the works, the SVM was used to separate healthy lymphocyte from ALL using PB pictures. From the cell nucleus, several traits were extracted, including fractal dimension, contour signature, fundamental form features, first-order statistics, GLCM, and mean color value based on RGB and HSV color spaces. With true positive accuracy rate of over 90%, the SVM demonstrated strong classification ability. Later, an ensemble classification strategy was performed and assessed using k-fold validation, yielding 94.73% accuracy.

2.15 SURVEY ON EXISTING METHOD IN BONE CANCER DIAGNOSIS USING AI, ML AND DEEP LEARNING MODELS

Prediction levels made before the metastatic stage account for a large portion of cancer deaths worldwide. All human bodily organs, including the breast, lung, prostate, and kidney, can develop rashes and abrasions, which account for 80% of all metastases to the bone.

It was hypothesized that in a few cases of bronchogenic cancer, bone scanning with 99m monodiphosphate found early bone metastases before these lesions became obvious clinically or radio graphically. A bone scan may reveal signs of bone metastases.

It is generally known that in previous approaches, radiation therapy was followed by monitoring, treatment, and assessment. These processes relied on the results of CT and MRI scans (Rajer & Kovac 2008 & Nestle *et al.* 2009). However, the primary advantage of these techniques, known as anatomical imaging, is that they analyze the anatomy in great detail and contribute to the development of extremely complex RT procedures.

Discrete Wavelet Transform (DWT), developed by Donoho & Johnstone in 1994, is a wavelet thresholding de-noising technique that is frequently used to denoise ECG signals. Kalman and Wiener filtering techniques were utilized by Sayadi & Shamsollahi (2008) to eliminate the extraneous material commotions. Harishchandra & Holambe provided a different approach to edge estimation for ECG signal de-noising using wavelet decomposition (2013). Using the most severe and smallest wavelet coefficients at each level, this approach records the threshold.

Wavelet provides an incredibly poor and useful description for images. A suggestion was provided on the most recent methods for wavelet-based mammography evaluation. According to Liu Sheng *et al.* (2001) research, the use of multi-determination mammography examinations improves the suitability of any analytic framework in light of wavelets coefficients.

A mark vector for the process of comparing anomalies in a mammogram may be constructed utilizing higher values of wavelet coefficients in the low recurrence (near estimate) of wavelets modification, according to Ferreira and Borges' 2003 research. In multilevel disintegration, Essam *et al.* (2007) estimate employing a multi-determination mammography examination concentrated some of the highest coefficients. By applying several picture-handling techniques, such as contrast enhancement, edge finding, and picture combining, Nisthula & Yadhu (2013) use a straightforward, efficient, and reliable way to identify cancerous bone tissue.

Many algorithms have been proposed for the detection of bone fissures. As of 2010 publications, Vijay Kumar et al. offered a filtering method for Gaussian interruption removal that first approximations the amount of disturbances from the noisy image before substituting the center pixel by the mean of the amount of the neighboring pixels dependent on a threshold value.

When compared to earlier filtering methods like mean, alpha trimmed mean, Wiener, K-means, bilateral, and trilateral, this approach offers the two crucial qualities of lower mean absolute error (MAE) and higher peak signal to noise ratio.

Another technique used in research, physical science, is to close estimate by wavelets. Wavelets were first conceptualized by Morlet *et al.* (1982) as a collection of capabilities that resulted from the elaboration and growth of a key capability known as mother wavelet.

Typically, salt and pepper noise has been introduced to the DICOM pattern's pictures. AlKhaffaf *et al.* (2008) predicted the K-fill algorithm's structure based on the number of pixel values in a matrix with a 3 3 window in order to reduce salt and pepper noise. The salt and pepper noise contaminates photographs as a result of the Poisson and Gaussian process combination.

This advancement makes it possible for the method to anticipate the Poisson model's scaling boundary as well as the Gaussian model's mean and consistency all at once. Chan & Fu (1999) proposed a method for extracting features by combining the wavelet, curvelet, and Haar transform approaches. Compared to wavelet and curvelet procedures, the Haar methodology offers the highest level of evaluation precision.

In the procedure tested by Tian in 2002, the neck shaft angle of the femur bone was evaluated to determine the fracture in that area. The method of employing Gabor, markov, and gradient concentration features that can be deleted from the X-ray pictures was suggested by Lim *et al.* (2004). And then the Support Vector Machines (SVM) classifiers get these characteristics as input. They discovered that merging three SVM classifiers can increase the algorithm's sensitivity and accuracy.

Mahendran & Baboo (2011) presented a classification approach based on the fusion process to automatically detect the presence of fractures in the Tibia bone. The preprocessing procedures the authors begin with include edge detection, noise reduction, binary data conversion, and picture splitting.

He ranks the three jointly produced classification algorithms using a smooth developed voting system- feed forward, back propagation Neural Networks (NN), Support Vector Machines (SVM), and Naive Bayes (NB) - into action in order to carry out the operation procedure. The splitting of the picture is done after that. An algorithm based on the GLCM approach that permits a long-term enhancement to separate the x-ray picture and identify bony sections of the soft tissue cells was tested by Chai *et al.* (2011).

The authors begin with preprocessing methods such as binary data conversion and edge detection, after which they extract attributes using the k-means segmentation algorithm and the Gray-Level Co-Occurrence Matrix (GLCM) method. Scanned area from X-ray should be automatically segmented, the data should be analyzed, and then the image should be divided to only include the bones in the carpal region, according to Hao *et al.* (2013). An automated method to determine the width of the joints in x-ray pictures of the hand was introduced by Bielecki *et al.* (2008).

Cheng *et al.* (1995) proposed a novel fuzzy co-occurrence matrix-based texture analysis method. This method deals with early and precise breast cancer identification by performing statistical analysis on the microscope slide biopsy images. After collecting the characteristics from the digitized photographs using a novel approach to feature extraction, the photos are classified into three risk categories using a multilayer back-propagation neural network.

It was determined that this technique performs better than the already used ways after evaluating the presentations of the predicted cancer diagnosis approaches and the future algorithm. The suggested method can be applied in a number of ways in the fields of pattern recognition and image processing.

A convolutional neural network (CNN) architecture developed by Claro *et al.* (2020) can distinguish between blood slides containing ALL, AML and healthy blood slides. 97.18% accuracy and 97.23% precision are provided by this framework.

This framework's accelerated processing speed is its primary benefit. This model is more appealing to employ in applications on mobile devices because it also has a smaller file size. However, this study's increased energy consumption is the only restriction found.

To detect ALL, AML, and MM, Baig *et al.* (2020) used deep learning (DL)-based CNN and hybridized two separate blocks of CNN, designated CNN-1 and CNN-2. This framework enhanced image contrast during pre-processing and segmentation by converting RGB color space to gray scale 8-bit mode. It did this by using an image intensity adjustment approach and an adaptive histogram equalization method.

The collected features are then fused using the Canonical Correlation Analysis (CCA) fusion technique to create features that stand out more. Five classification methods were used to evaluate the performance of feature extraction strategies: SVM, Bagging Ensemble, Total Boosts, RUSBoost, and Fine KNN. With a 97.04 percent accuracy rate, this framework has the best accuracy. Its increased computational complexity, however, is a disadvantage of this framework.

Bukhari *et al.* (2022) demonstrated an improved deep learning model based on squeeze and excitation learning to identify leukemia malignancy using a given microscopic blood sample from patients. By enabling it to carry out periodic channel-wise feature recalibration, this model enhances its representational capability at each level of feature representation.

The model is able to separate leukemic and normal cells using strong, pertinent, and discriminative properties that are extracted by the squeezing and excitation processes. Comparing this model to the conventional deep learning model, which has not been validated on publicly available datasets, yields encouraging results. But this framework's greater memory usage is a significant limitation.

In order to comprehend how deep neural networks are trained to converge, Mallick *et al.* (2022) developed a classification technique (DNN), the assumptions are taken as true because the inputs don't degenerate and the network is over-parameterized. Additionally, there are sufficient hidden neurons. The authors of this article used DNN to categorize the gene expression data.

The bone marrow expressions of 72 leukemia patients make up the dataset used in this study. To categorize ALL and acute myelocytic AML samples, a five-layer DNN classifier was created. The 20% of the data are utilized for validation once the network has been trained using 80% of the data. Comparing this DNN classifier to other classifiers, it is producing results that are satisfactory.

Two types of leukaemia may be classified with 98.2% accuracy, 96.59% sensitivity, and 97.9% specificity. The advantage of using a deep learning-based classifier is that classification accuracy can be increased with little additional processing work. However, this framework's high energy consumption represents a significant limitation that must be taken into account.

Shen *et al.* (2021) created a leukemia diagnosis system using CNN. By recognizing and discarding smashed and uncountable cells, the computer skillfully emulated a hematologist's operation. It then classified and counted the remaining cells to make a diagnosis.

CNN's performance in classifying WBCs received an F1 score of 82.02% and exhibited accuracy of 82.93% and precision of 86.07%. Additionally, the performance in identifying acute lymphoid leukemia was accurate 89% of the time, sensitive 86% of the time, and specific 95% of the time. An average accuracy of 82.93% is attained by the system when it comes to identifying lymphoma and neuroblastoma bone marrow metastases. The increased memory usage of this system as data size grows, however, is a significant disadvantage.

The major goal of Alagu *et al.* (2021) is to propose key features for the detection of ALL. An online database is used to provide the necessary input photos. To make all photos of the same size, resizing is used. U-Net segments the nucleus of blast and healthy cells. From the completely linked layer, several CNN models, including AlexNet, GoogleNet, and SqueezeNet, extract roughly 1000 deep features.

In order to concatenate all the features, deep feature fusion is used. By using a variety of feature selection techniques, including mutual information (MI), minimum recursive maximal relevance (mRmR), and recursive feature elimination, the prime features are chosen. The biggest problem is it takes more time to complete the task.

According to a novel ensemble gene selection technique introduced, the most well-liked classifiers are collected into an ensemble and utilized as a fitness function to PSO to discover the appropriate number of informatics genes to boost classification accuracy by Alrefai *et al.* (2019).

Kim *et al.* (2021) trained the Xception, VGG16, VGG19, and MobileNet models using the deep learning technique to improve the precision of medical picture detection. The training model can determine if the provided data is a benign ALL or a pro-B ALL by the use of medical imaging to find anomalies in the dataset. With a 98.5% accuracy rate in identifying anomalous regions from the dataset, this VGG16 demonstrated the best overall performance in terms of accuracy and precision. The results of anomalies were visualized in this study using the XAI approach in addition to a deep convolutional neural network.

Fauzi *et al.* (2021) examined the performance of the Fuzzy based SVM approach with and without PCA feature extraction for the accuracy of multi-class classification of leukemia cancer data. To improve the classification of leukemia cancer data, we employ the PCA as a feature selection technique.

In order to accurately classify leukemia cancer data into many classes, fuzzy-based SVM with PCA as the feature selection (60 feature extraction) achieves a 96.924% accuracy rate, while FSVM without feature selection achieves an 87.694% accuracy rate. Therefore, when classifying leukemia cancer data into many classes, FSVM plus PCA as the feature selection approach yields higher accuracy than FSVM alone. Deep convolutional neural network architecture for the automatic identification of white blood cell cancer from bone marrow microscopic images was presented by Kumar *et al.* (2020). Before creating the improved convolutional neural network structure, the model performs the photos and selects the best highlights. Finally, it makes a prediction regarding the type of cancer depicted in the image.

The accuracy of the model was assessed at 97.2%. This model can be effectively used as a tool to identify the kind of cancerous development in the bone marrow. This approach must acknowledge that a more extensive experimental investigation that takes into account the dependence on the size of the databases has not been carried out and provided here.

2.16   SUMMARY

This chapter covers the background research on leukemia, machine learning, deep learning, digital image processing, including color spaces, and picture segmentation. An extensive description of feature extraction is given because it is used in the work discussed here to detect acute leukemia blast cells. Several more ideas that are pertinent to this thesis were introduced in this chapter. We also investigated current approaches to acute leukemia diagnostic technologies that have been created to aid and enable hematologists in the precise identification of the illness.

CHAPTER 3

BONE MARROW CANCER CLASSIFICATION USING EXTREME LEARNING MACHINE ARCHITECTURE

3.1 OBJECTIVE

After incorporating machine learning techniques into the framework, tumor cell categorization and identification are carried out. For convenient tracking of the patient's health status, the suggested work classifies the tumor kind and stage. Then, in order to increase the procedure's precision for bone marrow malignancy prediction, LBP Extreme Learning is employed. This will allow for continuous patient monitoring and will ultimately increase prediction accuracy rates.

3.2 CAD FRAME WORK

Three processes involved in the Computer Aided Design (CAD) frameworks are pre-processing, feature extraction, and characterization. The diagnostic outline is shown in Figure 3.1.

Numerous strategies have been produced so as to build the recognition exactness rates of Bone Marrow tumor growth using CAD frameworks. For example, Von Boehmer *et al.* (2010) introduced a CAD framework for pneumonic tumor location in chest radiography.

The proposed framework is utilizing an informational collection that comprises of 167 chest radiography that contains 181 Bone Marrow tumors; the framework uses versatile separation based limit calculation for tumor division, from that point onwards, features are processed for every tumor utilizing geometric features, force features and slope features. In conclusion, a straight discriminate classifier is utilized to classity the computed features.

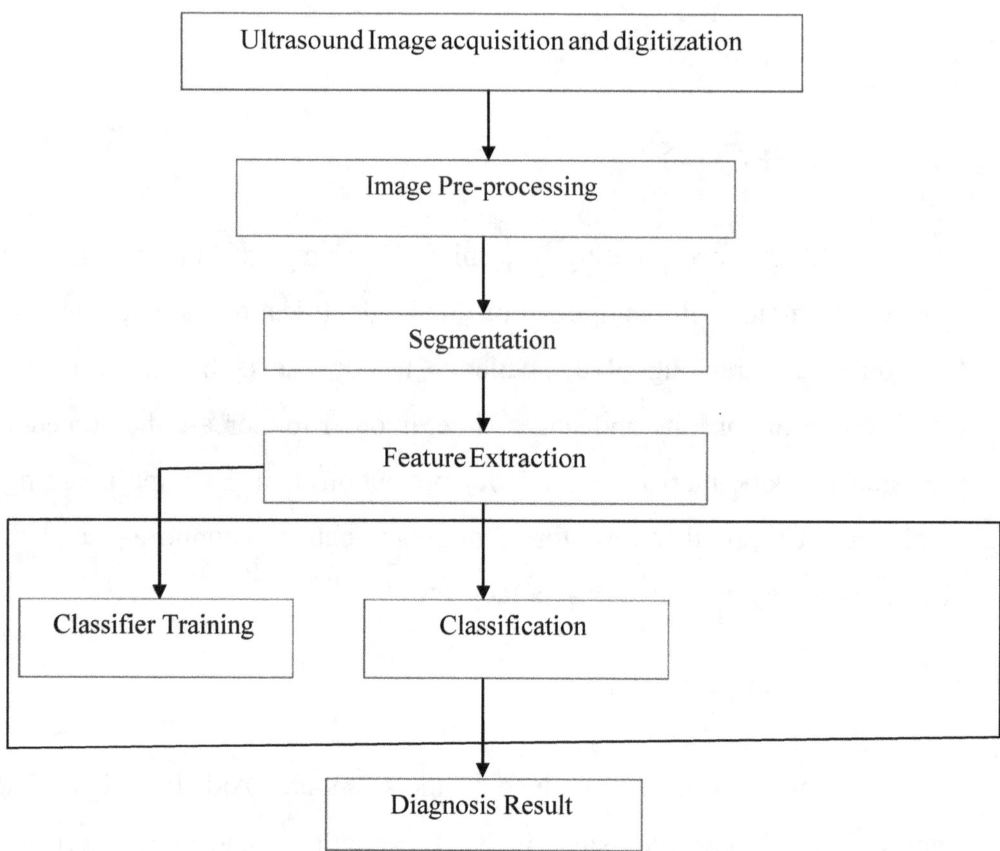

Figure 3.1 Diagnostic framework

A 78.1% accuracy rate is achieved using the framework. A bone marrow tumor identification technique based on a cluster classifier helped by bunching is proposed by Sant *et al.* (2010). To evaluate the approach, 6872 images from bone marrow sweeps of 32 individuals are used. 98.33% affectivity is added to the framework.

Another framework proposed by Ahmedin Jemal *et al.* (2009) is used to recognize bone marrow tumors by utilizing a shape-based hereditary calculation format coordinating method. A 3D geometric shape is chosen to acquire the wellness work in this system, and a pretreatment task for the upgrade is carried out using a round-arranged convolution-based separating plan. An informative index consisting of 70 CT images including 278 tumors are issued to evaluate the framework. 90% of 160 tumors could be recognized by the framework. Additionally, software is provided for identifying bone marrow tumor development.

The specificity has reached 73.15%, while the affectability is up to 67.84%. These are examples of frameworks designed to differentiate the development of bone marrow tumors. With current frameworks, there is a widespread issue with the high prevalence of false positives and false negatives. Because of this, it is essential to develop a PC-supported analysis to aid in the detection and prediction of bone marrow tumor progression.

Increasing the proportion of true positives and true negatives, this study helps to provide a classification framework for bone marrow tumors that is cutting-edge and persuasive. The suggested system, in particular, provides two steps of feature determination, resulting in the selection of only relevant characteristics that improve execution. The Cluster k-nearest neighbor computation is used in expansion, and it combines the K means clustering and K-Nearest Neighbor calculations. High accuracy can be expected from this classifier.

It is obvious that the condition is not one-and-only because there are many disorders associated with tumor growth that all include unregulated cell formation and expansion. With around 8 million fatalities each year, it is the second-leading cause of death worldwide.

In order to help patients to receive the appropriate therapeutic therapy, early diagnosis and disease type prediction are essential in cancer growth research. It is essential to precisely differentiate between benign and dangerous tumors in order to select the most appropriate course of therapy.

3.3 ORDER OF MACHINE LEARNING TECHNIQUES USED FOR CANCER DETECTION

Computational methods and systems have been built to perform fundamental tasks using microarray and cutting-edge sequencing. In cell research, there are a number of urgent problems that necessitate deep nonlinear connections amongst practical modules.

By maintaining information and yield running on the computer, the programme depicted in Figure 3.2 is produced using the machine learning methodology.The demand for human services is rising as a result of developments in social insurance and therapeutic innovation as well as population growth and maturation. Longer wait times may result in patients being checked at later stages of their illness, increasing the risk of death and necessitating more resources and spending in the human services sector.

For the medical service sector to become more effective, creative and modern solutions are required. Infections frequently lead to tumor development, and the most well-known tumor on the globe is bone marrow disease. Analyzing a patient's chance of survival as soon as a tumor first appears is crucial. The patient's chance of survival increases with the time it takes to identify and cure tumor development.

Bone marrow images, such as CT scans and normal X-rays, are routinely utilized to find bone marrow cancers. An experienced radiologist is required to translate restorative pictures, which is a challenging and time-consuming task.

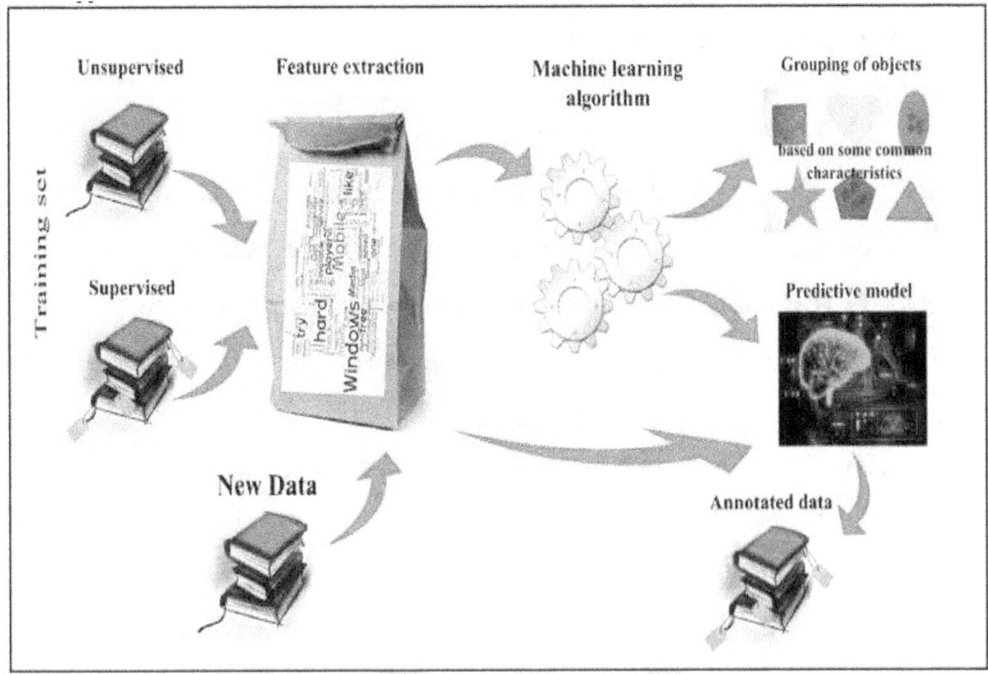

(Source : Ozaki *et al.* 2019)

Figure 3.2 Schematic representation of machine learning workflow

Self-governing finding structures can be used by clinicians as a decision support system, reducing both expenses for the medical services and patient suffering. The aim of this proposed work is to calculate if a grouping computation can efficiently discriminate between bone marrow tumor tissue and normal bone marrow tissue in CT scans.

3.4 ELM-BASED FRAMEWORK FOR PREDICTING BONE MARROW CANCER

The proposed framework's whole design is given in Figure 3.3. LBP recognizes edges, corners, elevated or flat regions, and hard liners in order to encode geometric aspects of an image and provide a feature vector representation of an image or collection of images. Preprocessing and feature extraction steps make the proposed ELM-based categorization system. Deep convolutional layers are used for data preparation, augmentation, segmentation, and feature extraction.

Features that are gathered during segmentation are used to train the networks. The proposed design substitutes feed forward networks, which are based on the theory of Extreme Learning Machines and traditional training networks (ELM). Extreme learning machines are a sort of neural network that Chand *et al.* (2019) recommended can be used. This type of neural network employs only one hidden layer and doesn't need to be tuned.

ELM performs better, faster, and has less computational cost than alternative learning algorithms like Support Vector Machines (SVM) (Paswan *et al.* 2018) and Random Forest (RF) (Mishra *et al.* 2016). To provide superior accuracy and improve efficiency, ELM employs the kernel function. The two key benefits of the ELM are reduced training error and enhanced approximation. ELM uses auto-tuning of the weight biases and non-zero activation functions, which has applications in classification and classification values. The ELM's complex method of operation is described in (Huang *et al.* 2012). The "L" neurons in the hidden layer must operate with an activation function that is substantially differentiable, for example, the sigmoid function; ELM does not require hidden layer be modified but tuning is necessary. The output layer in this type of system has a straight activation function.

Loads of the concealed layer and counting the bias loads are chosen at random. Contrary to popular belief, the hidden nodes are not useless; they do not need to be tweaked, and the parameters of a hidden neuron can even be constructed randomly beforehand. Specifically, before handling the training datasets.

The symbol for the output ELM function is

$$-\tag{3.1}$$

where X is the LBP, which has characteristics of bone marrow cancer cells.

The equation provides a system yield for an ELM with a single hidden layer (3.1)

$$\Sigma\tag{3.2}$$

where $x \rightarrow$ input

$\rightarrow$ It is presented as the following output weight vector

$$\tag{3.3}$$

H(x) $\rightarrow$ *The output hidden layer from the following equation*

$$\tag{3.4}$$

The hidden layers are represented as above, and the goal is to identify output vector O, also known as the target vector (3.5)

$$[\quad]\tag{3.5}$$

Simple non-linear least square algorithms, as shown in Equation (3.6), are used in the ELM's fundamental implementation

$$*\tag{3.6}$$

where $H* \rightarrow$ inverse of H known as Moore–Penrose generalized inverse.

Additionally, the following equation can be used.

$$-\tag{3.7}$$

Consequently, the output function may be calculated using above equation.

$$- \tag{3.8}$$

The following equation provides the Fitness Function (FF) for the proposed ELM network.

$$FF = Max\ (Accuracy,\ sensitivity,\ specificity) \tag{3.9}$$

Here is a list of the hyper-parameters chosen for the ELM network in Table 3.1. Algorithm-1 presents the training methods for assessing the ELM model.

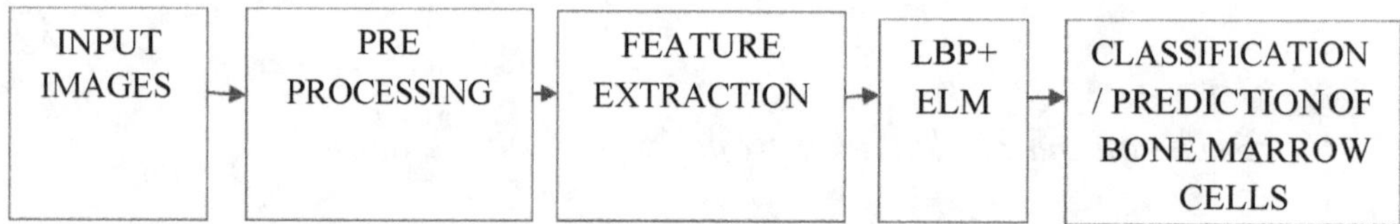

Figure 3.3   Detection of BONE MARROW CANCER using a proposed LBP-based ELM architecture

Table 3.1 LBP based ELM network's hyper -parameters

S.No	Hyper - parameters	Values
1	Learning rate	0.001
2	Batch size	30
3	Number of epochs	250
4	Hidden layers	4
5	Optimizer	Adam
6	Activation function Used	Relu
7	Loss function	MSE

S. No	Algorithm1 // Pseudo Code for the Proposed LBP based ELM network
01	Input = Hyper -parameters of the ELM training network
02	Output : Categorization of the normal and abnormal bone marrow cells
03	While (true)
04	Calculate the output value from the ELM network using Equation(3.5)
05	Calculate the FF using the Equation (3.9)
06	For t=1 to Max_iteration
07	Assign the bias weights and input layers
08	Calculate the FF from the network using Equation (3.2)
09	If (FF = = Maximum Accuracy)
10	Go to Step 14
11	Else
12	Go to Step 08
13	End
14	End

3.5 DETAILS OF THE EXPERIMENT

Tensorflow v.18, an end-to-end open-source Python platform, is used to carry out the proposed research. Using 1024 pictures over 1000 iterations, the multi-classification model is trained. To detect the BMC in the photos, the trained model is then used. The model is trained using an i7 CPU, 16GB of RAM, and an NVIDIA K80 GPU running at 2.5 GHz.

3.6 MEASUREMENTS OF PERFORMANCE AND EVALUATION

The proposed approach makes use of LBP-based ELM layers for better cancer cell classification in images of bone marrow. Given in Table 3.2 are the partitioned datasets used to train and test the network in Table

Table 3.2 Total number of datasets (after augmentation) used to train and test the proposed network

Sl.No	Total Images	Data under training (%)	Data under testing (%)
01	1024	70	30

The data are split 70:30 between training and testing data in order to accurately classify BMCs. The proposed architecture is evaluated in which the convolutional layers extract the visual characteristics and input them to the feed-forward training networks that classify the relevant categories.

3.7 SUMMARY

The method for identifying the sickness has a fundamental impact on locating bone marrow cancer cells. In order to solve the issue, it is crucial to disclose and predict the growth of bone marrow tumors first. This study uses the LBP based ELM network for improved categorization in order to locate cancer cells. Despite this framework produces improved accuracy of 80.34%, precision of 80%, recall of 78.8%, specificity of 77.9%, and F1-Score 79.6% values, it struggles to handle large-scale datasets. Therefore, optimization is needed to further improve the framework's suitability for any type of network. This indicates that the deep learning technique is crucial for achieving improved performance. The shortcomings of the current framework are overcome and discussed in Chapter 4 using deep learning based optimization networks.

CHAPTER 4

TRANSFER LEARNING AND OPTIMIZED -FIREFLY NEURAL NETWORKS FOR BONE MARROW CANCER PREDICTION

4.1   INTRODUCTION

This chapter utilizes Firefly-optimized pre-trained transfer learning for improved prediction of bone marrow malignancies from the input CT images and presents a new network for better segmentation. Reducing future computational complexity and over fitting issues are achieved by integrating capsule-based saliency segmentation.

Furthermore, the firefly optimization approach adjusts the hyper parameters of trained networks to increase prediction accuracy while reducing complexity. LUNA-16 and LIDC Bone Marrow Image datasets are used for extensive testing, and performance metrics like accuracy, precision, recall, specificity, and F1-score are analyzed.

4.2   PROPOSED METHODOLOGY-SYSTEM OVERVIEW

The full design is shown in Figure 4.1 for the suggested methodology. There are three crucial phases that make up the operation of the proposed deep learning-based diagnostic and classification system, which are preprocessing of the images, the augmentation method, and saliency segmentation are based on capsules. Before training the firefly-optimized

CNNs, accurate feature extraction is carried out by utilizing the previously taught transfer learning.

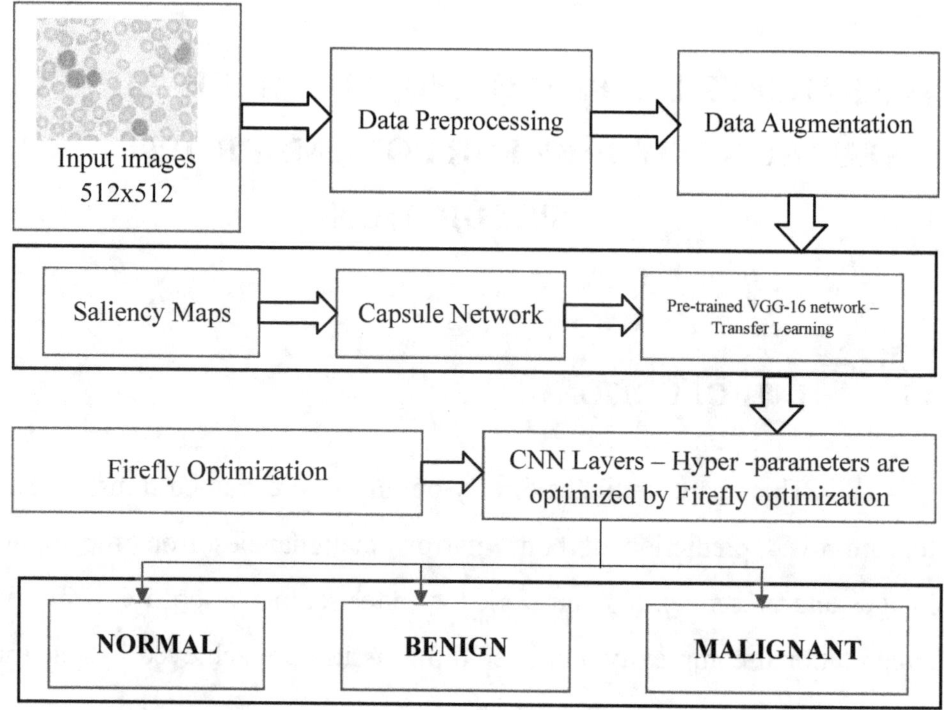

Figure 4.1 Overview of the proposed architecture

4.2.1   Data Preprocessing and Augmentation

Histogram Equalization (HOE) is used in the initial phase to separate the bone marrow pictures. Adjusting the picture intensities and contrast are done at the pre-processing stage. In order to apply HOE to image pre-processing, the following formula is given:

$$(4.1)$$

where T.N is the total number of pixels

N is one of the following values: 0, 1, 2, 3, etc.

P - Total Pixels.

An Adaptive Median Filter (AMF) is used to effectively denoise the pictures once preprocessing is complete. The appearance is enhanced by AMF, a category of bilateral pictures that produces "clean, sharp, and artifact-free edges."

The recommended design uses an image enhancement approach in the second step. Whenever there are not enough tagged data, Deep Neural Network (DNN) (Hasan *et al.* 2020) over fitting issues arise. Data augmentation is the most knowledgeable and effective approach to solve this issue.

Each picture is subjected to a series of adjustments during the data augmentation step, yielding a sizable quantity of freshly corrected training image samples. According to Boreiri *et al.* (2022) discussion, effective data augmentation makes use of an affine transformation.

Conversion, ascending, and spinning techniques for affine transformations are used. Inputs are linked to the augmentation step, which is retrieved prior to the training phase, to avoid the over-fitting issue. Figure 4.2 shows the various images of the bone marrow after applying the affine corrections.

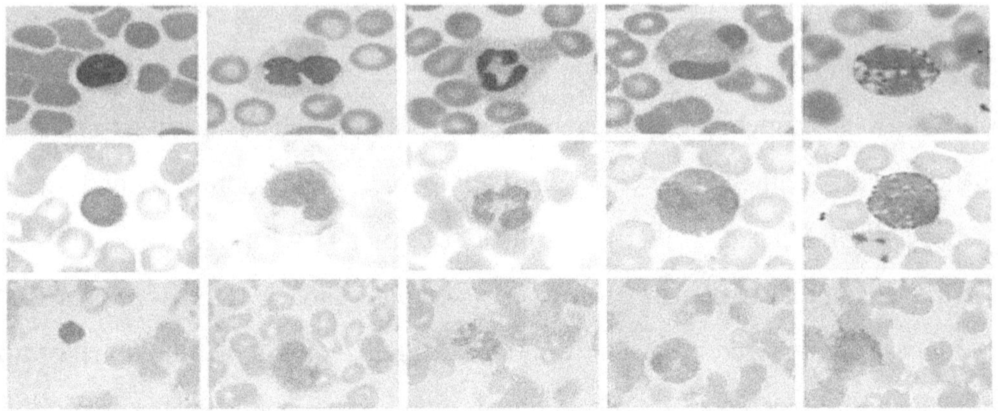

Figure 4.2 Examples of CT-Bone Marrow Images after Augmentation

4.2.2   Segmentation of Capsule Saliency

A technique for dividing pictures into various sizes of patterns and pixels is called segmentation. The photos are divided using a variety of approaches. Here, a structured method called capsule saliency is introduced. It totally separates the visuals into little and interesting sections. The number of extraneous components in the photographs will decrease.

Saliency models will be constructed. Each pixel is represented as a block in Iwashima *et al.* (2019) pixel-based processing, which applies color difference and spatial difference. In order to achieve this, picture pixels "X" are first divided into non-overlapping blocks of size nxn, where n is either 8 or 16 depending on the situation. The following mathematical formulas are used to calculate the saliency maps S(k).

$$\Sigma * \tag{4.2}$$

As stated in Banerjee *et al.* (2016), the final saliency maps are produced as the biased sum of the spatial and color saliency of the real (S(m)), preceding (S(m1)), and subsequent blocks (S(m2)). This is due to the fact that cancer cells are present in the same location, size, and shape in their adjacent slices,

$$* \qquad * \qquad * \tag{4.3}$$

Segmentation images must be improved using post-processing methods after the saliency maps are computed. Active contour techniques are used to find cancer cells in the blocks of twins that are spaced the closest. It is absolutely necessary to properly separate cancer cells from other bone marrow imaging components in order to obtain accurate results. Furthermore, since active contours are dependent on picture intensity, they presumably do not successfully distinguish between cancer cells. Additionally, these contour approaches demand longer calculation durations, which is seen to be a severe issue when processing bigger datasets. In order to address this drawback, this research suggests capsule networks with pre-trained optimal models to deliver high-performance and reliable identification of CT bone marrow cancer images.

The fundamental drawback of these strategies appears to be that they require significant fine-tuning and optimization to obtain such high-standard results, which is plainly impractical with large datasets and affects recognition rates. In contrast, the training process in the suggested system takes less time and improves the overall system performance.

4.2.3 Capsule Networks: A High-Level Summary

Capsule network is the brand-new network developed by Shah*et al.* (2021) will take the place of the existing models. The convolutional layer, hidden layer, primary caps layer, and digit caps layer are the four layers that make up the capsule network. For the provided training model, Figure 4.3 depicts the full working framework.

The various saliency maps in the photographs may be more effectively categorized using capsule networks. The suggested capsule networks receive the input of the preprocessed visual picture. Groups of cells called capsules are used to encrypt location information and the possibility that an object would appear in a picture; To reflect the crucial spatial association between the small and large-scale characteristics of the images, the input variable matrices and the weight matrices are combined and produced.

$$* \tag{4.4}$$

Equation (4.5) determines the overall weight that will be applied to updating the current capsule values and carrying the same ID to the next level of capsule determination.

$$\Sigma\ * \tag{4.5}$$

When applying non-linearity, the squash job is employed. The vector's direction are changed by the squashing tool into a vector with a minimum length of zero and an extreme length of one.

$$\tag{4.6}$$

4.2.4   Process of Segmentation

The architecture of the capsules used for the saliency segmentation is shown in Figure 4.3. Equation (4.2), which uses convolutional layers and capsule layers, is used to encode the previously processed pictures. First, the convolutional procedures are applied to the preprocessed pictures from the convolutional layers to the first capsule layers, later often to the upper capsule layers.

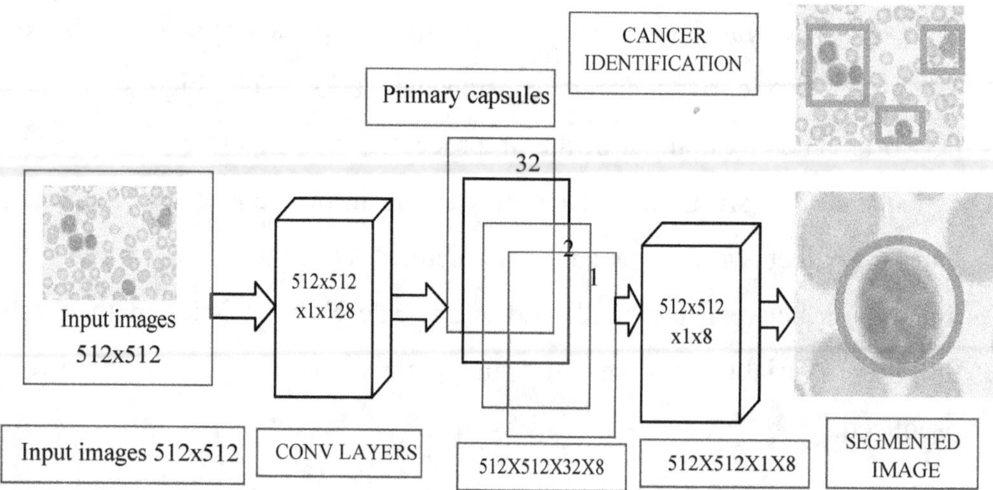

Figure 4.3 Architecture for a Saliency based Segmentation Capsule

4.2.5   Learning Transfer-Based Feature Extraction

Transfer learning is applied in this procedure for more efficient feature extraction and categorization. Convolutional neural networks that have already been trained and may be used for a variety of image categorization problems which are referred to as transfer learning techniques. The Inception V3 module is utilized in this study due to its exceptional accuracy and high flexibility. The unique Inception-V3 weights are pre-trained using ImageNet and accommodate all images, reshaped in the size of 150X150X3.

4.2.6   Classification Layers

Features are retrieved during segmentation and these features are subsequently utilized to train the networks. A pooling layer that determines the estimate and maximum of a frame of neurons is added to a CNN's numerous convolution layers, which have many convolution layers on their own.

With good accuracy and less over-fitting, this layer streamlines the yield saliency map (Iwashima *et al.* 2019; Shah *et al.* 2021). The last layers of a CNN are called densely integrated layer, which connect every cell from the layer such that the complex information gleaned from the convolution layer is globally connected.

Each completely linked layer has several kernels. These kernels are only once used on the input map in thick layers. Dense layers are computationally light due to the one-time usage of each kernel. The total architecture of CNN is shown in Figure 4.4. The suggested CNN architecture is fed the pre-trained vector matrix "Y." Let "K" be the set of "K" predetermined vectors that make up the input vector matrix. The following information is provided for every word's input vector matrix.

$$Y_{1:K} = Y_1 \oplus Y_2 \oplus Y_3 \oplus Y_4 Y_K \tag{4.7}$$

— $\oplus$ denotes the —concatenation operation‖. In the first stage, filter layers with dimension of $L \in Y_K$ where –Y‖ is y-dimensional pre trained vectors and k is size of each filter layers and also the number of vectors in input matrix. The input word matrix is convoluted with filter kernel k to get first set of features.

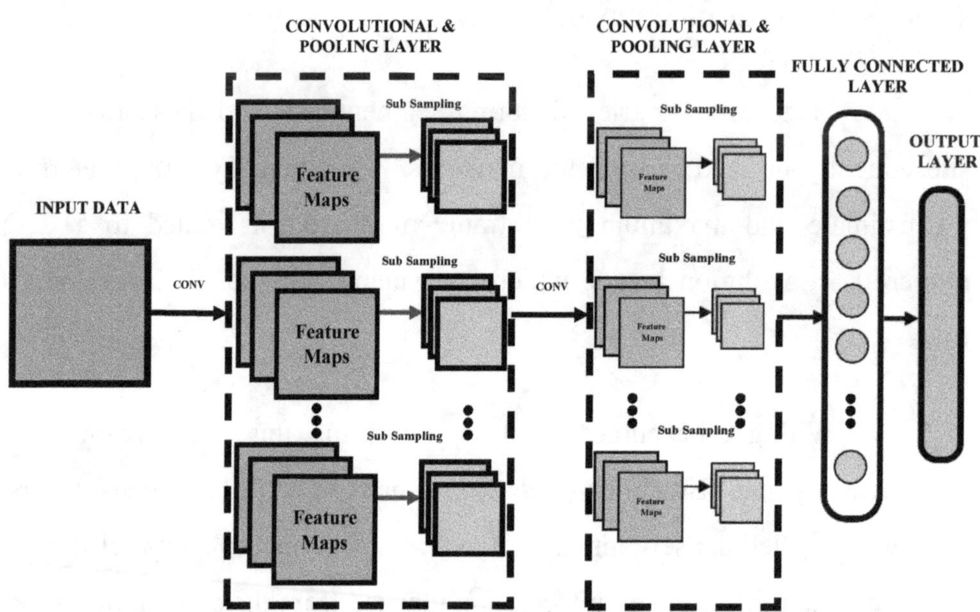

Figure 4.4 Network Architecture of Convolutional Neural Networks

Equation 4.1 captures spatial characteristics like corners and edges. Equation (4.8), which is presented here, yields the initial spatial characteristics.

$$A(i) = F(L * Y_K + O) \tag{4.8}$$

where "O" stands for the "bias factors," Next, filter "L" is applied to each potential word combination, and several feature vectors are provided as

$$A(i) = [A_1, A_2, A_3, A_4, \ldots\ldots\ldots\ldots\ldots\ldots A_L]$$

(4.9)

The generated feature maps are then supplied to the pooling layers, which use the average value of the $A(a_{avg})$ feature, which is thought to be the most crucial one because it is the feature that corresponds to the kernel of certain algorithms. To extract the feature from the max-pooling layer and for one filter, the entire cycle is used.

It takes several filter layers and pooling layers to create all the different feature maps. To automatically extract the unidentified characteristics from the dataset, a structure of five convolutional layers, four average pooling layers, and rectified linear unit (ReLU) activation units is utilized.

4.2.7 Firefly Optimized CNN

In this section, the firefly method for optimizing the CNN layers is covered. The Firefly algorithm, a subset of swarm intelligence algorithms, was created by Sarangi *et al.* (2016). During summer nights, one may frequently observe the fireflies - lighting bugs - flashing their lights in the sky. A mating partner might be attracted by a firefly's flashing behavior, or it can serve as protection from predators.

Another crucial feature of fireflies is that when they move farther from a brighter one, their light intensity not only dims but also becomes absorbed by the air, which makes it less intense. As a result, there is a direct correlation between light intensity and fitness value. The complexity of firefly behavior in their natural state, however, drives us to construct three assumptions in order to create an algorithmic working principle. The following assumptions are made:

- It is supposed that all fireflies are unisex and that all of them experienced attraction. The brightness of fireflies has a direct relationship to attractiveness, which decreases with increasing separation between them.

- The possible solutions of the objective function are used to calculate brightness, or light intensity.

The assumptions demonstrate an inverse relationship between distance r and the intensity of light I(r) emitted by fireflies, since it gets weaker as the distance grows and is absorbed by the air. As the coefficient of light absorption, y is employed as a notation. The fluctuation of the firefly light's intensity I(r) with respect to distance r is therefore shown by Equation (4.10).

$$I(r) = I_0 e^{-yr2} \tag{4.10}$$

Where I_0 - initial value of intensity at the source and the attractiveness parameter β can be defined in two different ways as shown in

$$e^{-yr2} \tag{4.11}$$

The attractive parameter is denoted as at the starting distance of zero

Given in the equation below is the behavioral rule for calculating firefly locations.

$$_{i+1} = _i + \tag{4.12}$$

The random number vector E and the randomization factor A are both drawn from the Gaussian distribution. $_i$ is the ith position of the firefly and $_{i+1}$second term represents the value of attraction.

4.2.8 Proposed Model

The weights of CNN networks are improved using the firefly optimization technique as mentioned in the preceding part. The major parameters employed to optimize the weights of CNN networks in this situation are several firefly criteria for finding and fixing the prey. A randomized weight matrix is typically given to CNN channels, which results in bias. The greatest accuracy index is referred to as the performance index.

The input bias and weights are chosen for each repeated one by using the numerical simulations. Using equations, the CNN system, which creates the exponential function, is then given these values. The repeat will end or continue depending on whether the output function equals the fitness value. Contrary to other meta-heuristic techniques, firefly adaptation has a slower convergence time, but it is quicker to hone and enhance reaction time.

The firefly optimized CNN is now used as the classification of Bone Marrow cancer images. Table 4.5 presents the optimized parameters used for training the network. The proposed framework working mechanism is presented in Algorithm - 2. Images of bone marrow cancer are categorized using the firefly-optimized CNN. The optimized parameters used to train the network are shown in Table 4.5.

The following pseudo code Algorithm - 2 outlines the suggested framework's functioning mechanism. The whole architecture of the optimized CNN for the classification and prediction of BMC is shown in Figure 4.5.

Table 4.2 Total number of Datasets (after Augmentation)

Sl.no	Total Number of Images	Training data (%)	Testing data (%)
01	1024	80	20

For the purpose of accurately classifying BMCs, the training and testing data are split as 80:20. Chapter 6 presents the exhaustive findings and discussions.

4.5   CHAPTER SUMMARY

In the second phase of the research, bone marrow images are used to identify and classify benign and malignant cancer cells. In order to identify the location of cancer cells, this work employs feature extraction based on transfer learning and capsule-based saliency segmentation. The suggested design also uses categorization layers based on fireflies to improve accuracy.

The provided tumor identification method is tested using the Tensorflow 1.8 tool with the Keras API and a number of performance measures, including accuracy (83.12%), precision (86.45%), recall (87.05%), specificity (87.95%), and F1-score (87.25%) which are used to calculate and examine.

The suggested method also requires improvement in terms of processing complexity, which, from the viewpoint of a radiologist, will be crucial for the study and identification of cancer cells. So, finally the hyper parameters of unique deep Convolutional Neural Networks are tuned by adaptive multi-objective cat algorithm which is presented in the next chapter.

CHAPTER 5

CAT- INSPIRED DEEP CONVOLUTIONAL NEURAL NETWORK FOR BONE MARROW CANCER CELLS DETECTION

5.1   INTRODUCTION

The unchecked proliferation of leukocytes, which are white blood cells, causes bone marrow cancer, which is thought to be the most severe and complicated illness among the several other illnesses. Considered to be significant bone cancer subtypes, Acute Lymphoblastic Leukemia (ALL) and Multiple Myeloma (MM) causes a higher concentration of cancer cells in the bone marrow, inhibiting the formation of healthy blood cells.

Deep learning in particular has made it possible for humans to analyze and diagnose these more complicated illnesses to a greater extent since the development of artificial intelligence and deep learning models. But the research still has question about how accurately the cancer cells can be identified and reduce the possibility of false alert rates.

In this chapter, innovative deep convolutional neural network is proposed, whose hyper- parameters are optimized via multi-objective adaptive cat algorithms. The proposed method first uses an optimized Convolutional Neural Network (OCNN) to train on pre-processed cell pictures, and then it uses that OCNN network to recognize the specific type of cancer cells observed in bone marrow.

procedure have a correlation. Figure 5.2 displays several cancer cell photos which are taken after the data augmentation process.

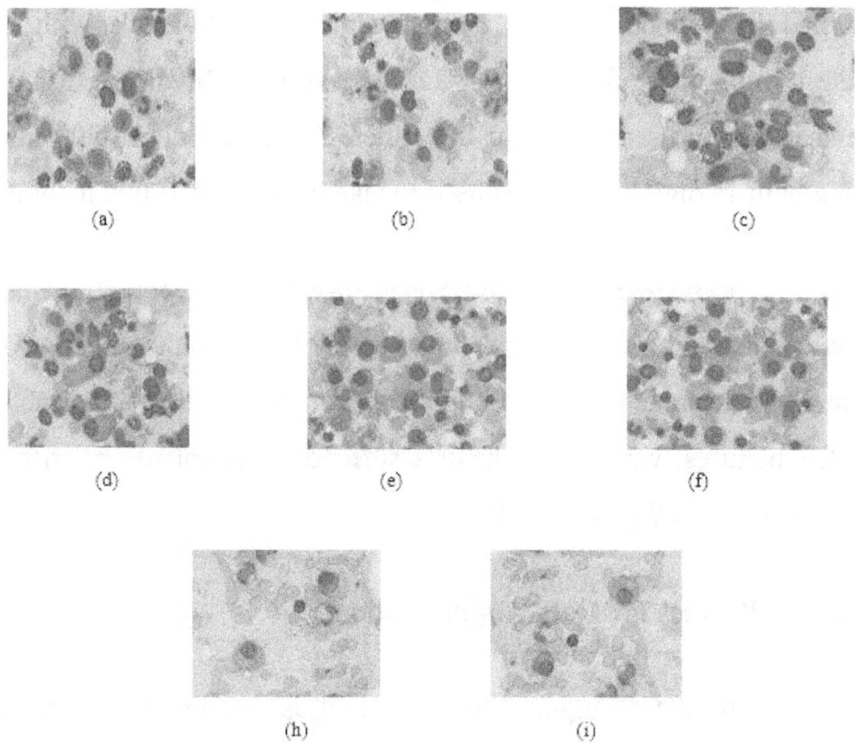

Figure 5.2   Augmented Cancer cell images: MM Cancer cell images (a-f) and ALL Cancer Cell Images (h&i)

5.2.3   Proposed Training Techniques

Convolutional Neural Network and cat optimization technique are covered in this part along with how they are utilized to adjust the hyper parameters.

5.2.3.1   Convolutional Neural Networks

Convolutional Layers (CL), Pooling Layers (PL), Fully Connected Layers (FCL), and Output Layers (OL) are the layers that make up the CNN architecture. The CL layers are in-charge of extracting various characteristics using various convolutional filters from the input cancer cell pictures. Each offset of the input pictures is subjected to these filters' convolutional procedures.

The features taken from the CL are concatenated and transferred into feature space using a non-linear activation unit (reLu). Utilizing the PL, the feature maps obtained from the CL are reduced in size while retaining the majority of the image's accessible data. The information included in the image is kept in the suggested architecture using Max-Pooling Layers. The final CNN layer, which is completely linked, assigns a specific class to the extracted feature maps.

CNN training entails adjusting the settings of the hidden neurons and convolutional kernels in the fully connected layers in order to lower the misclassification rate. To do so, the CL and fully connected layer parameters are tuned using the Stochastic Gradient Descent (SGD) training method. The main disadvantage of using SGD is that it has lot of hyper-parameters that might have an effect on how well the network performs. An illustration of a convolutional neural network's overall architecture is provided in Figure 5.3.

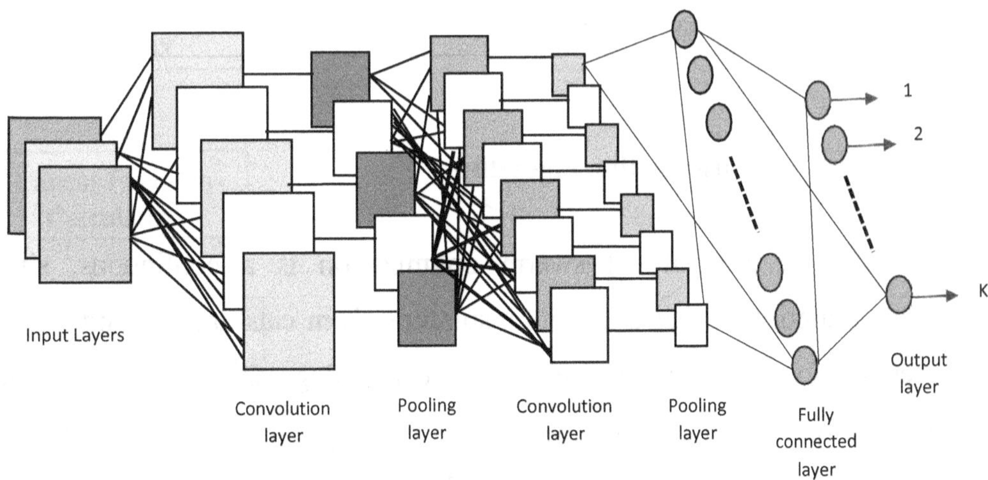

Figure 5.3 Convolutional Neural Network and Its Functioning layers

## 5.3	EXPERIMENTAL SET UP

### 5.3.1	Implementation Details

Tensorflow v.18, a complete open source Python platform, is used to implement the proposed model. The multi-classification model underwent 1000 rounds of training on 1024 photos. The networks' loss functions are optimized using the cat-optimizer to provide the lowest possible loss during iteration. The photos of the bone marrow malignancy are then used to train the model to recognize it. The model is trained using an i7 CPU, 16GB RAM, and a 2.5 GHz operating NVIDIA K80 GPU.

### 5.3.2	Performance Metrics

Table 5.4 shows the total number of datasets employed to train and test the proposed model. Performance metrics are accuracy, sensitivity, specificity, recall, and f1-score; they are computed and examined in order to assess the performance of the proposed architecture.

Table 5.4 Datasets Used for Training and Testing the Proposed Network (After Augmentation)

Sl.no	Total Number of Images	Training Data (%)	Testing Data (%)
01	1024	70	30

## 5.4	CHAPTER SUMMARY

The framework is designed to identify and categorize different types of bone marrow cancer cells from healthy cells using microscopic cancer pictures. The proposed model first uses an Optimized Convolutional Neural Network (OCNN) to train on preprocessed cell pictures before detecting the specific kind of cancer cells observed in the bone marrow.

In addition, the proposed architecture incorporates four convolutional layers and cat-swarm optimization is performed to optimize the hyper-parameters. Hence, this study employs the optimized hyper -parameters to lower the computational complexity, which has an impact on the performance of the training network.

In order to compare the proposed approach to other state-of-the-art deep learning architectures, Tensorflow 1.8 and Keras API are used in its development to compute the performance metrics. Multiple performance indicators, which are accuracy (99.59%), precision (99.23%), recall (99.47%), specificity (99.31%), and F1-score (99.90%), are computed and examined.

CHAPTER 6

RESULTS AND DISCUSSION

6.1   EXPERIMENTAL SETUP

Tensorflow v.18, a complete Python open source platform, is used to implement the proposed work. Using 1024 pictures over 1000 iterations, the multi-classification model is trained. The loss functions in the network are optimized using the cat optimizer, which results in the iteration's lowest loss. Finally, the BMC in the photos is recognized using the trained model. The model is trained using a 2.5 GHz operating-frequency NVIDIA K80 GPU, 16GB of RAM, and an i7 CPU is used. To validate the suggested learning model, the proposed work is put into practice using a Raspberry Pi Model B+.

Performance matrices which are "accuracy, precision, sensitivity or recall, specificity and F1-score" , are calculated to assess the performance of the proposed architectures . The mathematical formulas for computing the metrics used to assess the proposed architectures are shown in Table 6.1.

Table 6.1 Performance metrics using mathematical expressions

Sl.No	Performance metrics	Mathematical expression
01	Accuracy	——————————
02	Sensitivity or recall	——— x100
03	Specificity	———
04	Precision	———
05	F1-Score	—— * ——

Where, —TP‖ - True Positive Values, —TN‖ - True Negative Values, —FP‖- False Positive and —FN‖ - False Negative Values‖. The proposed work is implemented in three phases. In every phase around 7% performance enhancements in predicting the cancer cells are shown. Phase – III shows the superior performance.

6.2   PHASE I: LBP ENABLED ELM FRAMEWORK

This framework is compared to various current models as LBP+SVM, LBP+RF, LBP+KNN, GLCM+ELM, and LBP+DT in order to demonstrate the superiority of the proposed approach. The proposed LBP enabled ELM (LBP+ELM) framework performance is evaluated using following parameters presented in preceding sections.

6.2.1 Accuracy Analysis

In this subsection, the proposed LBP+ELM framework's performance is evaluated in terms of accuracy where two datasets namely ALL and MM are used for the evaluation.

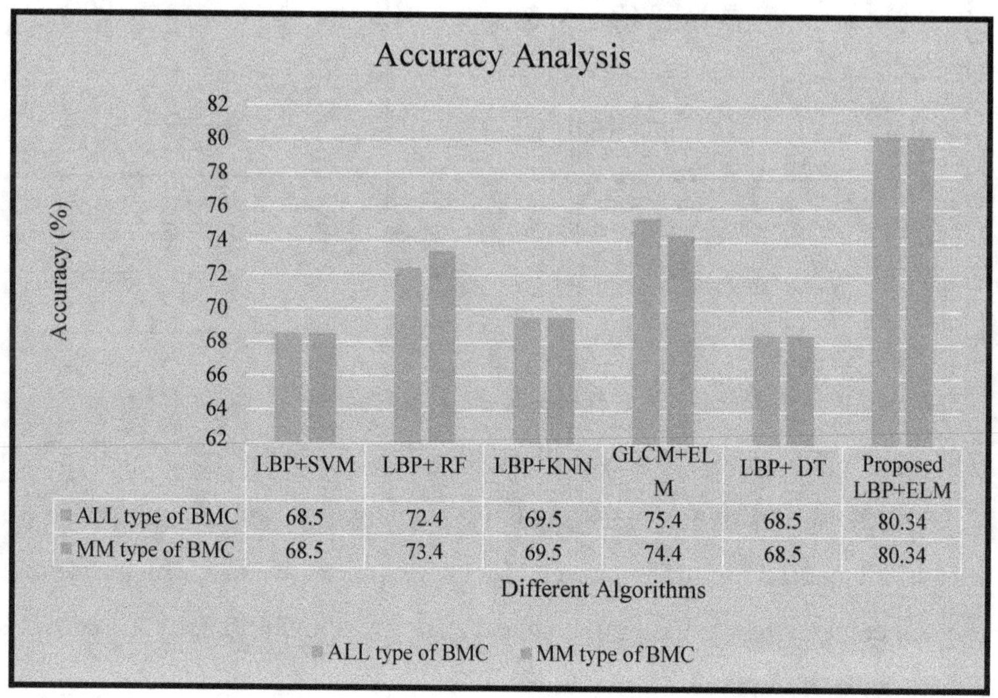

	LBP+SVM	LBP+ RF	LBP+KNN	GLCM+ELM	LBP+ DT	Proposed LBP+ELM
ALL type of BMC	68.5	72.4	69.5	75.4	68.5	80.34
MM type of BMC	68.5	73.4	69.5	74.4	68.5	80.34

Figure 6.1   Accuracy analysis of Proposed LBP+ELM framework with other algorithms

Figure 6.1 illustrates the accuracy analysis of the proposed LBP+ELM framework with other existing algorithms for the classification of ALL and MMM type of BMC. For the ALL type of BMC, the proposed LBP+ELM algorithm achieved 80.34% of accuracy, whereas the other algorithms such as LBP+SVM, LBP+RF, LBP+KNN, GLCM+ELM and LBP+DT algorithms achieved less accuracy of 68.5%, 72.4%, 69.5%, 75.4% and 68.5% respectively.

The proposed LBP+ELM algorithm maintained same performance that is 80% accuracy for another type of BMC namely MM. In this case the other existing algorithms produced less accuracy of 68.5%, 73.4%, 69.5%, 74.4%, 68.5% respectively.

6.2.2   Precision Analysis

In this subsection the proposed LBP+ELM framework's performance is evaluated in terms of Precision.

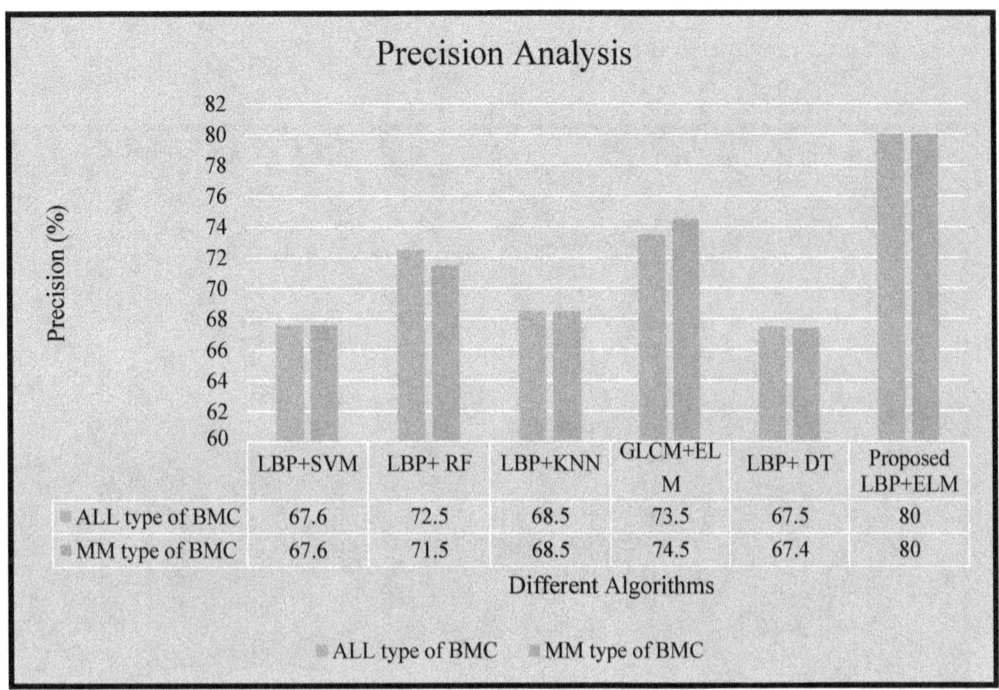

	LBP+SVM	LBP+ RF	LBP+KNN	GLCM+ELM	LBP+ DT	Proposed LBP+ELM
ALL type of BMC	67.6	72.5	68.5	73.5	67.5	80
MM type of BMC	67.6	71.5	68.5	74.5	67.4	80

Figure 6.2   Precision analysis of Proposed LBP+ELM framework with other algorithms

Figure 6.2 illustrates the precision analysis of the proposed LBP+ELM framework with other existing algorithms for the classification of ALL and MMM type of BMC. For the ALL type of BMC, the proposed LBP+ELM algorithm achieved 80 % of precision, whereas the other algorithms such as LBP+SVM, LBP+RF, LBP+KNN, GLCM+ELM and LBP+DT algorithms produced less precision of 67.6%, 72.5%, 68.5%, 73.5% and 67.5% respectively.

The proposed LBP+ELM algorithm maintained same performance that is 80% precision for another type of BMC namely MM. In this case the other existing algorithms are produced less precision of 67.6%, 71.5%, 68.5%, 74.5%, 67.4% respectively.

6.2.3   Recall Analysis

In this subsection the proposed LBP+ELM framework's performance is evaluated in terms of recall.

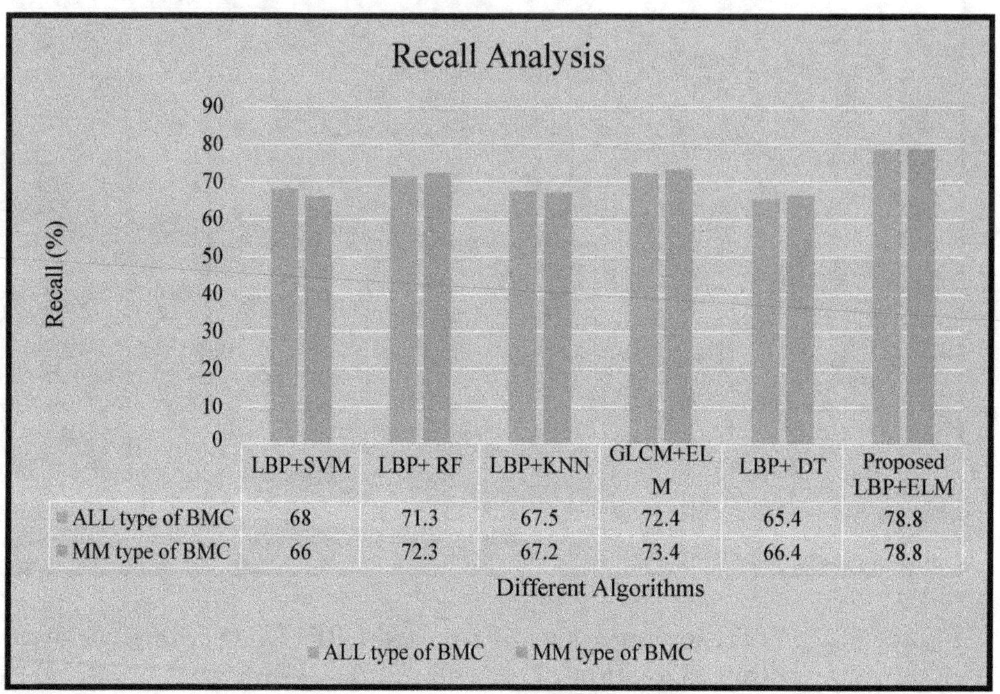

	LBP+SVM	LBP+ RF	LBP+KNN	GLCM+ELM	LBP+ DT	Proposed LBP+ELM
ALL type of BMC	68	71.3	67.5	72.4	65.4	78.8
MM type of BMC	66	72.3	67.2	73.4	66.4	78.8

Figure 6.3   Recall analysis of Proposed LBP+ELM framework with other algorithms

The recall analysis of the proposed LBP+ELM framework with other current methods for the classification of ALL and MMM type of BMC is shown in Figure 6.3. For the ALL type of BMC, the proposed LBP+ELM algorithm achieved 78.8 % of recall, whereas the other algorithms such as LBP+SVM, LBP+RF, LBP+KNN, GLCM+ELM and LBP+DT algorithms produced less recall of 68%, 71.3%, 67.5%, 72.4% and 65.4% respectively.

The proposed LBP+ELM algorithm maintained same performance that is 78.8 % recall for another type of BMC namely MM. In this case the other existing algorithms produced less recall of 66%, 72.3%, 67.2%, 73.4%, 66.4%.

6.2.4 Specificity Analysis

In this subsection the proposed LBP+ELM framework's performance is evaluated in terms of specificity.

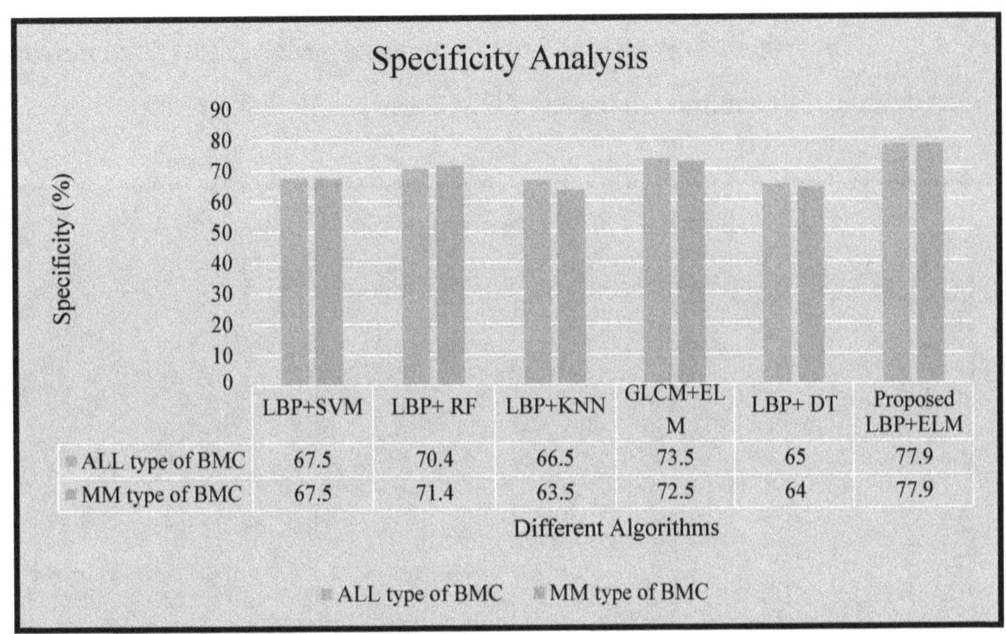

	LBP+SVM	LBP+ RF	LBP+KNN	GLCM+ELM	LBP+ DT	Proposed LBP+ELM
ALL type of BMC	67.5	70.4	66.5	73.5	65	77.9
MM type of BMC	67.5	71.4	63.5	72.5	64	77.9

Figure 6.4   Specificity analysis of Proposed LBP+ELM framework with other algorithms

Figure 6.4 illustrates the specificity analysis of the proposed LBP+ELM framework with other existing algorithms for the classification of ALL and MMM type of BMC. For the ALL type of BMC, the proposed LBP+ELM algorithm achieved 77.9 % of specificity, whereas the other algorithms such as LBP+SVM, LBP+RF, LBP+KNN, GLCM+ELM and LBP+DT algorithms achieved less specificity of 67.5%, 70.4%, 66.5%, 73.5% and 65% respectively.

The proposed LBP+ELM algorithm maintained same performance that is 77.9% specificity for another type of BMC namely MM. In this case the other existing algorithms achieved less specificity of 67.5%, 71.4%, 63.5%, 72.5%, 64% respectively. Because LBP and ELM were combined, the suggested LBP+ELM framework beat other algorithms in terms of specificity, according to the results. For both type of BMCs this framework provides good results in terms of specificity.

6.2.5   F1-Score Analysis

In this subsection the proposed LBP+ELM framework's performance is examined in terms of F1-Score.

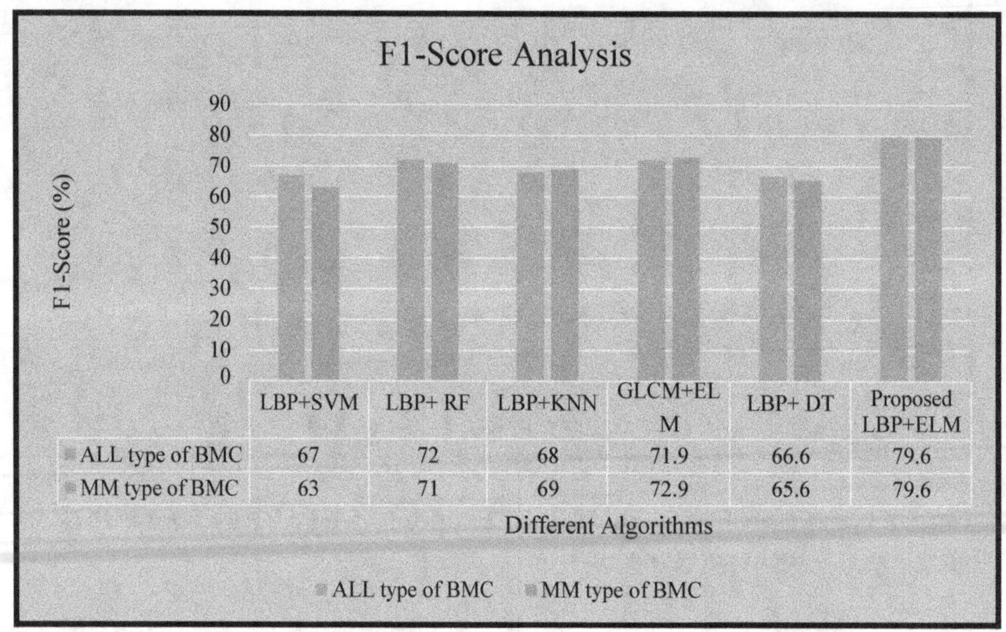

	LBP+SVM	LBP+ RF	LBP+KNN	GLCM+ELM	LBP+ DT	Proposed LBP+ELM
ALL type of BMC	67	72	68	71.9	66.6	79.6
MM type of BMC	63	71	69	72.9	65.6	79.6

Figure 6.5   F1-Score analysis of Proposed LBP+ELM framework with other algorithms

Figure 6.5 illustrates the F1-Score analysis of the proposed LBP+ELM framework with other existing algorithms for the classification of ALL and MMM type of BMC. For the ALL type of BMC, the proposed LBP+ELM algorithm achieved 79.6 % of F1-Score, whereas the other algorithms such as LBP+SVM, LBP+RF, LBP+KNN, GLCM+ELM and LBP+DT algorithms achieved less F1-Score of 67%, 72%, 68%, 71.9% and 66.6% respectively. The proposed LBP+ELM algorithm maintained same performance that is 79.6% F1-Score for another type of BMC namely MM.

In this case the other existing algorithms produced less F1-Score of 63%, 71%, 69%, 72.9%, and 66.6% respectively. The results strongly proved that the proposed LBP+ELM framework outperformed other algorithms due to the incorporation of LBP with ELM. For both type of BMCs this framework provides good results in terms of accuracy, precision, recall, specificity and F1-Socre.

Even though the proposed LBP+ELM framework established its better performance in terms of accuracy (80.34%), precision (80%), recall (78.8%), specificity (77.9%) and F1-Socre (79.6%), it struggles for large scale datasets. Hence, optimization is required to further enhance the performance matrices so as to make the framework more suitable for any kind of network. The next sub-section gives the second phase to countermeasure the drawback of Phase-I framework.

6.3 TRANSFER LEARNING + OPTIMIZED FIREFLY NEURAL NETWORKS

To establish the superiority of the proposed Transfer Learning + Optimized Firefly Neural Networks is compared with the other existing models such as Whale+VGG-19, ACO+VGG-19, PSO+VGG-19, GA+VGG-19, BCO+VGG-19. The proposed framework performance is evaluated using following parameters presented in preceding sections.

6.3.1 Accuracy Analysis

In this subsection the proposed Transfer Learning + Optimized Firefly Neural Networks framework's performance is evaluated in terms of accuracy.

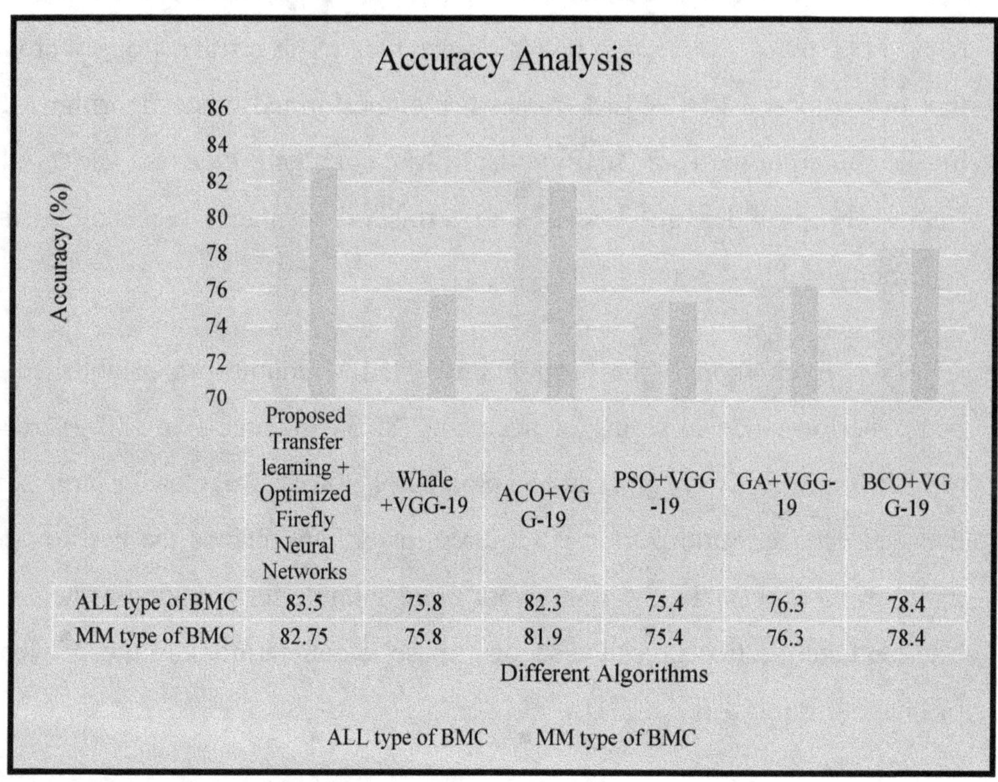

	Proposed Transfer learning + Optimized Firefly Neural Networks	Whale +VGG-19	ACO+VG G-19	PSO+VGG -19	GA+VGG- 19	BCO+VG G-19
ALL type of BMC	83.5	75.8	82.3	75.4	76.3	78.4
MM type of BMC	82.75	75.8	81.9	75.4	76.3	78.4

Figure 6.6   The accuracy analysis of proposed transfer learning + Optimized Firefly Neural Networks.

Figure 6.6 illustrates the accuracy analysis of Proposed Transfer Learning + Optimized Firefly Neural Network with other algorithms for the classification of ALL and MM types of BMC. For the ALL type of BMC, the proposed Transfer Learning + Optimized Firefly Neural Network achieved 83.5% of accuracy, whereas the other algorithms such as Whale +VGG 19, ACO+VGG-19, PSO+VGG-19, GA+VGG-19, BCO+VGG-19 algorithms produced   less accuracy of 75.8%, 82.3%, 75.4%, 76.3% and 78.4% respectively.

The proposed Transfer Learning + Optimized Firefly Neural Network almost maintained same performance that is 82.75% accuracy for another type of BMC namely MM. In this case, the other existing algorithms produced lesser accuracy of 75.8%, 81.9%, 75.4%, 68.5% and 78.4% respectively.

6.3.2　Precision Analysis

In this subsection the proposed Transfer Learning + Optimized Firefly Neural Networks framework's performance is evaluated in terms of Precision.

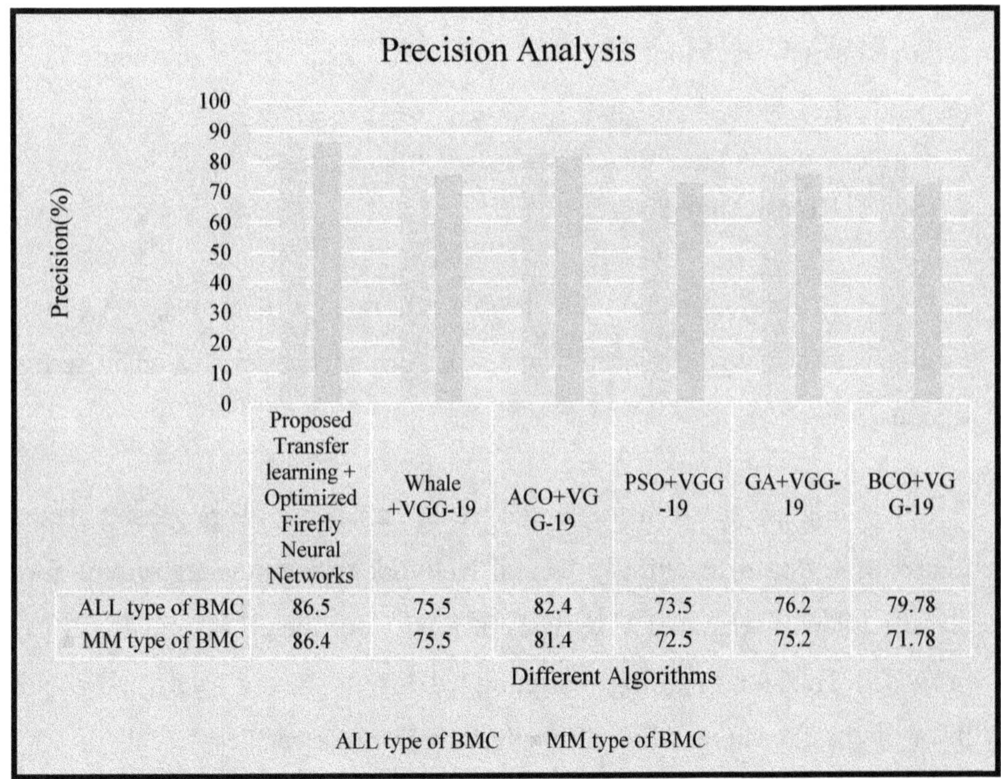

	Proposed Transfer learning + Optimized Firefly Neural Networks	Whale +VGG-19	ACO+VGG-19	PSO+VGG-19	GA+VGG-19	BCO+VGG-19
ALL type of BMC	86.5	75.5	82.4	73.5	76.2	79.78
MM type of BMC	86.4	75.5	81.4	72.5	75.2	71.78

Figure 6.7　Precision analysis of Proposed Transfer Learning + Optimized Firefly Neural Network with other algorithms

Figure 6.7 illustrates the precision analysis of Proposed Transfer Learning + Optimized Firefly Neural Network with other algorithms for the classification of ALL and MM types of BMC. For the ALL type of BMC, the proposed Transfer Learning + Optimized Firefly Neural Network achieved 86.5% of precision, whereas the other algorithms such as Whale +VGG 19, ACO+VGG-19, PSO+VGG-19, GA+VGG-19, BCO+VGG-19 algorithms produced less precision of 75.5%, 82.4%, 73.5%, 76.2% and 79.78% respectively.

The proposed Transfer Learning + Optimized Firefly Neural Network almost maintained same performance that is 86.4% precision for another type of BMC namely MM. In this case the other existing algorithms achieved less precision of 75.5%, 81.4%, 72.5%, 75.2% and 71.78% respectively.

6.3.3   Recall Analysis

In this subsection the proposed Transfer Learning + Optimized Firefly Neural Networks framework's performance is evaluated in terms of Recall.

Figure 6.8 illustrates the recall analysis of proposed Transfer Learning + Optimized Firefly Neural Network with other algorithms for the classification of ALL and MM types of BMC. For the ALL type of BMC, the proposed Transfer Learning + Optimized Firefly Neural Network achieved 87% of recall, whereas the other algorithms produced less recall of 73.3%, 83.2%, 72.4%, 76.4% and 78.8% respectively.

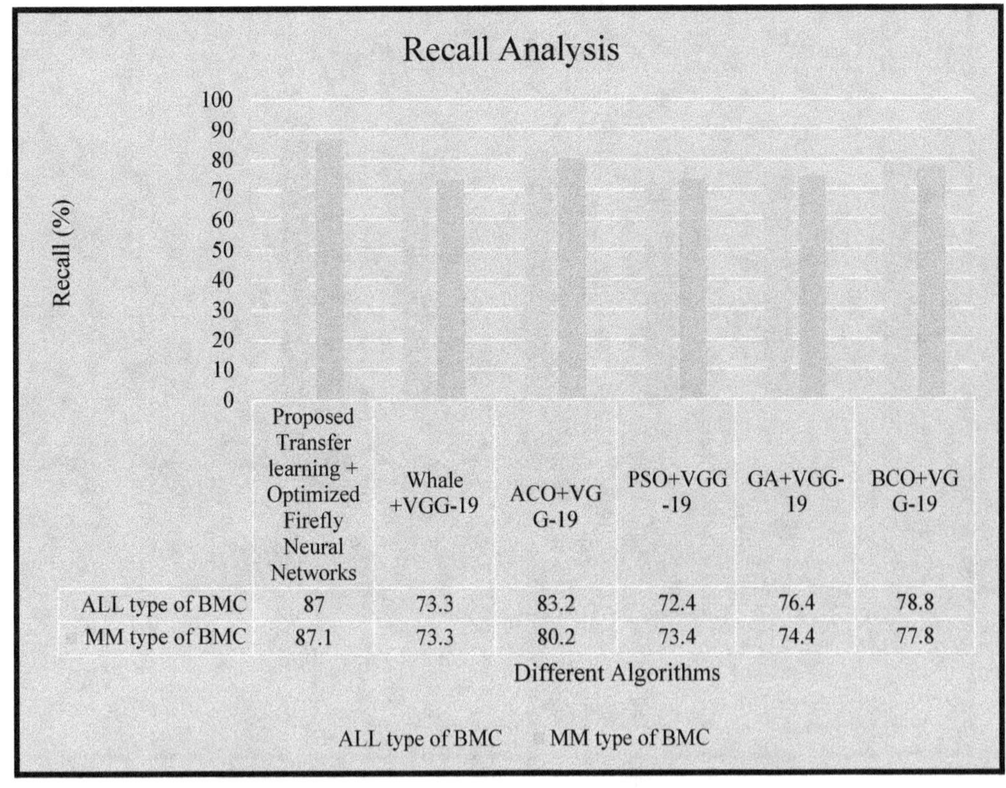

	Proposed Transfer learning + Optimized Firefly Neural Networks	Whale +VGG-19	ACO+VGG-19	PSO+VGG-19	GA+VGG-19	BCO+VGG-19
ALL type of BMC	87	73.3	83.2	72.4	76.4	78.8
MM type of BMC	87.1	73.3	80.2	73.4	74.4	77.8

Figure 6.8   Recall analysis of proposed Transfer Learning + Optimized Firefly Neural Network with other algorithms

The proposed Transfer Learning + Optimized Firefly Neural Network almost maintained same performance that is 87.1% recall for another type of BMC namely MM. in this case the other existing algorithms achieved less accuracy of 73.3%, 80.2%, 73.4%, 74.4% and 77.8 % respectively.

6.3.4   Specificity Analysis

In this subsection the proposed Transfer Learning + Optimized Firefly Neural Networks framework's performance is evaluated in terms of Specificity.

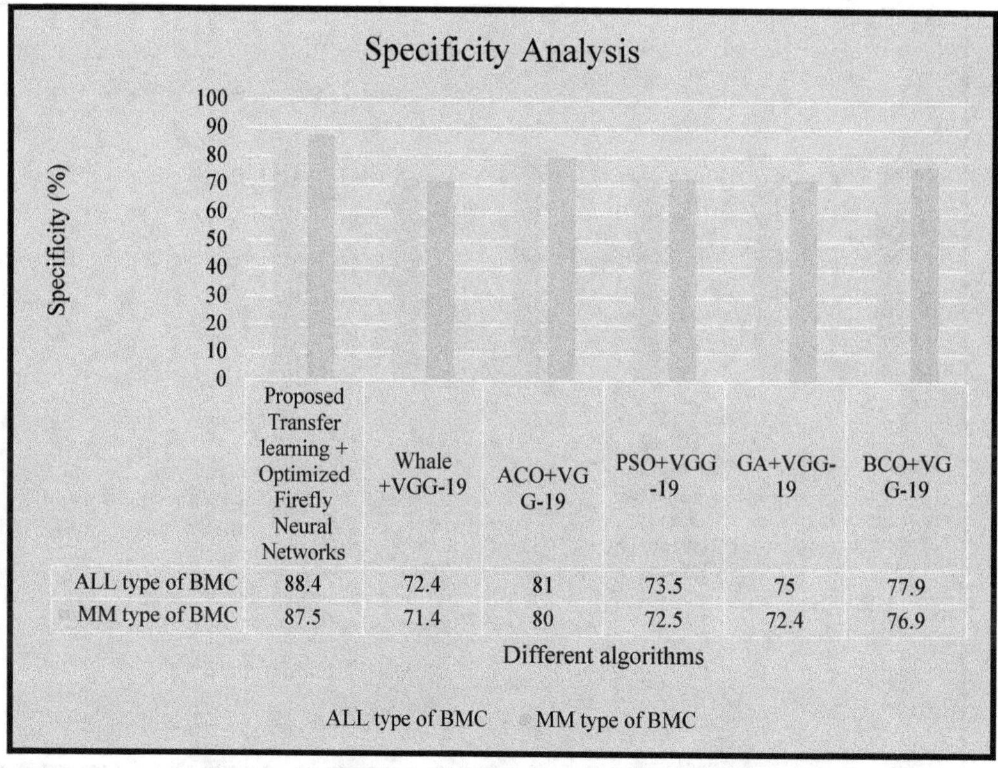

	Proposed Transfer learning + Optimized Firefly Neural Networks	Whale +VGG-19	ACO+VGG-19	PSO+VGG-19	GA+VGG-19	BCO+VGG-19
ALL type of BMC	88.4	72.4	81	73.5	75	77.9
MM type of BMC	87.5	71.4	80	72.5	72.4	76.9

Figure 6.9   Specificity analysis of Proposed Transfer Learning + Optimized Firefly Neural Network with other algorithms

Figure 6.9 illustrates the specificity analysis of proposed Transfer Learning + Optimized Firefly Neural Network with other algorithms for the classification of ALL and MM types of BMC. For the ALL type of BMC, the proposed Transfer Learning + Optimized Firefly Neural Network achieved 88.4% of specificity, whereas the other algorithms produced less specificity of 72.4%, 81%, 73.5%, 75% and 77.9% respectively.

The proposed Transfer Learning + Optimized Firefly Neural Network almost maintained same performance that is 87.5% specificity for another type of BMC namely MM. In this case the other existing algorithms achieved less accuracy of 71.4%, 80%, 72.5%, 72.4% and 76.9 % respectively.

6.3.5   F1-Score Analysis

In this subsection the proposed Transfer Learning + Optimized Firefly Neural Networks framework's performance is evaluated in terms of F1-Score.

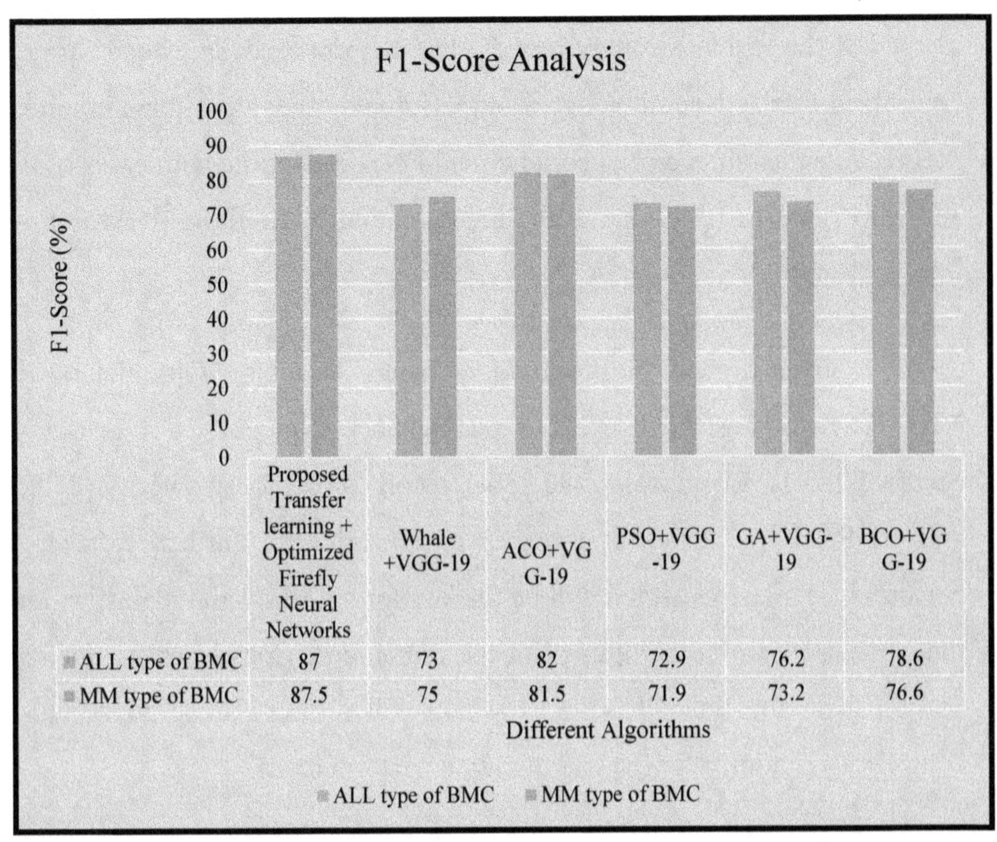

Figure 6.10 F1-Score analysis of Proposed Transfer Learning + Optimized Firefly Neural Network with other algorithms

Figure 6.10 illustrates the F1-Score analysis of proposed Transfer Learning + Optimized Firefly Neural Network with other algorithms for the classification of ALL and MM types of BMC. For the ALL type of BMC, the proposed Transfer Learning + Optimized Firefly Neural Network achieved 87% of F1-Score, whereas the other algorithms produced less F1-Score of 73%, 82%, 72.9%, 76.2% and 78.6% respectively.

The proposed Transfer Learning + Optimized Firefly Neural Network almost maintained same performance that is 87.5% F1-Score for another type of BMC namely MM. in this case the other existing algorithms achieved less F1-Score of 75%, 81.5%, 71.9%, 73.2% and 76.6% respectively.

The results strongly proved that the proposed Transfer Learning + Optimized Firefly Neural Network outperformed other algorithms in terms of accuracy, precision, recall, specificity and F1-Socre for the both cases of AAL and MM types of BMC due to the incorporation of firefly optimization with transfer learning.

Even though the proposed Transfer Learning + Optimized Firefly Neural Network established better performance than Phase - I in terms of accuracy (83.12%), precision (86.45%), recall (87.05%), specificity (87.95%) and F1-Socre (87.25%), it requires optimization to further enhance the performance matrices which will be the key for the study and identification of tumor cells based on the opinion of the radiologist. Consequently, upcoming section gives the final Phase – III which will further reduce computational complexity and improve the classification performance.

6.4 CAT OPTIMIZED CNN FOR BMC CLASSIFICATION

To prove the superiority of the cat- optimized CNN framework, the evaluation is carried out in terms of accuracy Vs number of iterations, confusion matrix, accuracy, precision, recall, specificity and F1-Score.

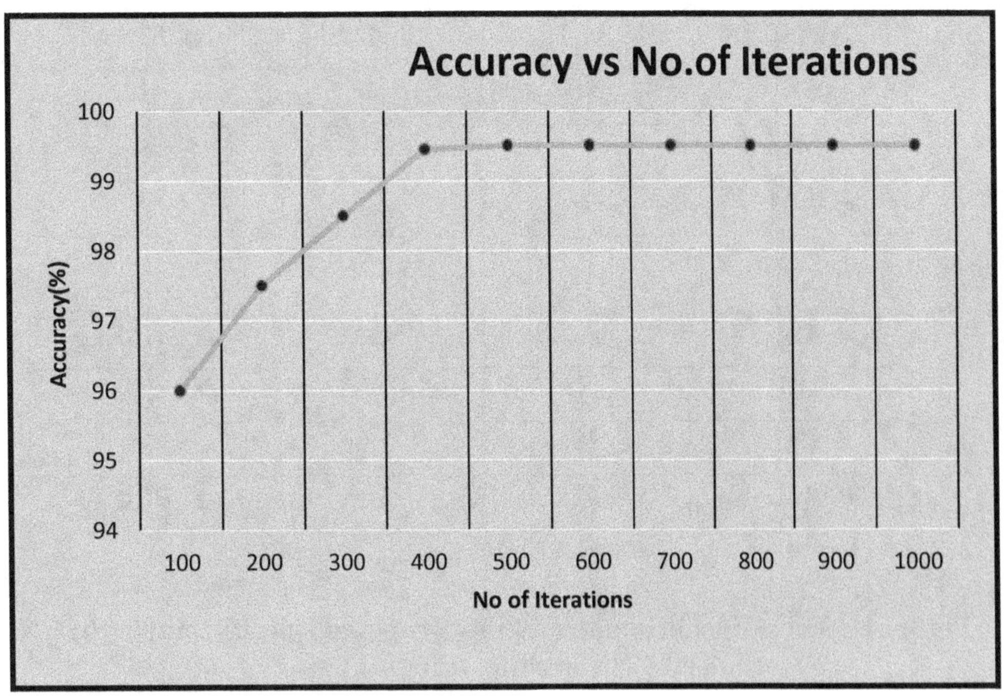

Figure 6.11 Accuracy in identifying ALL types of bone tumors using the proposed architecture

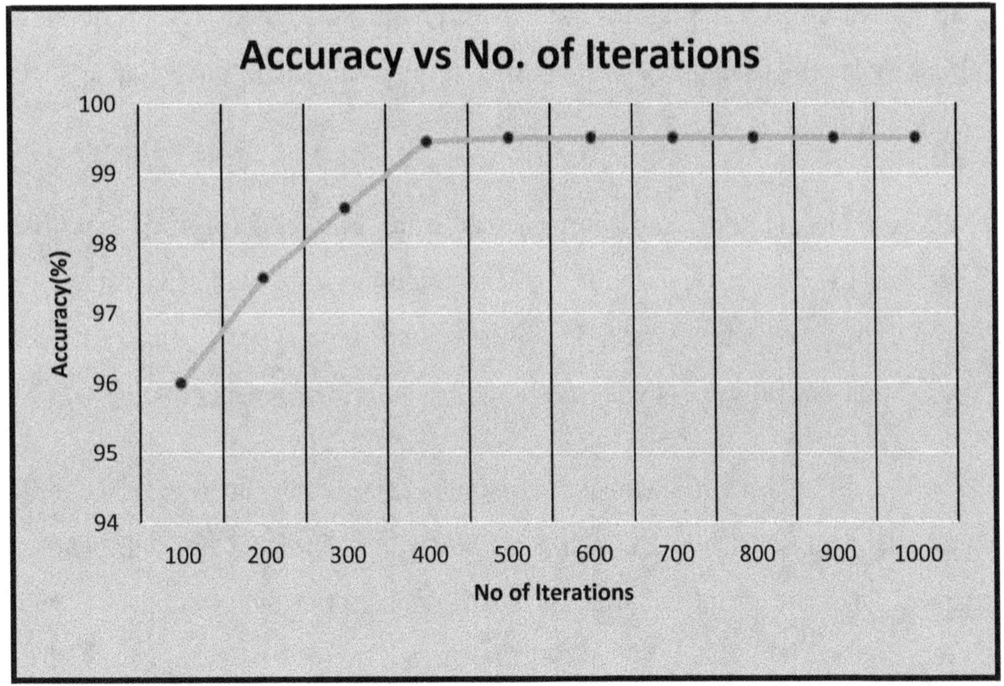

Figure 6.12 Accuracy of the proposed architecture for finding MM Type Bone Cancers

CLASSES	ALL	MM	NORMAL
ALL	341	0	1
MM	1	340	1
NORMAL	1	2	339

(a)

CLASSES	ALL	MM	NORMAL
ALL	281	30	29
MM	29	280	31
NORMAL	31	293	281

(b)

Figure 6.13   Confusion   matrices a)   Proposed   architecture   b)   Non-optimized CNN architectures

The accuracy of the proposed architecture in identifying the various cancer types is depicted in Figures 6.11 and 6.12 in relation with the number of iterations. According to Figure 6.11, the suggested design obtains its highest level of accuracy after 400 iterations and maintains that level until 1000 iterations.

Using the Confusion Matrix from Figure 6.13, it is possible to detect ALL cancer types with a 99.6% accuracy rate and MM cancer types with a 99.57% accuracy rate. The accuracy for both types of cancer detection in the non-optimized CNN layers is 92.0% and 92.1%, respectively.

The performance comparison between the non - optimized CNN and the proposed CNN algorithm is shown in Tables 6.2 and 6.3. Table 6.3 reveals that the proposed method has demonstrated the accuracy of 99.6%, precision of 99.2%, recall of 99.5%, and a high F1-Score of 99.89% in identifying ALL types of cancer cells.

Table 6.2 Metrics for the CNN's performance in predicting bone marrow malignancies (without optimization)

SL.NO	Type of Cancer	Performance Metrics (%)				
		Accuracy	Precision	Recall	Specificity	F1-Score
01	ALL	92.0%	92.4%	91.0%	91.4%	92.7%
02	MM	92.1%	91.25%	90.5%	90.3%	90.2%

Almost similar performance is found in MM type also. Further, it is observed from Table 6.2 and Table 6.3 that about 7% performance improvement is found between non optimized CNN architecture and the proposed optimized architecture.

Table 6.3 Performance metrics for the proposed Bone Marrow Cancer Prediction Algorithm (with optimization)

SL.NO	Type of Cancer	Performance Metrics (%)				
		Accuracy	Precision	Recall	Specificity	F1-Score
01	ALL	99.6%	99.2%	99.5%	99.3%	99.89%
02	MM	99.57%	99.25%	99.44%	99.32%	99.90%

6.4.1 Comparative Analysis

The proposed technique is compared to several current models, including CNN, Support Vector Machines (SVM), Naive Bayes (NB), Random Forest (RF), and Artificial Neural Networks, in order to demonstrate its superiority (ANN).

Table 6.4 Performance analysis of different algorithms for detection of ALL type of cancer cells

Sl.NO	Algorithms	Performance metrics (%)				
		Accuracy	Precision	Recall	Specificity	F1-Score
01	Alexnets	90%	89.5%	88.5%	88.45%	89.7%
02	U-Nets	84.5%	83.5%	84.5%	82.5%	80.4%
03	RESNETS	85%	84.3%	83.5%	84%	83.2%
04	VGG-16	91%	91.5%	92%	91.45%	92.4%
05	CNN	92.0%	92.4%	91.0%	91.4%	92.7%
06	SVM	78%	78.45%	77%	76.5%	75%
07	NB	70%	68.5%	75%	74.5%	74%
08	RF	68%	67.5%	67%	68%	67.5%
09	ANN	68.5%	68.4%	68.34%	68.25%	68%
10	Proposed Architecture	99.6%	99.2%	99.5%	99.3%	99.89%

Table 6.5 Performance Analysis of Different Algorithms for detection of MM type of Cancer Cells

Sl.No	Algorithms	Performance metrics (%)				
		Accuracy	Precision	Recall	Specificity	F1-Score
01	Alexnets	90%	89.5%	88.5%	88.45%	89.7%
02	U-Nets	84.5%	83.5%	84.5%	82.5%	80.4%
03	RESNETS	85%	84.3%	83.5%	84%	83.2%
04	VGG-16	91%	91.5%	92%	91.45%	92.4%
05	CNN	92.0%	92.4%	91.0%	91.4%	92.7%
06	SVM	78%	78.45%	77%	76.5%	75%
07	NB	70%	68.5%	75%	74.5%	74%
08	RF	68%	67.5%	67%	68%	67.5%
09	ANN	68.5%	68.4%	68.34%	68.25%	68%
10	Proposed Architecture	99.57%	99.25%	99.44%	99.32%	99.90%

Table 6.4 and Table 6.5 show a comparison of the results of the proposed and existing algorithms. It is clear from Tables 6.4 and 6.5 that the optimization technique used in the proposed architecture has demonstrated superior performance to other existing algorithms, outperforming them by 10% for Alexnets, 15%–16% for U-Nets and Resnets, 9%–10% for traditional CNN and VGG-16 nets, and even 15% for other cutting-edge learning models. As a result, the proposed system may identify cancer cells more accurately than other learning models already in use.

6.5 COMPARATIVE ANALYSIS OF PROPOSED FRAME WORKS Phase – I, II and III

Table 6.6 shows the comparative analysis of proposed frameworks. From the Table 6.6, it is obvious that the cat - optimized CNN framework produced better results in identifying the two types of cancer cells.

Table 6.6 Comparative analysis of proposed frameworks

Proposed Frameworks	Accuracy (%)	Precision (%)	Recall (%)	Specificity (%)	F1-Score (%)
LBP+ELM	80.34	80	78.8	77.9	79.6
Transfer learning + Firefly Neural Networks	83.12	86.45	87.05	87.95	87.25
Cat Optimized CNN	99.59	99.23	99.47	99.31	99.90

6.6 HARDWARE DEPLOYMENT AND VALIDATION OF THE PROPOSED RESEARCH WORK

The proposed Phase – III architecture, cat optimized CNN for BMC classification is deployed in embedded architecture for the validation of the software environment. Raspberry pi Model B+ with Quad Core Cortex architecture is taken for the validation. All the simulated algorithms in NVIDIA GPU are deployed on Embedded CPU architecture so that these algorithms can be deployed for real time applications.

The proposed architecture and algorithm can be ported in the hardware, Raspberry Pi Model B+ to validate the proposed architecture since the proposed research work is developed using TensorFlow 2.1. For Porting in the Raspberry Pi, Tensorflow model is converted in to Tensorflow lite version 2.1.

These models are trained in Raspberry pi model B+ and compared with the simulation experimentation of the proposed learning model. All the datasets used in simulation environment, are used as the training images in raspberry pi model b+ boards. 70% training and 30% are used for testing. All the performance metrics are measured during experimentation.

Averaging the proposed algorithm's performance is found to be 99.5% for Datasets-1 and 99.02% for Datasets-2. Table 6.7 presents the detailed comparative analysis of the algorithm in hardware and software environment.

It is found from the Table 6.7, average performance of the proposed algorithm in the embedded architecture has produced similar performance as in the software environment (error deviation is 0.54%). Hence the proposed model is validated with the hardware implementation and it is shown that the architecture has the ability to deploy in hardware environment also which can be applied for real time resource constraint devices.

Table 6.7 Comparison of software and hardware implementation performance metrics for Dataset-I and II.

Performance matrices	Software implementation		Hardware Implementation		Deviation	
	Data set - I	Data set - II	Data set - I	Data set - II	Data set - I	Data set - II
Accuracy	99.1%	99.57%	99.55%	99.02%	0.45%	0.55%
Precision	98.2%	99.25%	99.06%	98.7%	0.86%	0.55%
Recall	98.9%	99.44%	98.96%	98.66%	0.06%	0.78%
Specificity	98.1%	99.32%	99.5%	98.7%	0.40%	0.62%
F1-Score	99.1%	99.1%	99.4%	99.08%	0.30%	0.82%
Average divergence					0.54%	

6.7 CHAPTER SUMMARY

The research work is implemented in three phases; in every phase, performance enhancement is observed. It is obvious from the analysis that the optimized performance is achieved in the third phase to predict the cancer cells.

LBP enabled ELM classification approach is used for the BMC cell prediction in the first phase and got improved performance in terms of accuracy (80.34%), precision (80%), recall (78.8%), specificity (77.9%) and F1-Socre (79.6%) while comparing with other algorithms.

In the second phase of CNN, transfer learning and firefly optimization are used to address the shortcomings of Phase- I. With prediction accuracy of 83.12%, precision of 86.45%, recall of 87.05%, specificity of

87.95% and F1-Socre of 87.25% for the detection of BMC, the second phase performed better than the first phase.

Finally, cat-optimized hyper -parameters are employed in CNN in this phase. The third phase's performance metrics include prediction accuracy of 99.59% precision of 99.23%, recall of 99.47%, specificity of 99.31% and F1-Socre of 99.90% for the detection of BMC.

It is obvious that the proposed third phase architecture and algorithm perform better in detecting BMC cell types for both ALL and MM datasets, compared to other architectures and algorithms. For hardware realization, the Phase-III architecture, which uses a CNN that is cat-optimized for BMC classification, is deployed in the Raspberry Pi Model B+ with quad-core cortex architecture. As a result, the hardware design is used to validate the proposed software environment, which discovered an average divergence of 0.54%.

The conclusion of the research and future scope are presented in the next section.

CHAPTER 7

CONCLUSION

The proper identification of acute leukemia, a group of severe illnesses that affect people of all ages, is crucial for lowering morbidity and death. Despite recent technological advancements and investigation modalities like cytogenetic and flow cytometry, particularly for primary healthcare practitioners who are the initial point of contact for patients with haematology, the clinical diagnosis of acute leukemia continues to be difficult and vulnerable to inherent subjectivity.

In order to help general practitioners and clinical laboratory practitioners to diagnose leukaemia, CAD-AL has consequently been a significant area of research attention in recent years. This is done by providing quantitative, repeatable analysis of the PB smear. Quantitative outcomes, tracking patient follow-ups, and keeping track of therapy advancement can all be facilitated by CAD-AL.

The development of such a diagnostic system is currently ongoing, and this kind of CAD system has not yet been used in practice. A more accurate and reliable diagnostic system than what has so far been developed is required to enhance the prediction capability of acute leukemia.

This research effort presents novel ways to address the problem of forecasting the acute leukemia in order to enhance some of the existing approaches and develop new ideas for accurate and reliable categorization of acute leukemia. The proposed methodologies consist of a number of steps, including picture capture, image segmentation, feature extraction, feature selection, and classification. The only approach to lower the mortality rate is by early diagnosis of bone marrow malignancy.

However, early detection of bone marrow cancer nodules is difficult, nevertheless, as we accomplish the thesis, the contributions of the research work are explained as follows:

The chapter wise summary is presented as follows.

Chapter 1, It is described what bone marrow cancer is and its types in order to locate the bone marrow nodule region and carry out categorization. Here, the challenges of bone marrow cancer diagnosis are also discussed. Additionally, the significance of machine learning models is highlighted in the processing of medical images. The facts of the illness as well as the description and formulation of the obstacles are described because detecting bone marrow cancer poses a number of complications.

Chapter 2, Addressed the existing systems available to predict the bone morrow cancer, advantages and drawbacks of the current system for detecting bone marrow malignancy.

Chapter 3, employs LBP enabled ELM network for improved categorization in order to identify where cancer cells are located. The proposed approach is developed using Tensorflow 1.8 and the Keras API. The outcomes demonstrate that the suggested architecture produced better outcomes, compared to other architectures and algorithms. Despite producing better performance, this system struggles to handle huge datasets. In order to make the architecture more efficient and appropriate for any type of network, further optimization is necessary.

Chapter 4, employs feature extraction based on transfer learning and capsule-based saliency segmentation. The proposed design also uses categorization layers based on fireflies to improve the accuracy. Several performance metrics, including accuracy, precision, recall, specificity, and F1-score, are computed and tested for this tumor identification approach utilizing the Tensorflow 1.8 tool with the Keras API. The methodologies used in the Phase – II provide better results and performance enhancement than the previous methodologies provided in Phase – I. Furthermore, there is still scope for further performance enhancement, which would be crucial from a radiologist's point of view for the study and identification of cancer cells.

Chapter 5, deals with Cat-optimized for the categorization of pictures with high accuracy and minimal processing cost, CNN is proposed. The proposed solution is developed using Tensorflow 1.8 and the Keras API, and it is assessed and contrasted with other cutting-edge architectures.

Chapter 6, describes the classification of ALL and MM types of BMC, the results and discussions for three Phases – I, II and III namely LBP enabled ELM, Transfer learning + Firefly Neural Network, and Cat-optimized CNN are provided in this chapter. In Phase – I, the performance metrics are accuracy (80.34%), precision (80%), recall (78.8%), specificity (77.9%) and F1-Socre (79.6%) where LBP is integrated into the ELM architecture. Hence, its performance is better, still to improve the performance, Phase – II is proposed.

In Phase – II, the performance metrics are prediction accuracy of 83.12%, precision of 86.45%, recall of 87.05%, specificity of 87.95% and F1-Socre of 87.25% for the detection of BMC, the second phase performance is better than the first phase, it is due to the incorporation of firefly optimization with transfer learning. In phase – III, the performance metrics are prediction accuracy of 99.59% precision of 99.23%, recall of 99.47%, specificity of

99.31% and F1-Socre of 99.90% for the detection of BMC where cat optimized CNN architecture is used.

Phase – III architecture is able to achieve superior performance for larger datasets with almost similar computational complexity compared with Phase I and II. It is obvious from the analysis that three different architectures are developed to detect the BMC types and the performance is enhanced in each phase and the superior performance is achieved in Phase – III. The Phase-III architecture is deployed in Raspberry Pi Model B+ with quad-core cortex architecture. Thus, the proposed software environment is validated with the hardware implementation and 0.54% deviation is found between hardware implementation and software environment.

7.1 FUTURE RESEARCH DIRECTIONS

Larger real-time clinical datasets will need to be used in future testing in order to be more rigorous. Furthermore, there is room for improvement in the suggested algorithm with regard to classifying the pictures according to the malignant traits of bone marrow malignancies, since this would be crucial for the practical applications of bone marrow cancer detection and effective therapy. The following are the future scopes:

- To increase the precision of early bone marrow cancer detection and diagnosis, a variety of feature extraction approaches, segmentation methods, and enhanced classification models will be investigated and refined.

- Rigorous testing is to be carried out using real time clinical datasets and more hand held devices using embedded system architecture have to be developed for real time bio-medical applications.

REFERENCES

1. Akilandeswari, U, Nithya, R & Santhi, B 2012, _Review on feature extraction methods in pattern classification', European Journal of Scientific Research, vol. 71, no. 2, pp. 265-272.

2. Alagu, S, Ahana Priyanka N, Kavitha G & Bhoopathy Bagan K 2021, _Automatic Detection of Acute Lymphoblastic Leukemia Using UNET Based Segmentation and Statistical Analysis of Fused Deep Features', Journal of Applied Artificial Intelligence, vol. 35, no.15, pp. 1952-1969.

3. Al-Khaffaf, H, Talib, AZ & Salam, RA 2008, _Removing salt-and-pepper noise from binary images of engineering drawings', In Proceedings of 19th International Conference on Pattern Recognition ICPR, PP:1-12.

4. Almarzooqi, S, Crumbacher, J, Firgau, E & Kahwash, S 2011, _Comparison of Peripheral Blood versus Bone Marrow Blast Immunophenotype in Pediatric Acute Leukemias', Ibnosina Journal of Medicine and Biomedical Sciences, vol. 3, no. 6, pp. 195-204.

5. Alrefai, N 2019, _Ensemble Machine Learning for Leukemia Cancer Diagnosis based on Microarray Datasets', International Journal of Applied Engineering Research, vol. 14, no. 21, pp. 4077-4084.

6. American Cancer Society 2013, _Childhood Leukemia Retrieved 23/10/2013, from http://www.cancer.org/cancer/leukemiainchildren/ detailed guide/childhood leukemia-diagnosis, PP:1-13

7. American Childhood Cancer Organization. (2012). Childhood Cancer Statistics. Retrieved 19/3/2012, from http://www.acco.org/ Information/About Childhood Cancer/ChildhoodCancerStatistics.aspx

8. Angelescu, S, Berbec, NM, Colita, A, Barbu, D & Lupu, AR 2012, _Value of Multifaced Approach Diagnosis and Classification of Acute Leukemias', vol. 7, no. 3, pp. 254.

9. Baig R Rehman, A, Almuhaimeed, A, Alzahrani, A & Rauf, HT 2022, _Detecting Malignant Leukemia Cells Using Microscopic Blood Smear Images: A Deep Learning Approach', Applied Sciences, vol.12, no. 6317, pp. 1-26.

10. Bain, BJ 2010, Leukaemia Diagnosis: John Wiley & Sons.

11. Baptista, D, Ferreira, P & Rocha, M 2020, _Deep learning for drug response prediction in cancer', Brief. Bio inform., vol. 22, pp. 360–379.

12. Billard, M, Lainey, E, Armoogum, P, Alberti, C, Fenneteau, O & Da Costa, L 2010, _Evaluation of the Cella Vision DM automated microscope in pediatrics', International Journal of Laboratory Haematology, vol. 32, no. 5, pp. 530-538..

13. Boreiri, Z, Azad, AN & Ghodousian, A 2022, _A Convolutional Neuro-Fuzzy Network Using Fuzzy Image Segmentation for Acute Leukemia Classification', 2022 27th International Computer Conference, Computer Society of Iran (CSICC), pp. 1-7.

14. Boundless 2013, _Anatomy and Physiology: Boundless.

15. Briggs, C, Longair, I, Slavik, M, Thwaite, K, Mills, R, Thavaraja, V & Machin, SJ 2009, _Can automated blood film analysis replace the manual differential? An evaluation of the Cella Vision DM96 automated image analysis system', International Journal of Laboratory Haematology, vol. 31, no. 1, pp. 48-60.

16. Bukhari, M, Yasmin, S, Sammad, S & Abd El-Latif, AA 2022, _A Deep Learning Framework for Leukemia Cancer Detection in Microscopic Blood Samples Using Squeeze and Excitation Learning', Mathematical Problems in Engineering, pp. 1-18.

17. Burger, W & Burge, MJ 2009 _Digital image processing: an algorithmic introduction using Java: Springer'. , pp:1-11

18. Cairo, MS & Perkins, SL 2012, _Hematological Malignancies in Children', Adolescents and Young Adults: World Scientific, PP:1-13.

19. Castellano, G, Bonilha, L, Li, LM & Cendes, F 2004, _Texture analysis of medical images', Clinical Radiology, vol. 59, no. 12, pp. 1061-1069.

20. Celik, C, Aksel, J & Karaoglan, B 2006, ‚Comparison of the Orpington Prognostic Scale (OPS) and the National Institutes of Health Stroke Scale (NIHSS) for the prediction of the functional status of patients with stroke‘, Disability & Rehabilitation, vol. 28, no. 10, pp. 609-612.

21. Chai, HY, Wee, LK, Swee, TT & Hussain, S 2011, ‚GLCM based adaptive crossed reconstructed k-mean clustering hand bone segmentation‘, in Proceedings of 3rd WSEAS International conference on World Scientific and Engineering Academy and Society, PP:1-9.

22. Chan, KP & Fu, AWC 1999, ‚Efficient time series matching by wavelets‘, in Proceedings of 15th International Conference on Data Engineering, Sydney, PP:1-13.

23. Chand, S & Vishwakarma, VP 2019, ‚Leukemia Diagnosis using Computational Intelligence‘, International Conference on Issues and Challenges in Intelligent Computing Techniques (ICICT), pp. 1-7.

24. Chen, M & Decary, M 2019, ‚Artificial intelligence in healthcare: An essential guide for health leaders‘, Health Manag. Forum 2019, vol. 33, pp. 10–18.

25. Chen, Y, Li, Y, Narayan, R, Subramanian, A & Xie, X 2016, ‚Gene expression inference with deep learning‘, Bioinformatics 2016, vol. 32, pp. 1832–1839.

26. Cheng, C, Mu, J, Farkas, I, Huang, D, Goebl, MG & Roach, PJ 1995, ‚Requirement of the self-glucosylating initiator proteins Glg1p and Glg2p for glycogen accumulation in Saccharomyces cerevisiae‘, Molecular Cell Biology, vol. 15, no. 12, pp. 6632-6640

27. Chu, SC, Tsai, Pw & Pan, JS 2006, ‚Cat Swarm Optimization: Trends in Artificial Intelligence‘, Lecture Notes in Computer Science, Springer, Berlin, Heidelberg. https://doi.org/10.1007/978-3-540-36668-3_94, vol. 4099.

28. Ciesla, B 2007, ‚Haematology in Practice‘ book.

29. Claro, M, Vogado, L, Veras, R, Santana, A, Tavares, J, Santos, J & Machado, V 2020, ‚Convolution Neural Network Models for Acute Leukemia Diagnosis‘, IWSSIP International Conference on Systems, Signals and Image Processing, pp. 63-68.

30. COLORROTATE. (2012). Retrieved from http://learn.colorotate.org/colormodels/#.VJo8jeCAg

31. Costa, Ld. FD & Cesar Jr, RM 2000, ‚Shape analysis and classification: theory and practice: CRC Press'.

32. Diamond Diagnostics 2013, Sysmex KX21N Haematology Analyzer. Retrieved from http://www.diamonddiagnostics.com/ equipment/ Hem/Sysmex_KX21n.html

33. Ding, C & Peng, H 2005, ‚Minimum redundancy feature selection from microarray gene expression data', Journal of bioinformatics and computational biology, vol. 3, no. 02, pp. 185-205.

34. Döhner, H, Estey, EH, Amadori, S, Appelbaum, FR, Büchner, T, Burnett, AK & Larson, RA 2010, ‚Diagnosis and management of acute myeloid leukemia in adults', vol. 115, no. 3, pp. 453-474.

35. Donoho 1995, ‚De-noising by soft thresholding', IEEE Transactions on Information Theory, vol. 41, no. 3, pp. 613-627.

36. Duda, RO, Hart, PE & Stork, DG 2012, ‚Pattern classification: John Wiley & Sons.

37. Dugdale, DC 2010, ‚Bone Marrow Aspiration', Retreived from:- http://health.allrefer.com/pictures-images/bone-marrow-aspiration.html.

38. Ehrenstein, V, Nielsen, H, Pedersen, AB, Johnsen, SP & Pedersen, L 2017, ‚Clinical epidemiology in the era of big data: new opportunities, familiar challenges', Clinical Epidemiology, vol. 9, pp. 245–250.

39. Escalante, HJ, Montes-y-Gomez, M, González, JA, Gomez-Gil, P, Altamirano, L, Reyes, CA & Rosales, A 2012, ‚Acute leukemia classification by ensemble particle swarm model selection. vol. 55, no. 3, pp. 163-175.

40. Esposito, F & Malerba, D 2001, ‚Machine Learning in Computer Vision', An International Journal of Applied Artificial Intelligence, vol. 15, no. 8, pp. 693-705.

41.	Essam, AR, Ismail, A & Sherif, IZ 2007, ‗Multiresolution mammogram analysis in multilevel decomposition', vol. 28, no. 2, pp. 286-292.

42.	Esteridge, BH, Reynolds, AP & Walters, NJ 2000, ‗Basic medical laboratory techniques: Cengage Learning'.

43.	Estridge, BH & Reynolds, AP 2011, ‗Basic clinical laboratory techniques: Cengage Learning.

44.	Fabijanska, A & Sankowski, D 2009, ‗Computer vision system for high temperature measurements of surface properties', Machine Vision and Applications, vol. 20, no. 6, pp. 411- 421.

45.	Fauzi, I, R, Rustam, Z & Wibowo, A 2021, ‗Multiclass classification of leukemia cancer data using Fuzzy Support Vector Machine (FSVM) with feature selection using Principal Component Analysis (PCA)', Journal of Physics: Conference Series, vol. 1725, no.12.

46.	Ferreira, CBR & Borges, DL 2003, ‗Analyses of mammogram classification using a wavelet transform decomposition', vol. 24, no. 7, pp. 973-982.

47.	Ghaderzadeh, M, Rebecca, F & Standring, A 2013, ‗Comparing performance of different neural networks for early detection of cancer from benign hyperplasia of prostate', Applied Medical Informatics, vol. 33, pp. 45–54.

48.	Gokbuget, N & Hoelzer, D 2009, ‗Treatment of adult acute lymphoblastic leukemia', Paper presented at the Seminars in haematology, vol. 46, no. 1, pp. 64-75.

49.	Greer, JP, Arber, DA, Glader, B, List, AF, Means, RT, Paraskevas, F & Rodgers, GM 2013, ‗Wintrobe's Clinical Haematology (13th ed.): Wolters Kluwer.

50.	Gupta, P & Malhi, AK 2018, ‗Using deep learning to enhance head and neck cancer diagnosis and classification', IEEE International Conference on System, Computation, Automation and Networking (ICSCAN), pp. 1–6.

51.	Guyon, I & Elisef, A 2003, ‗An Introduction to Variable and Feature Selection', Journal of Machine Learning Research, vol. 3, no. 15, pp. 1157-1182.

52. Haggstrom, M 2009, MedicineNet.com Leukemia (cont.), Symptoms. Retrieved from http://upload.wikimedia.org/ wikipedia/ commons/3 /3a/Symptoms_of_leukemia.png

53. Hasan, MM, Srizon, AY, Sayeed, A & Hasan, MAM 2020, ‗Accurate Recognition of Leukemia Sub-types by Utilizing a Transfer Learned Deep Convolutional Neural Network‛, 11th International Conference on Electrical and Computer Engineering (ICECE), pp. 427-430.

54. Hao, S, Han, Y, Zhang, J & Ji, Z 2013, ‗Automatic isolation of carpal-bone in hand x-ray medical image‛, Informatics and Management Science, Springer.

55. Harishchandra Patil & Holambe, RS 2013, ‗New approach of threshold estimation for denoising ECG signal using wavelet transform‛, in Proceedings of India Conference Annual IEEE Conference.

56. Hegde, RB, Prasad, K, Hebbar, H, Singh, BMK & Sandhya, I 2019, ‗Automated decision support system for detection of leukemia from peripheral blood smear images‛, Journal of Digital Imaging, vol. 33, pp. 361-374.

57. Huang, GB, Zhou, H, Ding, X & Zhang, R 2012, ‗Extreme Learning Machine for Regression and Multiclass Classification‛, IEEE Transactions on Systems, vol. 42, no. 2, pp. 513-529.

58. Ichihashi, T, Naoe, T, Kuriyama, K, Sasada, M & Ohno, R ‗Acute Lymphocytic Leukemia‛, Retrieved from http://pathy.med.nagoya-u.ac.jp/atlas/img/t6/img028.jpg.

59. Intel Developer Zone 2012, ‗Color Models‛, Retrieved from https://software.intel.com/en-us/node/503873

60. Ismail, W, Hassan, R & Swift, S 2010, ‗Detecting Leukaemia (AML) Blood Cells Using Cellular Automata and Heuristic Search‛, Advances in Intelligent Data Analysis IX vol. 6065, pp. 54-66.

61. Iwashima, Y J. Wang & Y. Yashima, ‗Full Reference Image Quality Assessment by CNN Feature Maps and Visual Saliency‛, IEEE 8th Global Conference on Consumer Electronics (GCCE), pp. 203-207.

62. James, D, Clymer, BD & Schmalbrock, P 2001, ‗Texture detection of simulated micro calcification susceptibility effects in magnetic resonance imaging of breasts‛, Journal of Magnetic Resonance Imaging, vol. 13, no. 6, pp. 876-881.

63. Jemal, A et al. Cancer statistics, 2009 _A Cancer Journal for Clinicians is a peer-reviewed journal of the American Cancer Society', vol. 59, no. 4, pp. 225–249

64. Jiang, F, Jiang, Y, Zhi, H, Dong, Y, Li, H, Ma, S, Wang, Y, Dong, Q, Shen, H & Wang, Y 2017, _Artificial intelligence in healthcare: Past, present and future', vol. 2, pp. 230–243.

65. Johnson,P 2010, _History of Leukemia', Retrieved from http://www.buzzle.com/articles/history-of-leukemia.html

66. Jones, W, Alaso, K, Fishman, D & Parts, L 2017, _Computational biology: Deep learning', pp. 257–274.

67. Joshi, MMD & Karode, A 2013, _Detection of Acute Leukemia Using White Blood Cells Segmentation Based on Blood Samples', International journal of Electronics and Communication Engineering & Technology, vol. 4, no. 1, pp. 148-153.

68. Kawthalkar, SM 2012, _Essentials of haematology: Jaypee Brothers Medical P'.

69. Khashman, A & Al-Zgoul, E 2009, _Image segmentation of blood cells in leukemia patients', Proceedings of the 4th WSEAS international conference on Computer engineering and applications, Cambridge, USA.

70. Kim, N 2021, _Deep Learning Technology-based Model to Identify Benign and Pro-B Acute Lymphoblastic Leukemia (ALL): Xception + LIME', American Journal of Biomedical and Life Sciences. Vol. 9, No. 5, pp. 279-285. doi: 10.11648/j.ajbls.20210905.19.

71. Koh, PW, Pierson, E & Kundaje, A 2017, _Denoising genome-wide histone Chip-sequence with convolutional neural networks', Bioinformatics, vol. 33, pp. 225–233.

72. Kothari, R, Cualing, H & Balachander, T 1996, _Neural Network Analysis of Flow Cytometry Immunophenotype Data', IEEE Transactions on Biomedical Engineering, vol. 43, no. 8, pp. 803-810.

73. Kumar, D 2020, _Automatic Detection of White Blood Cancer from Bone Marrow Microscopic Images Using Convolutional Neural Networks', in IEEE Access, vol. 8, pp. 142521-142531.

74. Kuncheva, L 2004, _Combining Pattern Classifiers: Methods and Algorithms' by John Wiley & Sons.

75. Labati, RD, Piuri, V & Scotti, F 2011, _All-IDB: The acute lymphoblastic leukemia image database for image processing', 18th IEEE International Conference on Image Processing (ICIP), doi: 10.1109/ICIP.2011.6115881.

76. Lavelle, P 2004 Leukaemia retrieved from http://www. abc. net. au/ health/library/stories/2004/10/18/1830091.html

77. Liao, Q & Deng, Y 2002, _An accurate segmentation method for white blood cell images', IEEE International Symposium on Biomedical Imaging, Proceedings, pp. 245-248.

78. Libbrecht, M & Noble, WS 2015, _Machine learning applications in genetics and genomics', vol. 16, pp. 321–332.

79. Lim, G C C, Rampal, S & Yahaya, H 2008, _Cancer Incidence in Peninsular Malaysia, 2003-2005: The Third Report of the National Cancer Registry', National Cancer Registry.

80. Lim, SE, Xing, Y, Chen, Y, Leow, WK, Howe, TS & Png, MA 2004, _Detection of femur and radius fractures in X-ray images' 2nd International Conference on Advances in Medical Signal and Information Processing.

81. Liu Sheng, Charles Babbs & Edward Delp 2001, _Multiresolution detection of spiculated lesions in digital mammograms', IEEE Transactions on Image Processing , vol. 10, no. 6, pp. 874-884.

82. Lofsness 2008 _ Blood Cell Maturation' from http://www1.umn.edu/ hema /pages/matchart.html

83. Lynch, CJ & Liston, C 2018, _New machine-learning technologies for computer-aided diagnosis', Nat. Med, vol. 24, pp. 1304–1305.

84. Madhloom, H, Kareem, S & Ariffin, H 2012, _An Image Processing Application for the Localization and Segmentation of Lymphoblast Cell Using Peripheral Blood Images', Journal of Medical Systems, vol. 36, no. 4, pp. 2149-2158.

85.   Mahendran, S & Baboo, SS 2011, _An enhanced tibia fracture detection tool using image processing and classification fusion techniques in X-ray images', Global Journal of Computer Science and Technology, vol. 11, no. 14, pp. 23-28.

86.   Mallick, P, K, Mohapatra, S, K, Chae , G, S 2020 _Convergent learning–based model for leukemia classification from gene expression', Personal Ubiquitous Computing, https://doi.org/10. 1007/ s00779-020-01467-3.

87.   Markiewicz, T, Osowski, S, Marianska, B & Moszczynski, L 2005, _Automatic recognition of the blood cells of myelogenous leukemia using SVM', IEEE International Conference.

88.   Mishra, A & Suhas, MV 2016, _Classification of benign and malignant bone lesions on CT images using random forest', IEEE International Conference on Recent Trends in Electronics, Information & Communication Technology (RTEICT), pp. 1807-1810.

89.   Morlet, J, Arens, G, Fourgeau, E & Giard, D 1982, _Wave Propogation and Sampling Theory', Geophysics, vol. 7, no. 2, pp. 203-221.

90.   Namayandeh, SM, Khazaei, Z, Lari Najafi, M, Goodarzi, E & Moslem, A 2020, _GLOBAL Leukemia in children 0–14 statistics 2018, incidence and mortality and human development index (HDI): GLOBOCAN sources and methods', Asian Pacific Journal of Cancer Prevention, vol. 21, no. 5, pp. 1487–1494.

91.   Nasir, AA, Mashor, MY & Hassan, R 2013, _Classification of Acute Leukaemia Cells Using Multilayer Perceptron and Simplified Fuzzy ARTMAP Neural Networks', International Arab Journal of Information Technology, vol. 10, no. 5.

92.   Nee, LH, Mashor, MY & Hassan, R 2012, _White Blood Cell Segmentation for Acute Leukemia Bone Marrow Images', Journal of Medical Imaging and Health Informatics, vol. 2, pp. 278-284.

93.   Nisthula, P & Yadhu, RB 2013, _A Novel Method to Detect Bone Cancer Using Image Fusion and Edge Detection', International Journal of Engineering and Computer Science, vol. 2, no. 6, pp. 2012-2018.

94.   Obermeyer, Z & Emanuel, EJ 2016, _Predicting the future—big data, machine learning, and clinical medicine', New England Journal of Medicine, vol. 375, no. 13, pp. 1216–1219.

95. Osowski, S, Robert Siroi, c, Markiewicz, T & Siwek, K 2009, _Application of Support Vector Machine and Genetic Algorithm for Improved Blood Cell Recognition', IEEE Transactions on Instrumentation And Measurement, vol. 58, no. 7, pp. 2159-2168.

96. Ozaki, Y, Yamada, H, Kikuchi, H, Hirotsu, A, Murakami, T, Matsumoto, T., Kawabata, T, Hiramatsu, Y, Kamiya, K, Yamauchi, T, Goto, K, Ueda, Y, Okazaki, S, Kitagawa, M, Takeuchi, H & Konno, H 2019, _Label-free classification of cells based on supervised machine learning of sub cellular structures', vol. 14, no.1.

97. Paswan, S & Rathore, Y 2018, _Recognition and Arrangement of Blood Cancer from Microscopic Cell Pictures Utilizing Support Vector Machine K-Nearest Neighbor and Deep Learning', International Conference on Communication, Computing and Internet of Things (IC3IoT), pp. 525-530.

98. Paul D O, Malley 2006, _New developments in sickle cell disease research: Nova Publishers'.

99. Pise, SJ, Kekre, HB, Sarode, T, Thepade, S & Halarnkar P Kekre's 2010, _Fast codebook generation in VQ with various color spaces for colorization of grayscale images Thinkquest', pp. 102-108.

100. Piuri, V & Scotti, F 2004, _Morphological classification of blood leucocytes by microscope images', IEEE International Conference on Computational Intelligence for Measurement Systems and Applications.

101. Pommerville, JC 2009, _Alcamo's Fundamentals of Microbiology: Body Systems: Jones & Bartlett Publishers'.

102. Putzu, L & Di Ruberto, C 2013, _White Blood Cells Identification and Classification from Leukemic Blood Image', International Work-Conference on Bioinformatics and Biomedical Engineering.

103. Rajendran, S, Arof, H, Ibrahim, F & Yegappan, S 2008, _Review on Technical Aspects of Image Acquisition, Analysis and Retrieval for Leukaemia Cells', International Conference on Biomedical Engineering, vol. 21, pp. 230-233.

104. Rajer, M & Kovac, V 2008, _Malignant spinal cord compression, Radiology and Oncology', vol. 42, no. 1, pp. 23-31.

105. Reaman, GH 2011, Childhood Leukemia: A Practical Handbook: Springer.

106. Reddy, S, Fox, J & Purohit, MP 2018, ‚Artificial intelligence-enabled healthcare delivery', vol. 112, pp. 22–28.

107. Riley, RS, James, GW, Sommer, S & Martin, MJ 2012, ‚How to Prepare & Interpret Peripheral Blood Smears', Retrieved from http://www.pathology.vcu.edu/education/PathLab/pages/hematopath/pbs.html

108. Rodak, B, Fritsma, G & Doig, K 2007, ‚Haematology: Clinical Principles & Applications: Elsevier Health Sciences'.

109. Rodenacker, K & Bengtsson, E 2003, ‚A feature set for cytometry on digitized microscopic images', Analytical Cellular Pathology, vol. 25, no. 1, pp. 1-36.

110. Sabino, D, Costa, LdF, Martins, S, Calado, R & Zago, M 2003, ‚Automatic leukemia diagnosis', Acta Microscopica, vol. 12, no. 1, pp. 1-6.

111. Saeys, Y, Inza, I & Larrañaga, P 2007, ‚A review of feature selection techniques in bioinformatics', Bioinformatics, vol. 23, no. 19, pp. 2507-2517.

112. Sant, M, Allemani, C, Tereanu, C, De Angelis, R, Capocaccia, R, Visser, O, Marcos-Gragera, R, Maynadie, M, Simonetti, A, Lutz, JM, Berrino, F & Group, HW 2010, ‚Incidence of hematologic malignancies in Europe by morphologic subtype: results of the HAEMACARE project', vol. 116, no. 19, pp. 3724-3734.

113. Sarangi, SK, Panda, R, Priyadarshini, S & Sarangi, A 2016, ‚A new modified firefly algorithm for function optimization', 2016 International Conference on Electrical, Electronics, and Optimization Techniques (ICEEOT), pp. 2944-2949.

114. Scotti, F 2005, ‚Automatic morphological analysis for acute leukemia identification in peripheral blood microscope images', IEEE International Conference on Computational Intelligence for Measurement Systems and Applications, doi: 10.1109/CIMSA. 2005. 1522835.

115. Selvarajah, S & Kodituwakku, S 2011, _Analysis and comparison of texture features for content based image retrieval', International Journal of Latest Trends in Computing, vol. 2, no. 1.

116. Shah, A, Naqvi, SS, Naveed, K, Salem, N, Khan, MAU & Alimgeer, KS 2021, _Automated Diagnosis of Leukemia: A Comprehensive Review', in IEEE Access, vol. 9, pp. 132097-132124.

117. Shen, Q, Liu, B, Shi, L ,Wu, S, Dong, B, Wang, H, Yuan, J, Shen, S & Zhao, L 2021, _Development and Evaluation of a Leukemia Diagnosis System Using Deep Learning in Real Clinical Scenarios', Frontiers in Pediatrics, vol.9, pp.1-10.

118. Sinha, N & Ramakrishnan, A 2003, _Automation of differential blood count', Conference on Convergent Technologies for the Asia-Pacific Region, doi:10.1109/TENCON.2003.1273221

119. Srinivasan, G & Shobha, G 2008, _Statistical Texture Analysis', Proceedings of World Academy of Science: Engineering & Technology, p. 48-50.

120. Suematsu, N, Ishida, Y, Hayashi, A & Kanbara, T 2002, _Region-based image retrieval using wavelet transform', international conference on vision interface.

121. Supardi, NZ, Mashor, MY, Harun, NH, Bakri, FA & Hassan, R 2012, _Classification of blasts in acute leukemia blood samples using k-nearest neighbour', IEEE 8th International conference at the Signal Processing and its Applications (CSPA), Malaysia, doi: 10.1109/CSPA.2012.6194769

122. Theera-Umpon, N & Dhompongsa, S 2007, _Morphological Granulometric Features of Nucleus in Automatic Bone Marrow White Blood Cell Classification', IEEE Transactions on Information Technology in Biomedicine, vol. 11, no. 3, pp. 353-359.

123. Umbaugh, SE 2010, _Digital Imaging Processing and Analysis: Human and Computer Vision Applications with CVIP tools', Second Edition: CRC Press.

124. Ushizima, DM, Lorena, AC & De Carvalho, ACPLF 2005, _Support vector machines applied to white blood cell recognition'.

125. Vijaykumar, V, Vanathi, P & Kanagasabapathy, P 2010, ‚Fast and efficient algorithm to remove Gaussian noise in digital images', International Journal of Computer Science, vol. 37, no. 1, pp. 9-15.

126. Von Boehmer, H & Melchers, F 2010, ‚Checkpoints in lymphocyte development and autoimmune disease', vol. 11, no. 1, pp. 14-20.

127. Wainberg, MM, Merico, D, Delong, A & Frey, BJ 2018, ‚Deep learning in biomedicine', vol. 36, pp. 829–838.

128. Walsh, S, de Jong, EE, van Timmeren, JE, Ibrahim, A, Compter, I, Peerlings, J, Sanduleanu, S, Refaee, T, Keek, S, Larue, RT *et al.* 2019, ‚Decision Support Systems in Oncology', Cancer Information, vol. 3, pp. 1–9.

129. Wang, XM 2014, ‚Advances and issues in flow cytometric detection of immunophenotypic changes and genomic rearrangements in acute pediatric leukemia', Translational Pediatrics, vol. 3, no. 2, pp. 149-155.

130. Wen, J, Xu, Y, Li, Z, Ma, Z & Xu, Y 2018, ‚Inter-class sparsity based discriminative least square regression', Neural Networks, vol. 102, pp. 36–47.

131. Wilson, L & Moore, J 2010, ‚Design Matters: Creating Powerful Imagery for Worship: Abingdon Press'.

132. Wolach, O & Stone, RM 2017, ‚Mixed-phenotype acute leukemia', Current Opinion in Haematology, vol. 24, no. 2, pp. 139-145.

133. Wu, Yi-Ying, Huang, Tzu-Chuan, Ye, Ren-Hua, Fang, Wen-Hui, Lai, Shiue-Wei, Chang, Ping-Ying, Liu, Wei-Nung, Kuo, Tai-Yu, Lee, cho-hao, Tsai, Wen-Chiuan & Lin, Chin 2020, ‚A Hematologist-Level DL Algorithm (BMSNet) for Assessing the Morphologies of Single Nuclear Balls in Bone Marrow Smears: Algorithm Development', JMIR Medical Informatics, vol. 8, e15963. 10.2196/15963.

134. Xing, F & Yang, L 2016, ‚Robust nucleus/cell detection and segmentation in digital pathology and microscopy images: a comprehensive review', IEEE Reviews in Biomedical Engineering, vol. 9, pp. 234–263.

135. Yu, KH, Beam, AL & Kohane, IS 2018, ‚Artificial intelligence in healthcare', Nat. Biomed. Eng., vol. 2, pp. 719–731.

136. Zephyris, RW 2007, Microscope and Digital Camera Retrieved from http://commons.wikimedia.org/wiki/File:Microscope_ And_Digital_Camera.JPG

137. Zhang, D & Lu, G 2004, _Review of shape representation and description techniques‘, Pattern Recognition, vol. 37, no. 1, pp. 1-19.

138. Zhao, J, Zhang, M, Zhou, Z, Chu, J & Cao, F 2017, _Automatic detection and classification of leukocytes using convolutional neural networks‘, Medical & Biological Engineering & Computing, vol. 55, no. 8, pp. 1287–1301.

139. Zou, J, Huss, M, Abid, A, Mohammadi, P, Torkamani, A & Telenti, A 2018, _A primer on deep learning in genomics‘, Nat. Genet., vol. 51, pp. 12–18.